Metabotropic Receptors for Glutamate and GABA

Gregory Stewart, Julie Kniazeff, Laurent Prézeau,
Philippe Rondard, Jean-Philippe Pin and Cyril Goudet
Institut de Génomique Fonctionnelle,
CNRS UMR5203 - INSERM U661 - Universités Montpellier 1&2
France

1. Introduction

G protein-coupled receptors (GPCRs) are the largest superfamily of transmembrane proteins and due to their ubiquitous expression and vast array of functions they present attractive targets for the treatment of a wide number of diseases and disorders. Accordingly, they represent up to 30% of targets of current therapeutics (Overington et al., 2006). Despite the capacity of GPCRs to modulate many (patho-)physiological functions there is a high attrition rate with regard to new compounds entering clinical trials. There are many reasons for the number of failed drug-like compounds such as non-specificity, unfavourable pharmacokinetic profile and lack of clinical efficacy. In this regard, molecules targeting neurotransmitter receptors in the CNS traditionally have poor side-effect profiles due to the high concentrations required to pass the blood-brain barrier. There remain many specific challenges in drug discovery such as promiscuous GPCR-effector coupling; differential cell- and tissue-specific effects; ligand-induced changes in receptor trafficking; and protein-protein interactions and receptor oligomerisation (Galandrin et al., 2007; Hanyaloglu and von Zastrow, 2008; Kniazeff et al., 2011; Wettschureck and Offermanns, 2005).

GPCRs are divided into three main classes (A-C) based on structural homology; however all GPCRs possess a 7-alpha-helical transmembrane-spanning (7TM) domain, which facilitates the transduction of extracellular signals into intracellular responses. GPCRs recognise a myriad of different stimuli from photons, amino acids and biogenic amines to large peptides and proteins. Class A (rhodopsin-like) GPCRs are among the best characterised and consist of a relatively short N-terminal domain, a 7TM domain connected by extracellular and intracellular loops, and an intracellular C-terminal domain (Fredriksson et al., 2003). Class B (secretin-like) GPCRs have comparatively long N-terminal domains with similar 7TM and C-terminal topography as Class A receptors. By far and away, Class C (glutamate-like) GPCRs have the most distinct topography compared the other GPCRs; they possess large, structured N-terminal domains, which form a venus-fly trap-like structure known as the venus-fly trap (VFT) domain. The VFT domain is often (with exceptions) connected to the 7TM domain via a cysteine-rich domain, and further to this the C-terminal domain is often comparatively longer than those of Class A GPCRs. Structurally, all GPCRs are similar in their 7TM domains, yet the activation mechanisms, at least by the endogenous ligand varies greatly across the classes. The orthosteric (endogenous ligand) binding site in Class A GPCRs lies in the 7TM helical bundle (with exceptions, e.g. CXCR4 chemokine receptor and relaxin family receptors (Allen et al., 2007; Sudo et al., 2003)); class B receptor ligands tend to bind in the large N-terminal domain and have been postulated to possess a bimodal receptor activation mechanism, whereby after the ligand binding event the ligand-N-terminal complex inserts into the 7TM helical bundle to elicit receptor activation (Hoare, 2005); class C receptor orthosteric ligands bind in the VFT domain and, through a series of conformational changes, are able to induce receptor activation via the 7TM domain (Pin et al., 2004)(Figure 1).

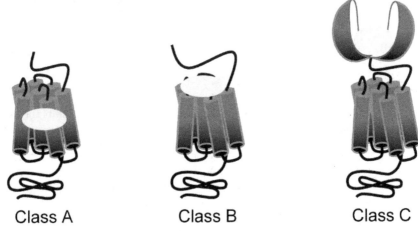

Fig. 1. Canonical orthosteric ligand-binding domains of the three classes of GPCRs. Highlighted in yellow are the typical binding regions of orthosteric ligands, in addition to the general architecture of the three major classes of GPCRs.

One large hindrance to drug discovery is the high degree of protein sequence and structural conservation between orthosteric sites of receptors of the same family, increasing the difficulty to specifically and selectively target a single receptor subtype. However, by their very nature GPCRs are highly dynamic proteins that are able to adopt a spectrum of conformational arrangements and it is this characteristic that allows GPCRs to be modulated by, not only a range of orthosteric ligands, but also ligands that bind in a topographically distinct region to the orthosteric binding pocket. These ligands are known as allosteric ligands and are able to modulate the affinity and/or efficacy of the orthosteric ligand, and indeed, possess their own efficacy in the absence of orthosteric ligand (Christopoulos and Kenakin, 2002; Conn et al., 2009a). This phenomenon presents a unique opportunity to exploit GPCRs as drug targets through offering novel and often less-conserved ligand binding sites across receptor subtypes.

Despite the best-characterised coupling partners of GPCRs being heterotrimeric G proteins, they are also well known to couple to a host of other intracellular proteins (e.g. arrestins and small G proteins (Burridge and Wennerberg, 2004; Lefkowitz, 1998)), thus adding an extra degree of complexity to the pluri-dimensional response of ligand-GPCR interactions. Furthermore, promiscuous coupling has been shown, in some cases, to be a concentration- and/or oligomerisation-dependent event (Sato et al., 2007; Scholten et al., 2011; Urizar et al., 2011).

Taken together, the ligand-receptor-effector combinations, receptor oligomerisation and allosteric modulation of GPCRs furnish a mode of fine-tuning functional outputs and potentially, therefore, clinical outcomes.

This chapter will focus on two major receptor types of Class C GPCRs, the metabotropic glutamate and metabotropic γ-amino-butyric acid (GABA) receptors, which are the GPCRs of the major excitatory and inhibitory neurotransmitters in the adult brain, respectively. These receptors represent major targets for many CNS disorders such as schizophrenia, Parkinson's disease, Alzheimer's disease, epilepsy and diseases of addiction (Conn et al., 2009a; Tyacke et al., 2010).

2. Metabotropic glutamate receptors

2.1 Phylogeny and structure/function of mGlu receptors

Metabotropic glutamate (mGlu) receptors are widely expressed in the CNS and are activated by the excitatory neurotransmitter, glutamate. These receptors play a vital role in the regulation on neuronal excitability and synaptic transmission (Conn and Pin, 1997). Consequently, these receptors are valuable targets for treating neurological disorders such as schizophrenia, Parkinson's disease and neuropathic pain, either by correcting neurological imbalances in non-glutamatergic systems or through treating disregulation of glutamatergic signalling.

The members of the mGlu receptor family are obligate dimers and long thought of as obligate homodimers, but have recently been demonstrated to selectively form heterodimers amongst other mGluR subtypes in HEK cells (Doumazane et al., 2011). This propensity may be of utility in texturing the glutamatergic response across diverse brain regions. mGlu receptors consist of 8 subtypes that are divided into three subgroups (I-III) based on sequence homology, function and pharmacological profile (Pin and Acher, 2002). Group I mGluRs ($mGlu_1$ and $mGlu_1$) are $G_{q/11}$-coupled thereby signalling through the phospholipase C-IP$_3$-Ca^{2+} axis; whereas Group II ($mGlu_2$ and $mGlu_3$) and Group III ($mGlu_4$, $mGlu_6$, $mGlu_7$ and $mGlu_8$) signal through inhibitory G proteins ($G_{i/o}$), which most likely serve as intermediaries between the receptor and ligand-gated ion channels, such as voltage-operated potassium channels (K_v2 channels) and voltage-operated calcium channels (Ca_v2 channels) (Doupnik, 2008; Herlitze et al., 1996; Peleg et al., 2002).

In drug discovery the understanding of the molecular mechanisms of ligand binding and receptor activation are paramount in order to investigate novel and improved methods for targeting these receptors therapeutically. In this regard, it is important to determine the overall receptor activation event by breaking it down into its fundamental component. Furthermore, to gather information about mGlu receptors, we must also use information gained from studies of other Class C GPCRs to form a global conformational image. Ligand binding in a VFT structure has been described with the periplasmic binding protein, which appears to be similar in class C receptors (O'Hara et al., 1993). The VFT remains in a state of equilibrium between two main conformations: open (o) and closed (c), known as the resting state. The orthosteric ligands bind primarily to the open VFT in lobe 1 and subsequently promote the closed conformation as interactions with lobe 2 stabilises this state. This suggests that, if agonists induce the closure of the VFT, orthosteric antagonists act to prevent the closure of the VFT, thereby blocking the appropriate mechanisms leading to 7TM activation (Bessis et al., 2000; Bessis et al., 2002; Kunishima et al., 2000; Tsuchiya et al., 2002). For a number of years, the question on how ligand binding in the VFT results in 7TM activation remained to be elucidated. The breakthrough came from the first crystal structures of a class C VFT dimer, from the mGlu1 receptor, crystallised in the presence and absence of glutamate (Kunishima et al., 2000). These structures confirmed the overall structure of the domain and, perhaps more importantly, the agonist binding mode in a single VFT domain. It also revealed large, structural rearrangements of the VFT dimer resulting in a change of the relative orientation of the two protomers. A general mechanism for VFT dimer conformational changes was proposed by the authors: two orientations of the VFT dimer exist and are in equilibrium: a resting (R) and an active (A) orientation. In the R orientation, the VFTs interact via lobe-I only, leaving the lobes-II separate from each other. In the A orientation, there is a reorganization of the VFTs relative orientation such that they also interact via each lobe-II. This large reorientation from R to A was proposed to induce the conformational changes required for 7TM activation. Resting and active designations were given to the different orientations as glutamate was proposed to stabilize the A form. The active and inactive property of the A and R orientations are further supported by mGlu1 structures obtained in the presence of an antagonist (MCPG) or in the presence of a potentiator (Gd^{3+}) in which the dimer orientation is R and A, respectively (Tsuchiya et al., 2002).

When considering the various conformations for the VFT and the VFT dimer, there are a total of six theoretical conformations that are possible: Roo, Rco and Rcc and Aoo, Aco and Acc, where A and R are indicative for the VFT dimer orientation and c and o for the VFT conformation. It is assumed that agonist binding to at least one of the VFT stabilizes the c form, which is the driving force leading to the VFT dimer reorientation from R to A. In agreement, only Roo, Rco, Aco and Acc are likely to exist. However, new crystal structures of the isolated VFT dimer in the 'forbidden' conformation Rcc (Muto et al., 2007) and Aoo (PDB accession number, 3KS9) were recently deposited in the protein data bank (PDB). In particular, the Aoo conformation appears to be highly unlikely to occur within a dynamic equilibrium as many residues of the same polarity from lobe 2 would be in close proximity to one another, so much so that this would likely destabilise this conformation through the repulsive forces exerted within lobe 2 (Tsuchiya et al., 2002). Whilst explanations for these surprising observations have not been provided, the absence of 7TM may have alleviated some conformational constraints that may otherwise be exerted on the VFT from the 7TM, acting as a structural tether that inhibits certain conformations.

A question arising upon closer analysis of the crystal structure is the number of agonists needed to activate a class C GPCR dimer. When considering the reorientation of the VFT from R to A as the sole mechanism responsible for 7TM activation, one may wonder whether there is a functional difference between Aco and Acc conformation. In other words, what would be the difference in binding one or two agonists? It was shown that in class C heterodimers a single subunit was responsible in binding the endogenous ligand (GABAB1 in GABAB receptor and T1R1 or T1R2 in the taste receptors)(Kniazeff et al., 2002; Nelson et al., 2001). This suggests that a single agonist molecule is sufficient to fully activate heterodimeric receptors in these cases.

As we have described above, an allosteric modulator binding in the 7TM affects both the G protein activation and agonist affinity for the VFT. Together with the fact that a conformational change in the VFT dimer activates the 7TM, this indicates that VFT and 7TM converse in both ways. The question that remains is how the stimulus is transduced through the VFT region to the 7TM domain?

In most of class C GPCRs, VFT and 7TM are connected with the CRD. The CRD is an 80 residues long domain containing 9 cysteines. This domain is present in mGlu, CaS, GPRC6A and T1R receptors, but not in GABA$_B$ receptors. The structure of this domain has been solved for mGlu$_3$ (Muto et al., 2007), and this domain appears to be a rigid 40Å long structure, which is most likely to form a physical gearing system between the VFT and 7TM domains. In agreement with these physical findings, both deletion of the CRD in mGlu or CaS receptors and mutations of T1R3 CRD abolish the agonist-induced receptor activation (Hu et al., 2000; Jiang et al., 2004). Furthermore, we have shown that the VFT and CRD domains in mGlu$_2$ are linked by a disulphide bridge between a cysteine at the bottom of the VFT and the only cysteine that is not engaged in intradomain disulphide bond within the CRD (Rondard et al., 2006). Rondard et al., had shown that the mutation of the residues involved in this interaction abolished agonist-mediated activation of the receptor. This supports the idea of a central role for the CRD in the transduction of the conformational changes from the VFT dimer to the 7TM in these receptors.

The exact mechanisms of 7TM activation Class C and indeed, mGlu receptors remain to be solved. This notwithstanding, there are approaches that can be employed in an attempt to determine the molecular mechanisms involved in the conformational changes that the 7TM domains undergoes upon activation. One of these approaches is entails the use of both positive and negative allosteric modulators. The first allosteric modulators of class C GPCRs to be described were found to be non-competitive antagonists or inverse agonists (Carroll et al., 2001; Litschig et al., 1999; Pagano et al., 2000). Other compounds have been described that potentiated the effect of the agonists (increased affinity and efficacy) (Felts et al., 2010; Hammond et al., 2010; Urwyler et al., 2001). These molecules are structurally distinct from the orthosteric agonists and antagonists, as reflected in their binding within the 7TM, in a binding region that is reminiscent of the orthosteric binding pocket in Class A receptors (Brauner-Osborne et al., 2007; Goudet et al., 2004). So far, no endogenous PAM or NAM binding in the 7TM pocket has been described. Selective pressure in the evolution of a site/pocket is often indicative of a biological function, but there is no conserved pocket located within the 7TM domain of mGluRs, making it less likely that there is an endogenous allosteric ligand that acts in that region. The absence of conservation allowed the discovery of molecules specific for a single subtype of mGlu receptor, as opposed to a ligand acting at the well conserved orthosteric binding site. If both PAM and NAM act at the 7TM, then their opposite effects are likely due to differences in the residues that the ligands are in contact with in the 7TM. Specifically, several studies indicate that PAM and NAM bind to overlapping but not identical sites (Miedlich et al., 2004; Petrel et al., 2004). Some of these interaction networks should stabilize the active conformation of the 7TM, whilst some others should lock the receptor in its inactive conformation. However, it was shown that structurally different molecules bind essentially at the same position in the 7TM, only the precise identity of the residues contacting the molecule may differ. It appears that the position of PAM/NAM binding site is largely conserved in the whole family and includes residues from TM3, 5, 6 and 7 (Hu et al., 2000; Miedlich et al., 2004; Pagano et al., 2000). However, in some cases, two distinct sites have been identified for PAMs, as exemplified at mGlu5 (Chen et al., 2008). See Figure 2 for a schematic overview of mGlu receptor architecture and binding domains.

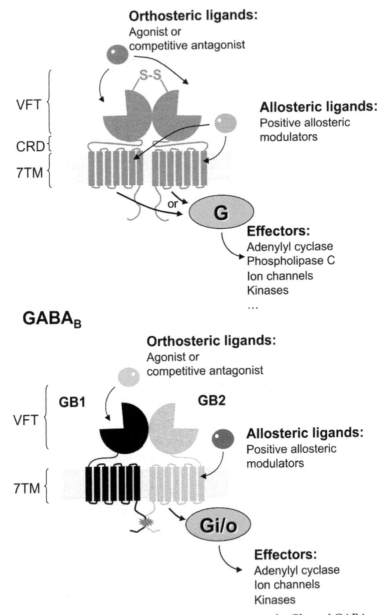

Fig. 2. Architecture, binding domains and dimerisation states of mGlu and GABAB receptors.

2.2 Protein-protein interactions of mGlu receptors

Studying molecular mechanisms and pharmacology of GPCRs in heterologous cells systems can be exceptionally useful due to the eradication of confounding factors such as multiple receptor subtypes; in addition the capacity to modulate receptor expression and function of specific signalling pathways with relative ease. However, these systems are rarely indicative of native systems and it needs to be recognised that various GPCR interactions exist *in vivo* that do not exist in heterologous cell systems for a myriad of reasons. One such interaction is that of protein-protein interactions, whereby the physical or functional interaction of a number of proteins can greatly alter its behaviour. An example of this occurrence is a fundamental component of some Class C GPCR pharmacology, such that receptor activity-modifying proteins (RAMPs) modulate the pharmacology of receptors such as the calcitonin and calcitonin receptor-like receptor (Sexton et al., 2006). mGlu receptors are also a family that are capable of interacting with non-mGluR proteins to form complexes.

2.2.1 mGlu$_1$–A$_1$ receptors

In cortical neurons, the simultaneous activation of adenosine A$_1$ and mGlu$_1$ receptors has been shown to synergistically decrease the neuronal toxicity due to application of NMDA (Ciruela et al., 2001). In astrocytes or in co-transfected HEK293 cells, activation of A$_1$ receptors elicits an increased mGlu$_1$ response via G$_{i/o}$ proteins (Ciruela et al., 2001; Toms and Roberts, 1999). That effect could be indicative of cross-talk and priming of the intracellular Ca^{2+} response; however, Hirono et al. (2001) did not observe any potentiation of the mGlu$_1$ response upon co-activation of the A$_1$ receptor in in cerebellar Purkinje cells, supporting the hypothesis of cooperativity (physical or otherwise) rather than cross-talk of the signalling pathways. Although both receptors are co-localized and coimmunoprecipitated from neurons and transfected HEK293 cells, the existence and the requirement of a direct physical interaction is yet to be clearly established (Ciruela et al., 2001).

2.2.2 mGlu$_5$–A$_{2A}$–D$_2$ receptors

The mGlu$_5$, adenosine A$_{2A}$ and dopamine D$_2$ receptors are highly expressed in the striatum. These receptors have been proposed to play vital roles in the dysregulation of the motor coordination observed in the Parkinson's disease. Indeed, antagonists of both mGlu$_5$ and A$_{2A}$ display anti-parkinsonian effects, while the dopamine D$_2$ receptor is the target of L-DOPA, which is used to treat parkinsonian symptoms. It has been suggested that these three receptors may act in concert in pairs or as a triplet via signalling cross-talk or otherwise, to influence the striatal function in motor coordination (Agnati et al., 2003; Cabello et al., 2009). Indeed, this cross-regulation was observed *in vivo*, where mGlu$_5$ antagonist-induced motor effects were augmented by A$_{2A}$ receptor antagonists; and conversely these effects were diminished in A$_{2A}$-D$_2$ receptor double knock-out mice (Kachroo et al., 2005). The exact molecular mechanisms of the cross-regulation are not well understood, but DARPP-32 (dopamine- and cAMP-regulated neuronal phosphoprotein) may play a pivotal role. Adenosine A$_{2A}$ receptors have been show to increase DARP-32 phosphorylation via the G$_s$ signaling axis, whilst D$_2$ receptors counteract this effect via the G$_{i/o}$ pathway (Agnati et al., 2003); Furthermore, the co-activation of adenosine A$_{2A}$ and dopamine D$_2$ receptors synergistically potentiated DARPP-32 phosphorylation *ex vivo* studies in striatum tissues. Notwithstanding, the regulation of intracellular Ca^{2+} and cAMP signals underpins other signalling interactions between these receptors (Ferre et al., 2002). Not only may this phenomenon be due to signalling cross talk amongst these receptors, but may be a result of physical interactions and allosteric regulation across heteromers. It A_{2A}–D_2 hetero-oligomers are mediated by electrostatic interactions between a basic-rich motif in the third intracellular loop of the D_2 receptor and an acidic/serine residue-containing motif in the C-terminus of the adenosine A_{2A} receptor (Azdad et al., 2009; Ciruela et al., 2004; Ferre et al., 2007). Additionally, are postulated to not only be co-expressed, but also to form hetero-oligomers in striatal neurons and in heterologous cells systems (Ferre et al., 2002). Recently, Cabello et al. (2009) demonstrated that $mGlu_5$, dopamine D_2 and adenosines A_{2A} receptors are localised within the same dendritic spines in glutamatergic striatal synapses, which led them to hypothesise that there may be hetero-oligomeric triplets of A_{2A}, $mGlu_5$ and D_2 receptors; this association was then investigated through the employment of various fluorescence techniques. Their data supported the formation of heterooligomers containing all three receptors and thus allosterically interacting with one another to influence either efficacy or affinity or both. It is noteworthy that additional cross-regulation between A_{2A} and $mGlu_5$ receptors has been reported in hippocampal neurons, where the inhibition of A_{2A} receptors decreased the $mGlu_5$-mediated potentiation of NMDA receptor responses (Tebano et al., 2006). However, the molecular mechanisms involved are yet to be elucidated.

2.2.3 mGlu$_2$–5-HT$_{2A}$ receptors

One of the best-characterized receptor complex involving a Class C GPCR is the complex between $mGlu_2$ and the serotonin 5-HT$_{2A}$ receptor. It is well documented that these receptors are both targeted by antipsychotic drugs such as 5-HT$_{2A}$ receptor inverse agonists and $mGlu_2$ receptor agonists and PAMs (Benneyworth et al., 2008; Benneyworth et al., 2007). Furthermore, 5HT$_{2A}$ receptors are the target of hallucinogenic substances, for example LSD and psilocybin, which induce hallucinogenic episodes that are thought to be similar to some of the symptoms in schizophrenics (Aghajanian and Marek, 1999). Indeed, non-hallucinogenic 5HT$_{2A}$ agonists (5-HT included) activate the G_q signalling axis, whilst hallucinogenic compounds are proposed to additionally activate $G_{i/o}$ and Src tyrosine kinase pathways, in cortical neurons (Gonzalez-Maeso et al., 2007; Gonzalez-Maeso et al., 2003). Activation of $mGlu_2$ receptors in the prefrontal cortex by the $mGlu_2$ PAM, biphenyl-indanone A (BINA), abrogated the hallucinogenic effects of compounds such as (-)2,5-dimethoxy-4-bromoamphetamine, [(-)DOB] (Benneyworth et al., 2007); suggesting functional antagonism between $mGlu_2$ and 5HT$_{2A}$ receptors in prefrontal cortex, an interaction that is possibly altered in schizophrenics (Gonzalez-Maeso et al., 2007). In fact, co-expression of both receptors revealed that the hallucinogen-induced G_i coupling of 5-HT$_{2A}$ is ameliorated by $mGlu_2$ in basal conditions, but abolished when $mGlu_2$ is activated. The mechanism of this complex cross-talk remains to be fully unraveled, but it has been proposed to be the result of $mGlu_2$–5-HT$_{2A}$ receptor oligomerisation. In cortical neurons, these receptors co-localise and co-immunoprecipitate (Gonzalez-Maeso et al., 2008). Indeed, biophysical approaches have been employed to demonstrate that these GPCRs are in fact in close enough proximity to be compatible with a physical association (Gonzalez-Maeso et al., 2008). Moreover, by adopting a chimeric approach between $mGlu_2$ and $mGlu_3$ (TM4 and TM5 substitution), the authors were able to demonstrate that $mGlu_3$ receptors with substituted TM domains were able to oligomerise with the 5-HT$_{2A}$ receptor, further to exhibiting functional cross-talk (Gonzalez-Maeso et al., 2008). This supports the potential relationship between receptor oligomerisation and functional cross-talk. The study of the precise mechanism of this phenomenon is still ongoing, and can perhaps furnish novel approaches for targeting these receptors for the treatment of schizophrenia and other neuronal disorders.

2.2.4 mGlu5-NMDA receptors

Another important interaction that further implicates the role of the glutamatergic system in schizophrenia is the interaction of the N-methly-D-aspartate (NMDA) receptor and mGlu5. This GPCR-ion channel interaction has been relatively well characterised from a functional stand point, but the molecular mechanisms of the interaction are only beginning to be unfolded.

Indeed, in hippocampal neurons, mGlu5a co-localises with NMDA receptors, which mediates a slow excitatory postsynaptic current (Collingridge et al., 1983; Oliet et al., 1997). The activation of mGlu5 receptors enhances the NMDA-evoked responses in different regions of the brain, such as the hippocampus, the striatum, the cortex, or the spinal cord (Aniksztejn et al., 1992; Harvey and Collingridge, 1993). Recently, Perroy et al., (2008) have shown that both receptors, indeed, interact via the C-terminal domain of mGlu5a. Through use of the bioluminescence resonance energy transfer (BRET) approach, they demonstrated that a significant and specific BRET signal can be measured between the two receptors, and moreover that this signal was transiently increased by activation of either the mGlu5a receptor or the NMDA receptor; this suggests an allosteric interaction and ligand-dependent conformational rearrangement of the opposite protomer in the hetero-oligomer. Interestingly however, when co-expressed, the functional response of the either receptor was reduced, compared to the response when either receptor was expressed in isolation. Thus suggesting a reciprocal and constitutive suppression of the signalling between NMDA and mGlu5a receptors, which was suggested to be independent of the G protein coupling of mGlu5a. The inhibitory reciprocal effect was dependent on the physical interaction between these receptors, given that the inhibition was abolished upon suppression of the C-terminal domain involved in receptor hetero-oligomerisation (Perroy et al., 2008).

2.3 Localisation and physiological function

Group I mGlu receptors (mGlu1 and mGlu5) are extensively expressed throughout neurons in the CNS and, in addition, mGlu5 is expressed in glial cells. mGlu1 is most abundantly expressed in Purkinje cells of the cerebellar cortex and in the olfactory bulb, in addition to strong expression in the hippocampus, substantia nigra and globus pallidus (Baude et al., 1993; Martin et al., 1992); and mGlu5 is greatly expressed in corticolimbic regions, such as the striatum, hippocampus and cerebral cortex (Ferraguti and Shigemoto, 2006). For example in the hippocampus, mGlu1 has been demonstrated to be involved in synaptic transmission and plasticity, in addition to neuronal excitability (Bortolotto et al., 1999), whilst in both mGlu1 and mGlu5 are required for the induction of long-term depression (LTD) in corticostriatal synapses (Sung et al., 2001). Through the use of knockout (KO) mice the putative function of mGluRs can be elucidated and, indeed, mGlu1 and mGlu5 KO mice have been studied. In mGlu1 KO animals is a marked deficits in long-term potentiation (LTP) in hippocampal slices and in context-dependent fear conditioning task (Aiba et al., 1994a); suggesting reduced hippocampal-mediated learning and memory. Furthermore, these mice are also cerebellar-LTD deficient, suggesting that mGlu$_1$ receptors are important for LTD induction in the cerebellum and subsequently motor learning, as demonstrated by the ataxic gait of the mGlu$_1$ KO mice (Aiba et al., 1994b). Recently, mice have been generated whereby the mGlu$_5$ gene can be selectively disrupted in the central nucleus of the amygdala; these mice exhibited a lack of mechanical hypersensitivity induced by peripheral inflammation (Kolber et al., 2010), strongly suggesting a role of mGlu$_5$ in the regulation of inflammatory pain transmission. Both mGlu$_1$ and mGlu$_5$ KO mice exhibit deficiencies in prepulse inhibition of the startle reflex, which is an indicator of sensorimotor gating that is impaired in schizophrenic patients, a trait that can be reversed through treatment with antipsychotics (Brody et al., 2003; Brody et al., 2004).

mGlu$_2$ and mGlu$_3$ (Group II) are widely expressed in the CNS, of which mGlu$_2$ is more limited in expression compared to mGlu$_3$. mGlu$_2$ expression has been observed in Golgi cells of the cerebellar cortex and in mitral cells of the accessory olfactory bulb (Ohishi et al., 1998; Ohishi et al., 1994). mGlu$_3$ receptors have been observed in the olfactory tubercle, neocortex, limbic cortex, and is also present in Golgi cells of the cerebellar cortex (Tamaru et al., 2001). Similar to Group I mGlu receptors, KO mice have also been generated for Group II mGluRs, with both mGlu$_2$ and mGlu$_3$ KO mice exhibiting a loss of mGlu$_{2/3}$ agonist, LY354740-induced anxiolytic behaviour in an elevated plus maze test (Linden et al., 2005). Further to this, mGlu$_2$, but not mGlu$_3$ KO mice displayed a loss of Group II agonist-mediated antipsychotic behaviour (Fell et al., 2008; Woolley et al., 2008), highlighting the role of mGlu$_2$ in anxiety and psychotic behaviours. Interestingly, in addition to these functions, Group II mGlu receptors have also been demonstrated to modulate the release of other neurotransmitters, for example, LY354740 reduced KCl-induced [^{3}H]-GABA release in rat primary cortical cultures, this effect was then reversed with the mGlu$_{2/3}$ antagonist, LY341495 (Schaffhauser et al., 1998).

Group III mGluRs (consisting of mGlu$_4$, mGlu$_6$, mGlu$_7$ and mGlu$_8$) are mainly expressed on presynaptic neurons throughout the CNS, with the exception of mGlu$_6$, which is expressed postsynaptically on retinal ON bipolar cells (Nakajima et al., 1993). mGlu$_4$ is highly expressed in the cerebellum and consequently, mGlu$_4$ KO mice experience deficits in spatial memory (Gerlai et al., 1998) and learning of complex motor tasks (Pekhletski et al., 1996). mGlu$_6$ KO display deficits in ON response to light stimulation, yet the OFF response remained unchanged (Masu et al., 1995), highlighting the importance of mGlu$_6$ in synaptic neurotransmission in retinal ON bipolar cells. mGlu$_7$ deficient mice display learning and memory deficits, in addition to exhibiting an epileptic phenotype (Bushell et al., 2002; Sansig et al., 2001). Both mGlu$_7$ and mGlu$_8$ KO animals display increase anxiety (Cryan et al., 2003; Duvoisin et al., 2005).

As previously mentioned, the mGluR family of receptors are expressed widely through the CNS and exhibit a wide number of functions; moreover through KO studies, we can deduce the key roles played by each mGluR subtype and subsequently tailor our pharmacological armamentarium accordingly.

2.4 Pharmacology and clinical relevance

2.4.1 Ligands for group I mGlu receptors

The first selective orthosteric agonist at mGlu$_1$ and mGlu$_5$ receptors is (S)-3,5-dihydroxyphenylglycine, [(S)-3,5-DHPG], and this remains the case given that ligands such as quisqualate and [(1S,3R)-ACPD] also bind to ionotropic glutamate and other mGluR subtypes, respectively (Niswender and Conn, 2010). A range of other orthosteric ligands have been generated, but have limited use due to their low affinity and/or potency. As previously discussed, mGlu receptor subtype selectivity is difficult to obtain due to the high degree of sequence and structural homology between subtypes.

Therefore, one approach is to target non-canonical ligand-binding sites; from this strategy a major breakthrough in Group I mGlu receptor pharmacology was made, with the discovery of CPCCOEt, which was the first $mGlu_1$ negative allosteric modulator (NAM)(Annoura et al. 1996). CPCCOEt was later discovered to bind to an allosteric domain and this highlighted the capacity of ligands to bind in allosteric binding modes, thereby modulating orthosteric ligand function (Litschig et al., 1999). Thereafter, structurally distinct NAMs for $mGlu_1$ were also discovered such as BAY36-7620 and FTIDC (Carroll et al., 2001; Suzuki et al., 2007). $mGlu_5$ selective NAMs were also identified of which the two flagship molecules were MPEP and MTEP, both providing good potency and selectivity (Anderson et al., 2002; Gasparini et al., 1999).

In addition to NAMs, a wide variety of PAMs have also been identified and characterised. Two of these PAMs, Ro 67-4853 and Ro 01-6128 both potentiated DHPG-mediated VOCC inhibition responses in CA3 neurons, but did not exhibit any agonist activity of their own, suggesting their main characteristic is the allosteric potentiation of orthosteric ligand binding and/or efficacy (Knoflach et al., 2001). Interestingly, these PAMs were found to bind to a topographically distinct domain to the NAM binding region, when they failed to displace the well-characterised allosteric antagonist, R214127 (Hemstapat et al., 2006). These data suggest that $mGlu_1$ possesses multiple allosteric binding sites, in addition to its orthosteric ligand-binding site. Similar to $mGlu_1$, $mGlu_5$ PAMs have also been discovered, such as DFB, CPPHA, CDPPB, VU29, and ADX47273, with CDPPB also having some PAM activity at $mGlu_1$ (Conn et al., 2009b; Hemstapat et al., 2006).

2.4.2 $mGlu_1$ in anxiety and depression

Anxiety and depression are two of the most common mental disorders, with a lifetime prevalence of approximately 17% and 12%, respectively (Andrade et al., 2003; Depping et al., 2010). It has now been well documented that $mGlu_1$ receptors and the glutamatergic system represent tractable targets for treating these common disorders (Bittencourt et al., 2004; Paul and Skolnick, 2003).

Anxiety results from an imbalance between GABAergic and glutamatergic systems, either from overactive glutamatergic neurotransmission or inadequate GABAergic activity in hypothalamus, periaqueductal gray, hippocampus and prefrontal cortex (Engin and Treit, 2008). It is hypothesised that the antagonism of $mGlu_1$ receptors is capable of augmenting the GABAergic response, whilst concomitantly decreasing the NMDA receptor-mediated glutamatergic response in key brain regions involved in anxiety. It has been demonstrated that intraperitoneal administration of the $mGlu_1$ antagonist, 1-aminoindan-1,5-dicarboxylic acid (AIDA), rats exhibited anxiolytic-like behaviours in the conflict drinking test and in elevated plus maze tests (Klodzinska et al., 2004). This reinforces the results seen by Chojnacka-Wojik et al., (1997) where intrahippocampal injection of the Group I mGlu receptor antagonist, (S)-4-carboxy-3-hydroxyphenyl-glycine (S-4C3H-PG), reduced anxiety-like behaviours in rats. The anxiolytic actions of $mGlu_1$ blockade were further confirmed through the study of the $mGlu_1$-selective antagonist, JNJ16259685 (Steckler et al., 2005). This study demonstrated that treatment with JNJ16259685 alleviated the suppression of the licking response in a conflict drinking test, which is consistent with other well characterized anxiolytic drugs (Petersen and Lassen, 1981). However, JNJ16259685 treatment did not induce anxiolytic-type behaviour in elevated plus maze tests, the authors thus postulating that the effects of JNJ16259685 be context specific (Steckler et al., 2005).

Depression is a complex disorder involving the interplay between different neurotransmitters, including noradrenaline, serotonin, dopamine and glutamate (Paul and Skolnick, 2003). Drugs for the treatment for depression are generally based on increasing the lifetime of biogenic amines, such as noradrenaline and serotonin, in the synaptic cleft, for example fluoxetine and escitalopram, which are inhibitors of serotonin- and serotonin and noradrenaline-reuptake transporters, respectively. Over the past decade, it has become more recognised that the glutamatergic system may also play a vital role in the regulation of depression, specifically NMDA receptors, where NMDA receptor expression was reduced in post-mortem depressive brains (Feyissa et al., 2009). This theory was retrospectively reinforced by evidence that NMDA receptor antagonists produce anti-depressant effects, whereby competitive and non-competitive antagonists of NMDA receptors, 2-amino-7-phosphonoheptanoic acid (AP-7) and Dizolcipine (MK-801) emulated anti-depressant effects of gold standard anti-depressants (Trullas and Skolnick, 1990). Given the regulatory link between $mGlu_1$ and NMDA receptors it was postulated that $mGlu_1$ receptor antagonists or NAMs could mimic the anti-depressant effect of NMDA receptor inhibitors. The $mGlu_1$ antagonist, JNJ-16567083 has been shown to be efficacious in despair-based animal models of depression, specifically forced swim test and tail suspension test (Belozertseva et al., 2007; Molina-Hernandez et al., 2008).

2.4.3 mGlu$_5$ and schizophrenia

Schizophrenia is a complex multi-faceted disease that manifests itself as a host of symptoms such as paranoia, social withdrawal and delusions, along with a number of cognitive deficits. Given that there is no single causative factor, there is some difficulty in finding a suitable target. Current first-line treatment involves broad-spectrum biogenic amine (e.g. dopamine, serotonin, acetylcholine) receptor antagonists, but these to not satisfactorily treat the cognitive symptoms. The underlying rationale of this approach is to decrease dopaminergic neurotransmission in thalamocortical and limbic circuits. One potential mode of treating schizophrenia lies within targeting GABAergic and glutamateric interneuons in pivotal cortical and limbic regions, specifically, the disregulation of the disinhibition of glutamatergic neurotransmission (Chavez-Noriega et al., 2002; Coyle, 2006). The blockade of N-methly-D-aspartate (NMDA) receptors on these interneurons results in a glutamatergic disinhibition, which in turn leads to an overexcitability of thalamocortical neurons, which is mostly mediated by DL-a-amino-3-hydroxy-5-methylisoxasole-4-propionate (AMPA) receptors in thalamocortical synapses. Within these regions NMDA and mGlu$_5$ receptors have been demonstrated to functionally and physically interact, i.e. the activation of mGlu$_5$ receptors increases the activity of NMDA receptors on GABAergic and glutamatergic neurons (Conn et al., 2009b); it is thus postulated that the activation of mGlu$_5$ can be employed as a means to decrease neuronal excitability in thalamocortical regions. This hypothesis is reinforced through knockout studies, whereby the knockout of mGlu$_5$ resulted in NMDA-dependent cognitive and learning deficits (Lu et al., 1997). Therefore, adopting an mGlu$_5$ agonist or PAM could alleviate the cognitive symptoms in schizophrenic patients; moreover, the use of a PAM will allow relatively specific mGlu$_5$ in the afflicted region whilst maintaining the spatio-temporal regulation of other mGlu$_5$-containing neurons. Indeed, the abovementioned mGlu$_5$ PAM, CDPPB, which has a suitable potency and solubility profile for *in vivo* studies, has been demonstrated to decrease amphetamine-induced disruption of prepulse inhibition (PPI) startle response and locomotor activity (Kinney et al., 2005); and to increase hippocampal synaptic plasticity, an important feature in cognition (Ayala et al., 2008; Conn et al., 2009b).

2.4.4 Group II mGlu receptor pharmacology

Group II mGlu receptors (mGlu$_2$ and mGlu$_3$) are generally localised presynaptically and negatively regulate cAMP signalling, and moreover, VOCCs. As with nearly all orthosteric mGlu pharmacological agents there is the underlying issue of selectivity. DCG-IV and LY379268 are reference Group II mGlu agonists, BINA and LY487379 are highly potent PAMs and the recently discovered MNI series of compounds (MNI-135, MNI-136 and MNI-137) are potent negative allosteric modulators (Galici et al., 2006; Hemstapat et al., 2006; Johnson et al., 2003; Linden et al., 2005; Schweitzer et al., 2000). Despite the large array of pharmacological tools available for Group II mGlu receptors, there remains a paucity of ligands that selectively differentiate between mGlu$_2$ and mGlu$_3$, which is due to the high degree of sequence homology between the two. Of lesser therapeutic relevance, there are also Group II mGlu receptor antagonists, such as 2S-2-amino-2-(1S,2S-2-carboxycyclopropan-1-yl)-3-(xanth-9-yl)propionic acid (LY341495) and (1R,2R,3R,5R,6R)-2-amino-3-(3, 4-dichlorobenzyloxy)-6-fluorobicyclo[3.1.0] hexane-2,6-dicarboxylic acid (MGS0039), which have been suggested to have some anti-depressant and anti-obsessive-compulsive characteristics; however they are mostly used and pharmacological tools (Palucha and Pilc, 2005; Shimazaki et al., 2004). Given the lack of selectivity across Group II mGlu receptors it is difficult to pharmacologically distinguish the roles of each receptor in various animal models of disease states without the use of knockout animals.

2.4.5 Group II mGlu receptors in addiction

Addiction is a unique disorder in that it is not only a physiological dependence, but is also a psychological dependence on, canonically, drugs of abuse. It is believed that mGlu$_2$/mGlu$_3$ receptor ligands could be capable of treating addiction to such substances as cocaine and nicotine. In fact, not only is it that mGlu$_2$/mGlu$_3$ receptor activation is involved in recovery of a dysfunctional system in the corticolimbic system, but it has been shown that the function of Group II mGlu receptors is impaired, either by receptor downregulation or dampening of the G protein-mediated signalling, after acute and chronic stimulation by nicotine, cocaine and ethanol (Bowers et al., 2004; Kenny and Markou, 2004; Neugebauer et al., 2000). Indeed, mechanistically, the decrease in function is hypothesised to be due to an alteration in expression of the activator of G protein signalling 3 (AGS3), whereby AGS3 is overexpressed during withdrawal of repeated dosing of cocaine (Bowers et al., 2004). The authors went on to postulate that AGS3 gates expression of cocaine-induced plasticity in prefrontal cortex, via the regulation of G protein signalling. Furthermore, the downregulation of mGlu$_2$/mGlu$_3$ receptors has been observed during cocaine withdrawal periods, specifically these receptors were downregulated in the shell and core of the nucleus accumbens (Ghasemzadeh et al., 2009). These alterations in expression and function in turn results in an impairment of long-term depression (LTD) in nucleus accumbens and prefrontal cortex in response to chronic morphine and cocaine exposure, respectively (Moussawi and Kalivas, 2010); similarly, a reduced activation of $mGlu_2/mGlu_3$ receptors resulted in a decrease in long-term potentiation (LTP) after self-administered cocaine withdrawal (Moussawi et al., 2009). Indeed, it is well documented that $mGlu_2/mGlu_3$ function is altered in the case of substance withdrawal, however the system is regulated in a manner of ways. Explicitly, Group II mGlu receptors are involved in the circuitry that leads to reward processing and addictive behaviour. The activation of $mGlu_2/mGlu_3$ receptors with the orthosteric agonist, LY379268 resulted in the attenuation of the reinstatement of cocaine-seeking behaviour after exposure, compared to a conventional reinforcer (in this case, sweetened condensed milk) (Baptista et al., 2004). The authors proposed that this was a cocaine-specific effect and was most likely related to the mechanism of action of cocaine itself. Functionally, this regulation may lie in the pre-activation of $mGlu_2$ receptors, whereby in $mGlu_2$ knockout mice there was an increased release of glutamate and dopamine in response to cocaine, in the nucleus accumbens (Morishima et al., 2005). Whilst this does provide some evidence on how glutamate is involved in reward circuitry, one must remain circumspect on their conclusions given any compensatory mechanisms are not accounted for.

2.4.6 Group III mGlu receptors and their ligands

For many years, much of the drug discovery efforts have been directed towards Group I and II receptors to exploit their roles in central nervous disorders such as schizophrenia and neuropathic pain. However, of late, efforts have been turned to developing selective ligands for Group III as novel targets for disorders, for example, Parkinson's disease. The prototypical Group III-selective orthosteric agonist is L-amino-4-phosphonobutyrate (L-AP4), yet this ligand is only selective for Group III mGlu receptors, not within the group. In an attempt to ameliorate the affinity and potency, a series of constrained cyclic forms of glutamate were generated and so was created aminocyclopentane-1,3,4-tricarboxylate (ACPT-I), which showed mildly enhanced potency at $mGlu_4$ and $mGlu_8$ compared to $mGlu_5$ and $mGlu_6$ (Acher et al., 1997; Schann et al., 2006). Similar to the agonists, there are only selective antagonists for Group III mGlu receptors, but not within the group. For example, there are the α-methyl analogues of L-AP4 and L-SOP, specifically MAP4 and MSOP, respectively, with affinity in the micromolar range (Wright et al., 2000). In addition to these, there are the hallmark antagonists of mGlu receptors such as DCG-IV and LY341495, which both have reasonable affinity for Group III mGlu receptors, but also have strong affinity at Group I and Group II receptors, respectively; notably, DCG-IV is also a Group II mGlu receptor agonist (Brabet et al., 1998). Allosteric modulators that act in the 7TM domain Group III mGlu receptors have also been characterised, specifically N-Phenyl-7-(hydroxyimino)cyclopropa[b]chromen-1acarboxamide (PHCCC) and cis-2-([(3,5-Dichlorophenyl)amino]carbonyl)cyclohexanecarboxylic acid (VU0155041), which are both PAMs at $mGlu_4$ (Niswender et al., 2008); 6-(4-Methoxyphenyl)-5-methyl-3-(4-pyridinyl)-isoxazolo[4,5-c]pyridine-4(5H)-one hydrochloride (MMPIP), a NAM for $mGlu_7$ (Niswender et al., 2010); however there remains a relative paucity of allosteric modulators for $mGlu_6$ and $mGlu_8$.

One pharmacological avenue that is only beginning to be explored at Class C GPCRs is that of extracellular domain allosteric modulators. For the umami taste receptors, it has been long known that purinergic ribonucleotides, such as inosine- and guanine-monophosphate molecules (IMP and GMP) were potent positive allosteric modulators of the L-glutamate action at the umami receptor (Yamaguchi and Ninomiya, 2000). Interestingly, mutants that altered the effects of glutamate effect were also enhanced by IMP and GMP (Zhang et al., 2008). By employing a chimeric approach along with mutagenesis and molecular modelling, sweet-umami receptors were analysed and the mode of binding and action of IMP was postulated; specifically, the residues lining the IMP binding pocket at the sweet-umami taste receptor, T1R1, were determined (Zhang et al., 2008). It was demonstrated that IMP binds to a novel site that is adjacent to the glutamate binding pocket, the authors thus proposed a model for ligand cooperativity for the mechanism of action of IMP in the T1R1 VFT. The binding of L-glutamate close to the hinge region of the VFT would stabilize the closed conformation of the domain; moreover, binding of 5' ribonucleotides to an adjacent site closer to the putative entrance of the VFT would further stabilize the closed conformation, thereby potentiating the affinity and/or efficacy of L-glutamate. At mGlu receptors, the glutamate-binding pocket is well conserved across the mGlu subtypes, encumbering the discovery selective orthosteric agonists and antagonists (Brauner-Osborne et al., 2007). However, recently, long alkyl chain containing derivatives of (R)-PCEP, a molecule discovered by virtual screening on the VFT of mGlu receptors, revealed a new binding pocket in mGlu$_4$ (Selvam et al., 2010). Indeed, these compounds not only bind in the glutamate-binding pocket itself, but may also interact with a novel, putative binding pocket adjacent to the glutamate-binding site. Given this new interacting region is formed with residues that are less conserved across the eight mGlu subtypes, this mode of targeting mGlu receptors may furnish compounds with greater selectivity. One such compound may already exist in LSP1-2111, with its L-AP4-like moiety and a 4-hydroxy-3-methoxy-5-nitro-phenyl moiety, it is possible that this molecule bridges across two distinct binding domains, in a similar fashion to bitopic ligands at muscarinic receptors (Antony et al., 2009; Valant et al., 2008; Valant et al., 2009). Accordingly, this ligand has superior selectivity at mGlu$_4$ and mGlu$_6$ over mGlu$_7$ and mGlu$_8$ (Beurrier et al., 2009).

For an overview of chemical structures of a small range of classical orthosteric mGlu receptor ligands, refer to Figure 3 below.

2.4.7 Group III mGlu receptors and Parkinson's disease

Parkinson's disease is one of the most common of neurological disorders, which is largely characterised by its effects on motor function, such as bradykinesia and dyskinesia; further to other non-motor symptoms, for example pain and gastrointestinal dysfunction. Parkinson's disease arises mostly due to a progressive degeneration of dopaminergic neurons in the substantia nigra, leading to excessive cholinergic neurotransmission in the striatum (Pisani et al., 2003). Subsequently, the inhibitory effect that dopamine provides in these circuits augments GABAergic firing in the striatopallidal pathway leading to excessive inhibition of GABAergic neurons in the subthalamic nucleus, in turn leading to the abnormal enhancement of glutamatergic neurons (Hirsch, 2000). Currently, the frontline treatment is levo-dopa, which compensates for the diminished dopaminergic function. However, the activation of presynaptic mGlu$_4$ specifically, may result in the diminution of

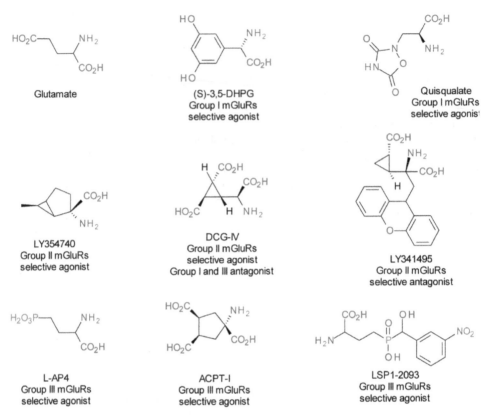

Fig. 3. Highlighting the structural diversity of agonist and antagonists of mGlu receptors.

increased GABAergic firing in striatopallidal projections. Indeed, compounds that have relatively good selectivity for mGlu4 have been demonstrated to depress the GABA-mediated inhibitory synaptic transmission and relive motor symptoms in animal models of Parkinson's disease (Beurrier et al., 2009; Valenti et al., 2003). Given that the dopaminergic dysfunction in the substantia nigra and inhibition of GABA signalling by mGlu4 in the globus pallidus are not inextricably linked there is potential that prolonged mGlu4 receptor activation will result in less compensatory over-activation of the dopaminergic system, therefore maintaining the therapeutic activity of mGlu4 targeting ligands (Nicoletti et al., 2011). Indeed, it has been shown that the *in vivo* treatment with the mGlu4 PAM, PHCCC, reduced dopaminergic neurodegeneration in substantia nigral projections in an MPTP-induced Parkinsonism model (Battaglia et al., 2004; Maj et al., 2003). Along with PHCCC, a more recent PAM of mGlu4 has been characterised and has demonstrated anti-parkinsonian effects (Niswender et al., 2008). VU0155041 is an allosteric agonist and positive allosteric modulator with potency nearly 10-fold of that of PHCCC, moreover, VU0155041 concentration-dependently diminished haloperidol-induced catalepsy and reversed reserpine-mediated akinesia in mice, with an effect that persisted longer than that of the reference Group III orthosteric agonist, L-AP4 (Niswender et al., 2008).

Despite receiving much of the attention within Group III mGlu receptors, mGlu$_4$ is not alone in its involvement in Parkinson's disease. There remains the possibility that post-synaptic mGlu$_7$ and mGlu$_8$ have some effect on the neuronal circuitry in question. The mGlu$_7$ allosteric agonist, N,N'-dibenzhydryl-ethane-1,2-diamine dihydrochloride (AMN082) may inhibit the release of [^{3}H]-D-aspartate in substantia nigral slices, suggesting that selective targeting of mGlu$_7$ may yield similar results to those at mGlu$_4$ (unpublished data; Duty, 2010). Despite there being a large amount of doubt surrounding the therapeutic potential of mGlu$_8$ for the treatment of Parkinson's disease, where the semi-selective mGlu$_8$ agonist was failed to reverse haloperidol-induced catalepsy (Lopez et al., 2007); administration of the mixed AMPA antagonist/mGlu$_8$ agonist, (R,S)-3-4-DCPG, decreased amphetamine- but not phencyclidine-induced hyperactivity (Ossowska et al., 2004). Concomitantly, (R,S)-3-4-DCPG actually enhanced haloperidol-induced catalepsy and induced catalepsy when administered alone. Taken together, and despite similar expression and function compared to mGlu$_4$, does not appear to be a good candidate target for the treatment of Parkinson's disease. Indeed, this scenario highlights the inherent difficulties that are encountered in the search for mGlu receptor subtype-selective therapeutics.

Taken together, it seems that the most appropriate and effective methods for targeting mGlu receptors is via their allosteric ligand-binding site, which increases subtype selectivity and does not impede normal neurotransmission. Refer to Figure 4 for the chemical structures of some allosteric ligands for mGlu receptors.

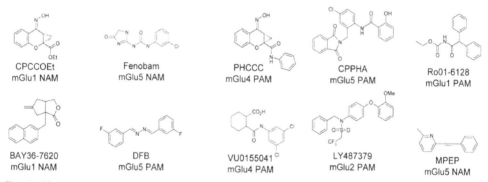

Fig. 4. Chemical structures of mGlu receptor allosteric ligands.

2.4.8 Clinical trials for mGlu receptor ligands

It is now well established that mGlu receptors are major targets for numerous central disorders and even for some in the periphery. Accordingly, there are a large number of clinical programs that are running at any one time (Table 1).

Gastro-(o)esophageal reflux disease (GERD) is a chronic condition, in which the major symptom is the abnormal reflux of stomach contents into the oesophagus. The inhibition of mGlu$_5$ is predicted to improve the tone of the cardiac sphincter, thus reducing reflux (Lehmann, 2008). In a recent phase II clinical study performed by Addex pharmaceuticals, reflux and other GERD symptoms are efficiently reduced by a NAM of mGlu$_5$. The same molecule has also entered into a different phase II study targeting migraine, which also yielded beneficial results. Since glutamate is the main neurotransmitter of the migraine circuit, then inhibition of postsynaptic mGlu5 receptors that are present in this circuit would decrease glutamatergic neurotransmission and hence may pose a useful approach in migraine therapy. However, due to liver toxicity after long-term treatment with this particular molecule, the study was discontinued. Fragile X syndrome is the most common form of inherited mental retardation. Preclinical studies indicate that fragile X phenotypes are linked to an overactivity of mGlu5 (Dolen et al., 2010), suggesting that antagonism of this receptor could be of therapeutic interest. Recently, fenobam, an mGlu5 NAM also known for its anxiolytic properties, entered phase II clinical studies, which so far have demonstrated potential therapeutic benefits on Fragile X symptoms (Berry-Kravis et al., 2009).

Target	Ligand	Company	Trial Phase	Indication
mGlu$_{1/5}$	Antagonist	Forest Laboratories	Preclinical	Anxiety/Depression
mGlu$_2$	TS-032 (Agonist)	Pfizer	Preclinical	Schizophrenia
mGlu$_{2/3}$	ADX1149 (PAM)	Addex Pharmaceuticals	Phase I	Schizophrenia/ Alzheimer's/ Depression
mGlu$_{2/3}$	LY2140023 (Agonist)	Eli Lily	Phase II	Schizophrenia
mGlu$_{2/3}$	Agonist	Eli Lily	Phase III*	Anxiety
mGlu$_4$	PAM	Merck	Preclinical	Parkinson's disease
mGlu$_5$	ADX48621 (Antagonist)	Addex Pharmaceuticals	Phase I	Parkinson's disease
mGlu$_5$	AZD2516 (Antagonist)	Astra Zeneca	Phase I	Chronic pain
mGlu$_5$	AZD2066 (Antagonist)	Astra Zeneca	Phase II	Chronic pain/GERD
mGlu$_5$	NPL-2009	Neuropharm	Phase II	Fragile X syndrome

Table 1. mGlu receptor ligands currently undergoing clinical trials. Sources: ClinicalTrials.gov and EvaluatePharma.com. * - Trial discontinued.

mGlu2 and mGlu3 receptors are a major target for the treatment of anxiety and schizophrenia (Conn and Jones, 2009; Conn et al., 2009b). As a result, the activation of these receptors has been exploited for the treatment of said diseases in several clinical studies. Non-selective mGlu2/mGlu3 agonists have reached phase II clinical studies for the treatment of generalised anxiety disorders, but the trial was terminated due to risks of seizure observed in animals (Dunayevich et al., 2008). Allosteric ligands represent an alternative to the use of orthosteric ligands, since they do not interfere with the spatiotemporal profile of the endogenous ligand; therefore they are more targeted and usually produce less deleterious side effects. Recently, a phase I study on anxiety was started by Ortho-McNeil-Janssen Pharmaceuticals Inc. and Addex pharmaceuticals using ADX71149, an mGlu2 PAM, but the conclusions remain known. Altered glutamatergic neurotransmission is also linked in part to schizophrenia and through a phase II study by Eli Lilly, the improvement of symptoms of schizophrenia with an $mGlu_2/mGlu_3$ agonist was similar to that demonstrated with olanzapine, a common antipsychotic drug; this drug was also tolerated by patients (Patil et al., 2007).

Preclinical studies strongly suggest that Group III mGlu receptors may play a vital role in the symptomatic control of Parkinson's disease. In particular, increasing $mGlu_4$ activity within the basal ganglia appears to be an interesting approach to reduce akinetic symptoms associated with Parkinson's disease (Beurrier et al., 2009; Lopez et al., 2007). However, to our knowledge, none of these compounds have reached phase I clinical trials.

3. Metabotropic GABA receptors

3.1 Structure/function of GABA$_B$ receptors

The metabotropic GABA (GABA$_B$) receptor is the only known GPCR that is responsive to GABA. Architecturally, it is not composed in the same manner as many other Class C GPCRs. Specifically, it consists of a ligand binding GB_1 subunit and a G protein coupling GB_2 subunit (Galvez et al., 2001; Kaupmann et al., 1998; Margeta-Mitrovic et al., 2001; White et al., 1998); each subunit consisting of a VFT and 7TM domains, but converse to mGlu receptors they lack a CRD (refer to Figure 2 for schematic overview). The two subunits are not covalently associated, but do interact via a coiled-coil domain in their C-terminal tails, which provides a solid hydrophobic interaction to maintain the integrity of the dimer (Kammerer et al., 1999). Through the use of circular dichroism spectroscopy the authors proposed a region in the C-terminal domains of GB_1 and GB_2 of approximately 30 amino acids, composed of roughly 5-7 heptads.

Discerning the number of ligands that bind to any one dimer at any one moment is often difficult, especially if there is the possibility for receptors to form higher-order oligomers. It has been shown that in class C heterodimers a single subunit was responsible for the binding of the endogenous ligand, in this case GB_1 in the GABA$_B$ receptor (Kniazeff et al., 2002). This suggests that a single agonist molecule is sufficient to fully activate heterodimeric receptors, but does not discount multiple binding sites on the same protomer. However, nearly nothing is known of the conformational movement of the GB_2 subunit, making it nearly impossible to distinguish between the conformational rearrangement and functional responses of Aco and Acc combinations. The only insights come from the GABA$_B$ receptor, whereby the introduction of several large residues, such as tryptophan in the crevice of GB_2 VFT leads to a decrease in G protein-mediated functional responses (Kniazeff et al., 2002).

It has always been questioned whether GPCRs remain in simple monomeric and dimeric forms or whether they self-associate into higher-order oligomers and, if so, what are the molecular determinants of these interactions. Recently, it has been demonstrated that GABA$_B$ are indeed capable of forming tetrameric complexes, which interact via their GB_1 subunits (Comps-Agrar et al., 2011; Maurel et al., 2008). By employing the use of a binding-null GB_1 subunit Comps-Agrar et al., (2011) demonstrated that GABA$_B$ receptor tetramers could be disrupted and that the resultant complexes are capable of binding approximately twice as much radioligand compared to the wild-type; in addition to increasing the apparent E_{max} in functional tests. The synthesis of this study was that GABA$_B$ receptors that are associated into a tetrameric assembly have reduced binding capacity and functional capability compared to GABA$_B$ receptors in dimeric form. Comps-Agrar et al., (2011) attempted to more precisely examine the structural determinants of the molecular construction of the GABA$_B$ receptor tetramer. They resolved that an important interaction between the VFTs of the GB$_1$ subunits occurs, and then experimentally demonstrated the disruption of this interaction through mutation and insertion of an N-glycosylation site (G^{380}N) increases the apparent B_{max} of fluorescent ligand binding and maximal function effect in intracellular calcium mobilisation assays. It is noteworthy that this study demonstrated that there is tetramerisation of GB$_{1A}$ subunit-containing GABA$_B$ receptors, but not GB$_{1B}$ subunit-containing receptors.

Stimulation of GABA$_B$ receptors results in the activation and dissociation of G$_{i/o}$ family G proteins, which in turn inhibit the function adeylyl cyclase thereby decreasing intracellular cAMP levels; activate Kir3 channels and inhibit Ca$_v$2 channels (Dunlap and Fischbach, 1981; Leaney and Tinker, 2000; Nishikawa et al., 1997). One of the major actions of GABA$_B$ receptor activation is the opening of Kir3 channels, where the increase in K$^+$ permeability through these channels hyperpolarises the cell thereby inhibiting the propagation of action potentials (Dascal, 1997; Misgeld et al., 1995).

Many GPCRs undergo rapid receptor phosphorylation and subsequent sequestration from the cell surface, commonly in an arrestin-dependent manner, followed by the recruitment of scaffolding proteins and by clathrin-mediated endocytosis (Shenoy and Lefkowitz, 2005). One interesting feature that is dissimilar to many GPCRs and is the subject of much debate is that GABA$_B$ receptors do not appear to undergo activation-dependent phosphorylation and internalisation. Indeed, it has been reported that these receptors are not phosphorylated by the canonical G protein-coupled receptor kinases (GRKs), yet are desensitised by GRK4 in the absence of any apparent phosphorylation (Perroy et al., 2003). It has been demonstrated in chick neurons that upon activation, GABA$_B$ receptors form a complex with Ca$_v$ channels and arrestins, then are consequently internalised as a mechanism of rapid desensitisation of GABA$_B$ receptor signalling (Puckerin et al., 2006). This however, is conflicting with evidence provided by Fairfax et al., (2004) whereby GABA$_B$ receptors did not associate with arrestins and, indeed, the cAMP-dependent kinase- (PKA) mediated phosphorylation of the GABA$_B$ receptor at position Ser892 on the GB$_2$ subunit increases its cell-surface stability; rather than impeding its cellular function. It would appear in these cases that the phosphorylation state and the subsequent events may very well be cell type specific, which may be yet another degree of complexity for texturing GABA$_B$ receptor-mediated signalling. Interestingly, despite the lack of consistent evidence that GABA$_B$ receptors are phosphorylated as a consequence of receptor activation, there is an accumulating body of evidence that these receptors are phosphorylated mostly by second-messenger kinases. For example, protein kinase C (PKC) has been described to phosphorylate the GB$_1$ subunit GABA$_B$ receptors after the dissociation of the chaprone protein, N-ethylmaleimide-sensitive fusion (NSF) protein, in Chinese hamster ovary (CHO) cells (Pontier et al., 2006). More recently, there have been new developments on how GABA$_B$ receptors are phosphorylated and dephosphorylated in neurons. Recent evidence suggests that NMDA receptors can also act as regulators of GABA$_B$ receptor function, such that NMDA receptor activation, via calcium/calmodulin-dependent protein kinase, phosphorylates the GB$_1$ subunit at position Ser867, resulting in rapid receptor internalisation from dendritic spines and shafts in the hippocampus (Guetg et al., 2010). Similarly, prolonged NMDA receptor activation results in the rapid phosphorylation of Ser783 on GB_2 in an 5' adenosine-monophosphate-dependent protein kinase- (AMPK) dependent manner (Terunuma et al., 2010). The rapid phosphorylation by AMPK altered the endocytic sorting pathway from receptor recycling to endosomal degradation, Ser783 was then slowly dephosphorylated by protein phosphatase 2A, returning the system back to its receptor recycling processes. Although the modes of which $GABA_B$ receptors are phosphorylated and there consequences are not entirely clear, recently there has been a great deal of progress made in understanding how $GABA_B$ receptor phosphorylation is affected by distinct signalling systems and their consequences on receptor function.

3.2 Localisation and physiology of $GABA_B$ receptors

The $GABA_B$ receptor is extensively expressed throughout the central nervous system, specifically, hippocampus, cortex, thalamus and cerebellum (Bettler and Tiao, 2006; Billinton et al., 1999); and in parts of the peripheral nervous system. They are located both pre- and post-synaptically where they mediate activity of Ca_v and Kir3 channels, respectively (Dutar and Nicoll, 1988; Lopez-Bendito et al., 2004; Luscher et al., 1997). Presynaptic $GABA_B$ receptors can be found at both homo- and hetero-autoreceptors on GABA and, for example, glutamate nerve terminals, respectively (Thompson et al., 1993). Activation of these receptors leads to a hyperpolarisation of the nerve terminal thereby inhibiting further neurotransmitter release. Postsynaptically, $GABA_B$ receptors have been demonstrated to mediate slow inhibitory postsynaptic potentials (IPSPs) through the operation of Kir3 channels. It is noteworthy that in the human brain, there are two major isoforms of the $GABA_B$ receptors, those that contain a GB_{1A} subunits, and those that possess GB_{1B} subunits, notwithstanding there is no apparent difference in pharmacology or physiology between the two receptors in heterologous cell systems (Ulrich and Bettler, 2007). Despite a lack of obvious differences in function and pharmacology, there is indeed a differential expression pattern, such that GB_{1A} and GB_{1B} are both expressed on GABAergic nerve terminals, yet only GB_{1A} subunits are expressed on glutamatergic synaptic terminals (Kulik et al., 2003). By using different sets of complementary approaches, the authors showed that GB_{1A}-containing heterodimers mainly control presynaptic release of glutamate, whereas receptors possessing GB_{1B} subunits predominantly mediate post-synaptic inhibition.

3.3 $GABA_B$ receptor pharmacology and clinical relevance

Similar to mGlu receptors, $GABA_B$ receptors have two main ligand-binding domains, the orthosteric ligand-binding pocket located within the VFT of GB_1; and the allosteric ligand-binding domain, which is within the 7TM region, most likely within the 7TM bundle. There are surprisingly few $GABA_B$ receptor full agonists aside from GABA itself and the well-known baclofen (refer to Figure 5). There are some other agonists such as CGP27492, the tritiated form of which replaced [^{3}H]-baclofen as the radioligand agonist of choice, but was surrounded by controversy when it failed to reproduce the same physiological effects in some key assays (Froestl et al., 1995). A number of $GABA_B$ receptor partial agonists have been identified, the most famous of which is the endogenous metabolite of GABA, γ-hydroxybutyric acid (GHB), synthesised from GABA transaminase and semialdehyde reductase. Other partial agonists include CGP44532 and CGP35024, the latter is also a

GABA$_C$ receptor antagonist (Chebib et al., 1997). The number of antagonists is much greater than that of agonists, among these ligands there are the baclofen derivatives, saclofen and 2-OH saclofen; CGP54626, the most common of the antagonists; and CGP71872; the former two possessing high micromolar affinity, whilst the latter two exhibit low nanomolar affinity (Kaupmann et al., 1997).

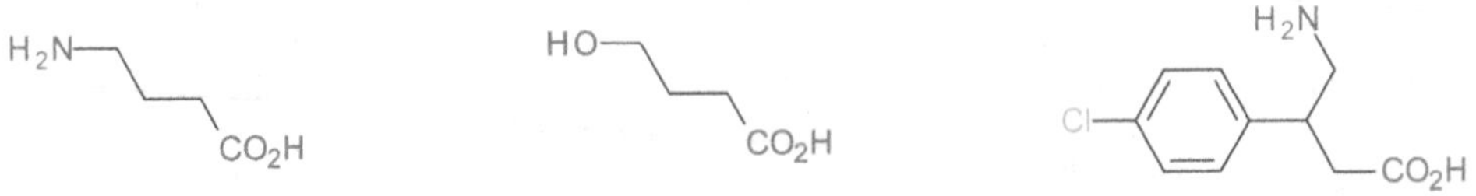

| GABA | GHB | Baclofen |

Fig. 5. Structural similarities across common GABA$_B$ receptor agonists.

As with many Class C GPCRs, there exist a number of allosteric modulators available for the GABA$_B$ receptor, yet all known modulators are PAMs, with no known NAMs, to date. Some PAMs of the GABA$_B$ receptor are CGP7930, GS39783 and the more recent, rac-BHFF (Malherbe et al., 2008; Pin and Prezeau, 2007)(Figure 6). These PAMs increase orthosteric agonist potency and maximal response in a system-dependent manner, whilst possessing partial agonism in their own right. Given that many PAMs will most often on activate their target receptor when the endogenous or orthosteric ligand is present, they offer an ideal approach for drug discovery given they maintain region-dependent transmission patterns, therefore theoretically limiting off-target effects and side effect profile.

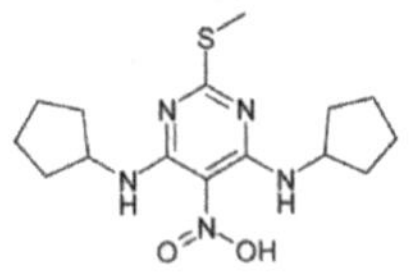

GS39783
GABAb PAM

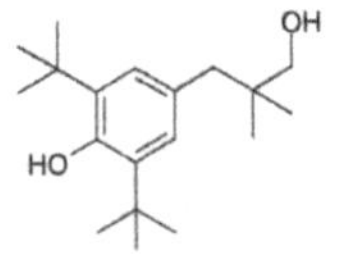

CGP7930
GABAb PAM

Fig. 6. Two of the best characterised positive allosteric modulators at the GABA$_B$ receptor.

3.3.1 Addiction and GABA$_B$ receptors

Today, there are two GABA$_B$ receptor ligands on the market, both agonist, but both treat largely different disorders. Baclofen, originally developed to treat epilepsy in the 1920s, was largely unsuccessful for the treatment of epileptic symptoms, but its potential was realised outside of epileptic patients. Among the more common uses for baclofen is the treatment of addiction of abusive substances. Specifically, alcohol dependence has received much attention with regard to GABAB receptors, such that baclofen administration in open-label trials reduced the number of heavy-drinking days and increased the number of abstinence days, in addiction to decreasing biological markers such as alanine aminotranferase and gamma glutamyl-transpeptidase, in some patients (Addolorato et al., 2000; Flannery et al., 2004). Baclofen was not only useful for the management of alcohol addiction, but may also be employed as a strategy against withdrawal and relapse (Addolorato et al., 2006). When compared with treatment of diazepam, baclofen was only slightly less efficient at reducing the symptoms of alcohol withdrawal, such as sweating, anxiety and agitation; however this suggests baclofen may be a useful treatment for alcohol withdrawal in patients that abuse other substances, for example, benzodiazepines.

Baclofen has also been investigated for its effects on relieving addiction to cocaine. In one study, users of freebase or crack cocaine who self-administered through inhalation of the drug (Haney et al., 2006). Users who were either treated with methadone or not were given varying doses of baclofen and subsequently were asked to choose to take either the available dose of cocaine or five dollar merchandise voucher. The group who were administered 60mg of baclofen and non-methadone treated demonstrated a decrease in the craving for the low dose of cocaine (12mg), whilst there was no change in the methadone-treated group. Interestingly, baclofen also decreased the effect of cocaine on heart rate, however the personal evaluation of the 'high' remained unchanged. These results suggest that in some specific cases that baclofen would have a positive effect on addiction, however these situations are also often confounded by psychological dependence and are by and large heavily dictated by the patient.

3.3.2 GHB and current therapeutic indications

As previously mentioned, GHB is a minor metabolite of GABA; however in the 1960s GHB was first developed as a therapeutic as a CNS depressor (Laborit et al., 1960). At the time, it was also used as an adjuvant for anesthetics and is still used in some countries as an intravenous anesthesia (Kleinschmidt et al., 1997). Nowadays, the therapeutic indications for GHB are cataplexy and excessive daytime sleepiness associated with sleep disorder narcolepsy. Narcolepsy is the condition characterised by interrupted nighttime sleep and excessive daytime sleep, in addition to this, approximately 70% of narcoleptics suffer from cataplexy, which is a sudden loss of muscle tone. The evidence of clinical efficacy of GHB is largely empirical through a number of studies on narcoleptic patients, daily doses of GHB was able to reduce the number of nocturnal sleep/awake transitions, cataplexy episodes and the frequency between wakefulness and REM sleep during the daytime (Pardi and Black, 2006; Scrima et al., 1990). Despite clinical evidence supporting the therapeutic benefits of GHB for these conditions, there is still much debate over the molecular mechanism of action of GHB. There is known to be at least two GHB-binding sites, a high-affinity site on an unidentified protein; and a low-affinity site, which is at the GABAB receptor (Kaupmann et al., 2003). However, there is evidence that the effects of GHB on stabilising patterns of somnolence are due to the subsequent actions at the GABAB receptor. Recently, Vienne et al., (2010) provided evidence that the effects on somnolence and circadian sleep organisation are dependent on GABAB receptors, whereby GHB and baclofen stabilised sleep/wake regulation in wild-type mice; these effects were lost in both GB1-/- and GB2-/- mice. This study suggests that the therapeutic benefits of GHB in narcoleptic patients may be mostly due to GHB-mediated activation of GABAB receptors.

3.3.3 GABA_B receptors in pain

The importance of GABA_B receptors in nociceptive processing was well documented in the early 90's in a series of preclinical studies in which the GABA_B receptor agonist, baclofen, exhibited antinociceptive properties in models of acute (Malcangio et al., 1991) and chronic pain (Dirig and Yaksh, 1995; Smith et al., 1994). These effects are likely mediated by spinal and supraspinal GABA_B receptors; where the supraspinal effects appear to reflect depression of ascending adrenergic and dopaminergic input to the brainstem, and facilitation of descending noradrenergic input to the spinal cord dorsal horn (Sawynok, 1984). Baclofen-induced antinociception at spinal cord level is attributed, at least partly, to the activation of presynaptic GABA_B receptors localised on the nerve terminals of peptidergic primary afferents fibers (Price et al., 1984). In the substantia gelatinosa of the spinal cord, baclofen exhibits a greater effect on C-fibers than Aδ-fiber-evoked glutamate release, suggesting a preferential GABA_B expression in C fibers afferent terminals (Ataka et al., 2000). Furthermore, baclofen inhibits electrically-evoked release of calcitonin gene-related peptide (CGRP) (Malcangio and Bowery, 1995) and substance P (Marvizon et al., 1999) from rat spinal cord slices. The decrease of dorsal horn neurons excitability and the regulation of intrinsic neuronal properties suggest additional postsynaptic sites for the action of baclofen on pain (Derjean et al., 2003; Kangrga et al., 1991). Taken together, the effects of activation of GABA_B receptors on the inhibition of pain signalling suggest that it is a tractable target for combating neuropathic and potentially other types of pain.

4. Concluding remarks

The treatment of neurological disorders is perhaps one of the most difficult tasks in modern day medicine; the multi-factorial nature of disease and the availability of appropriate therapeutics continually hamper the drug discovery process. The initial step in surmounting these obstacles is the validation of a target, which is perpetually being revised and, has now furnished two invaluable targets in the mGlu and GABA_B receptors. Both receptors, which present the major excitatory and inhibitory GPCR conduits, could be targeted for the treatment of a myriad of central and peripheral disorders. To better understand the function and physiology of these receptors it is paramount that we elucidate molecular mechanisms of receptor activation and ligand binding. There exists a large body of work the pharmacology of mGlu and GABA_B receptors, yet we are only now scratching the surface, as recently there has been an influx on novel receptor-selective pharmacophores, especially for mGlu receptors. With a better pharmacological armamentarium we will be better equipped to delineate (patho)physiological phenomena as we progress development of better therapeutics.

5. References

Acher FC, Tellier FJ, Azerad R, Brabet IN, Fagni L and Pin JP (1997) Synthesis and pharmacological characterization of aminocyclopentanetricarboxylic acids: new tools to discriminate between metabotropic glutamate receptor subtypes. *J Med Chem* 40(19):3119-3129.

Addolorato G, Caputo F, Capristo E, Colombo G, Gessa GL and Gasbarrini G (2000) Ability of baclofen in reducing alcohol craving and intake: II--Preliminary clinical evidence. *Alcohol Clin Exp Res* 24(1):67-71.

Addolorato G, Leggio L, Abenavoli L, Agabio R, Caputo F, Capristo E, Colombo G, Gessa GL and Gasbarrini G (2006) Baclofen in the treatment of alcohol withdrawal syndrome: a comparative study vs diazepam. *Am J Med* 119(3):276 e213-278.

Aghajanian GK and Marek GJ (1999) Serotonin and hallucinogens. *Neuropsychopharmacology* 21(2 Suppl):16S-23S.

Agnati LF, Ferre S, Lluis C, Franco R and Fuxe K (2003) Molecular mechanisms and therapeutical implications of intramembrane receptor/receptor interactions among heptahelical receptors with examples from the striatopallidal GABA neurons. *Pharmacol Rev* 55(3):509-550.

Aiba A, Chen C, Herrup K, Rosenmund C, Stevens CF and Tonegawa S (1994a) Reduced hippocampal long-term potentiation and context-specific deficit in associative learning in mGluR1 mutant mice. *Cell* 79(2):365-375.

Aiba A, Kano M, Chen C, Stanton ME, Fox GD, Herrup K, Zwingman TA and Tonegawa S (1994b) Deficient cerebellar long-term depression and impaired motor learning in mGluR1 mutant mice. *Cell* 79(2):377-388.

Allen SJ, Crown SE and Handel TM (2007) Chemokine: receptor structure, interactions, and antagonism. *Annu Rev Immunol* 25:787-820.

Anderson JJ, Rao SP, Rowe B, Giracello DR, Holtz G, Chapman DF, Tehrani L, Bradbury MJ, Cosford ND and Varney MA (2002) [3H]Methoxymethyl-3-[(2-methyl-1,3-thiazol-4-yl)ethynyl]pyridine binding to metabotropic glutamate receptor subtype 5 in rodent brain: in vitro and in vivo characterization. *J Pharmacol Exp Ther* 303(3):1044-1051.

Andrade L, Caraveo-Anduaga JJ, Berglund P, Bijl RV, De Graaf R, Vollebergh W, Dragomirecka E, Kohn R, Keller M, Kessler RC, Kawakami N, Kilic C, Offord D, Ustun TB and Wittchen HU (2003) The epidemiology of major depressive episodes: results from the International Consortium of Psychiatric Epidemiology (ICPE) Surveys. *Int J Methods Psychiatr Res* 12(1):3-21.

Aniksztejn L, Otani S and Ben-Ari Y (1992) Quisqualate Metabotropic Receptors Modulate NMDA Currents and Facilitate Induction of Long-Term Potentiation Through Protein Kinase C. *Eur J Neurosci* 4(6):500-505.

Annoura H, Fukunaga A, Uesugi M, Tatsuoka T and Horikawa Y (1996) A novel class of antagonists for metabotropic glutamate receptors, 7-(hydroxyimino)cyclopropa[b]chromen-1a-carboxylates. *Bioorg. Med. Chem. Lett.* 6, 763-766

Antony J, Kellershohn K, Mohr-Andra M, Kebig A, Prilla S, Muth M, Heller E, Disingrini T, Dallanoce C, Bertoni S, Schrobang J, Trankle C, Kostenis E, Christopoulos A, Holtje HD, Barocelli E, De Amici M, Holzgrabe U and Mohr K (2009) Dualsteric GPCR targeting: a novel route to binding and signaling pathway selectivity. *Faseb J* 23(2):442-450.

Ataka T, Kumamoto E, Shimoji K and Yoshimura M (2000) Baclofen inhibits more effectively C-afferent than Adelta-afferent glutamatergic transmission in substantia gelatinosa neurons of adult rat spinal cord slices. *Pain* 86(3):273-282.

Ayala JE, Niswender CM, Luo Q, Banko JL and Conn PJ (2008) Group III mGluR regulation of synaptic transmission at the SC-CA1 synapse is developmentally regulated. *Neuropharmacology* 54(5):804-814.

Azdad K, Gall D, Woods AS, Ledent C, Ferre S and Schiffmann SN (2009) Dopamine D2 and adenosine A2A receptors regulate NMDA-mediated excitation in accumbens neurons through A2A-D2 receptor heteromerization. *Neuropsychopharmacology* 34(4):972-986.

Baptista MA, Martin-Fardon R and Weiss F (2004) Preferential effects of the metabotropic glutamate 2/3 receptor agonist LY379268 on conditioned reinstatement versus primary reinforcement: comparison between cocaine and a potent conventional reinforcer. *J Neurosci* 24(20):4723-4727.

Battaglia G, Busceti CL, Molinaro G, Biagioni F, Storto M, Fornai F, Nicoletti F and Bruno V (2004) Endogenous activation of mGlu5 metabotropic glutamate receptors contributes to the development of nigro-striatal damage induced by 1-methyl-4-phenyl-1,2,3,6-tetrahydropyridine in mice. *J Neurosci* 24(4):828-835.

Baude A, Nusser Z, Roberts JD, Mulvihill E, McIlhinney RA and Somogyi P (1993) The metabotropic glutamate receptor (mGluR1 alpha) is concentrated at perisynaptic membrane of neuronal subpopulations as detected by immunogold reaction. *Neuron* 11(4):771-787.

Belozertseva IV, Kos T, Popik P, Danysz W and Bespalov AY (2007) Antidepressant-like effects of mGluR1 and mGluR5 antagonists in the rat forced swim and the mouse tail suspension tests. *Eur Neuropsychopharmacol* 17(3):172-179.

Benneyworth MA, Smith RL and Sanders-Bush E (2008) Chronic phenethylamine hallucinogen treatment alters behavioral sensitivity to a metabotropic glutamate 2/3 receptor agonist. *Neuropsychopharmacology* 33(9):2206-2216.

Benneyworth MA, Xiang Z, Smith RL, Garcia EE, Conn PJ and Sanders-Bush E (2007) A selective positive allosteric modulator of metabotropic glutamate receptor subtype 2 blocks a hallucinogenic drug model of psychosis. *Mol Pharmacol* 72(2):477-484.

Berry-Kravis E, Hessl D, Coffey S, Hervey C, Schneider A, Yuhas J, Hutchison J, Snape M, Tranfaglia M, Nguyen DV and Hagerman R (2009) A pilot open label, single dose trial of fenobam in adults with fragile X syndrome. *J Med Genet* 46(4):266-271.

Bessis AS, Bertrand HO, Galvez T, De Colle C, Pin JP and Acher F (2000) Three-dimensional model of the extracellular domain of the type 4a metabotropic glutamate receptor: new insights into the activation process. *Protein Sci* 9(11):2200-2209.

Bessis AS, Rondard P, Gaven F, Brabet I, Triballeau N, Prezeau L, Acher F and Pin JP (2002) Closure of the Venus flytrap module of mGlu8 receptor and the activation process: Insights from mutations converting antagonists into agonists. *Proc Natl Acad Sci U S A* 99(17):11097-11102.

Bettler B and Tiao JY (2006) Molecular diversity, trafficking and subcellular localization of GABAB receptors. *Pharmacol Ther* 110(3):533-543.

Beurrier C, Lopez S, Revy D, Selvam C, Goudet C, Lherondel M, Gubellini P, Kerkerian-LeGoff L, Acher F, Pin JP and Amalric M (2009) Electrophysiological and behavioral evidence that modulation of metabotropic glutamate receptor 4 with a new agonist reverses experimental parkinsonism. *FASEB J* 23(10):3619-3628.

Billinton A, Upton N and Bowery NG (1999) GABA(B) receptor isoforms GBR1a and GBR1b, appear to be associated with pre- and post-synaptic elements respectively in rat and human cerebellum. *Br J Pharmacol* 126(6):1387-1392.

Bittencourt AS, Carobrez AP, Zamprogno LP, Tufik S and Schenberg LC (2004) Organization of single components of defensive behaviors within distinct columns of periaqueductal gray matter of the rat: role of N-methyl-D-aspartic acid glutamate receptors. *Neuroscience* 125(1):71-89.

Bortolotto ZA, Fitzjohn SM and Collingridge GL (1999) Roles of metabotropic glutamate receptors in LTP and LTD in the hippocampus. *Curr Opin Neurobiol* 9(3):299-304.

Bowers MS, McFarland K, Lake RW, Peterson YK, Lapish CC, Gregory ML, Lanier SM and Kalivas PW (2004) Activator of G protein signaling 3: a gatekeeper of cocaine sensitization and drug seeking. *Neuron* 42(2):269-281.

Brabet I, Parmentier ML, De Colle C, Bockaert J, Acher F and Pin JP (1998) Comparative effect of L-CCG-I, DCG-IV and gamma-carboxy-L-glutamate on all cloned metabotropic glutamate receptor subtypes. *Neuropharmacology* 37(8):1043-1051.

Brauner-Osborne H, Wellendorph P and Jensen AA (2007) Structure, pharmacology and therapeutic prospects of family C G-protein coupled receptors. *Curr Drug Targets* 8(1):169-184.

Brody SA, Conquet F and Geyer MA (2003) Disruption of prepulse inhibition in mice lacking mGluR1. *Eur J Neurosci* 18(12):3361-3366.

Brody SA, Dulawa SC, Conquet F and Geyer MA (2004) Assessment of a prepulse inhibition deficit in a mutant mouse lacking mGlu5 receptors. *Mol Psychiatry* 9(1):35-41.

Burridge K and Wennerberg K (2004) Rho and Rac take center stage. *Cell* 116(2):167-179.

Bushell TJ, Sansig G, Collett VJ, van der Putten H and Collingridge GL (2002) Altered short-term synaptic plasticity in mice lacking the metabotropic glutamate receptor mGlu7. *ScientificWorldJournal* 2:730-737.

Cabello N, Gandia J, Bertarelli DC, Watanabe M, Lluis C, Franco R, Ferre S, Lujan R and Ciruela F (2009) Metabotropic glutamate type 5, dopamine D2 and adenosine A2a receptors form higher-order oligomers in living cells. *J Neurochem* 109(5):1497-1507.

Carroll FY, Stolle A, Beart PM, Voerste A, Brabet I, Mauler F, Joly C, Antonicek H, Bockaert J, Muller T, Pin JP and Prezeau L (2001) BAY36-7620: a potent non-competitive mGlu1 receptor antagonist with inverse agonist activity. *Mol Pharmacol* 59(5):965-973.

Chavez-Noriega LE, Schaffhauser H and Campbell UC (2002) Metabotropic glutamate receptors: potential drug targets for the treatment of schizophrenia. *Curr Drug Targets CNS Neurol Disord* 1(3):261-281.

Chebib M, Vandenberg RJ, Froestl W and Johnston GA (1997) Unsaturated phosphinic analogues of gamma-aminobutyric acid as GABA(C) receptor antagonists. *Eur J Pharmacol* 329(2-3):223-229.

Chen Y, Goudet C, Pin JP and Conn PJ (2008) N-{4-Chloro-2-[(1,3-dioxo-1,3-dihydro-2H-isoindol-2-yl)methyl]phenyl}-2-hy droxybenzamide (CPPHA) acts through a novel site as a positive allosteric modulator of group 1 metabotropic glutamate receptors. *Mol Pharmacol* 73(3):909-918.

Chojnacka-Wojcik E, Tatarczynska E and Pilc A (1997) The anxiolytic-like effect of metabotropic glutamate receptor antagonists after intrahippocampal injection in rats. *Eur J Pharmacol* 319(2-3):153-156.

Christopoulos A and Kenakin T (2002) G protein-coupled receptor allosterism and complexing. *Pharmacol Rev* 54(2):323-374.

Ciruela F, Burgueno J, Casado V, Canals M, Marcellino D, Goldberg SR, Bader M, Fuxe K, Agnati LF, Lluis C, Franco R, Ferre S and Woods AS (2004) Combining mass spectrometry and pull-down techniques for the study of receptor heteromerization. Direct epitope-epitope electrostatic interactions between adenosine A2A and dopamine D2 receptors. *Anal Chem* 76(18):5354-5363.

Ciruela F, Escriche M, Burgueno J, Angulo E, Casado V, Soloviev MM, Canela EI, Mallol J, Chan WY, Lluis C, McIlhinney RA and Franco R (2001) Metabotropic glutamate 1alpha and adenosine A1 receptors assemble into functionally interacting complexes. *J Biol Chem* 276(21):18345-18351.

Collingridge GL, Kehl SJ and McLennan H (1983) Excitatory amino acids in synaptic transmission in the Schaffer collateral-commissural pathway of the rat hippocampus. *J Physiol* 334:33-46.

Comps-Agrar L, Kniazeff J, Norskov-Lauritsen L, Maurel D, Gassmann M, Gregor N, Prezeau L, Bettler B, Durroux T, Trinquet E and Pin JP (2011) The oligomeric state sets GABA(B) receptor signalling efficacy. *EMBO J* 30(12):2336-2349.

Conn PJ, Christopoulos A and Lindsley CW (2009a) Allosteric modulators of GPCRs: a novel approach for the treatment of CNS disorders. *Nat Rev Drug Discov* 8(1):41-54.

Conn PJ and Jones CK (2009) Promise of mGluR2/3 activators in psychiatry. *Neuropsychopharmacology* 34(1):248-249.

Conn PJ, Lindsley CW and Jones CK (2009b) Activation of metabotropic glutamate receptors as a novel approach for the treatment of schizophrenia. *Trends Pharmacol Sci* 30(1):25-31.

Conn PJ and Pin JP (1997) Pharmacology and functions of metabotropic glutamate receptors. *Annu Rev Pharmacol Toxicol* 37:205-237.

Coyle JT (2006) Glutamate and schizophrenia: beyond the dopamine hypothesis. *Cell Mol Neurobiol* 26(4-6):365-384.

Cryan JF, Kelly PH, Neijt HC, Sansig G, Flor PJ and van Der Putten H (2003) Antidepressant and anxiolytic-like effects in mice lacking the group III metabotropic glutamate receptor mGluR7. *Eur J Neurosci* 17(11):2409-2417.

Dascal N (1997) Signalling via the G protein-activated K+ channels. *Cell Signal* 9(8):551-573.

Depping AM, Komossa K, Kissling W and Leucht S (2010) Second-generation antipsychotics for anxiety disorders. *Cochrane Database Syst Rev*(12):CD008120.

Derjean D, Bertrand S, Le Masson G, Landry M, Morisset V and Nagy F (2003) Dynamic balance of metabotropic inputs causes dorsal horn neurons to switch functional states. *Nat Neurosci* 6(3):274-281.

Dirig DM and Yaksh TL (1995) Intrathecal baclofen and muscimol, but not midazolam, are antinociceptive using the rat-formalin model. *J Pharmacol Exp Ther* 275(1):219-227.

Dolen G, Carpenter RL, Ocain TD and Bear MF (2010) Mechanism-based approaches to treating fragile X. *Pharmacol Ther* 127(1):78-93.

Doumazane E, Scholler P, Zwier JM, Eric T, Rondard P and Pin JP (2011) A new approach to analyze cell surface protein complexes reveals specific heterodimeric metabotropic glutamate receptors. *FASEB J* 25(1):66-77.

Doupnik CA (2008) GPCR-Kir channel signaling complexes: defining rules of engagement. *J Recept Signal Transduct Res* 28(1-2):83-91.

Dunayevich E, Erickson J, Levine L, Landbloom R, Schoepp DD and Tollefson GD (2008) Efficacy and tolerability of an mGlu2/3 agonist in the treatment of generalized anxiety disorder. *Neuropsychopharmacology* 33(7):1603-1610.

Dunlap K and Fischbach GD (1981) Neurotransmitters decrease the calcium conductance activated by depolarization of embryonic chick sensory neurones. *J Physiol* 317:519-535.

Dutar P and Nicoll RA (1988) Pre- and postsynaptic GABAB receptors in the hippocampus have different pharmacological properties. *Neuron* 1(7):585-591.

Duty S (2010) Therapeutic potential of targeting group III metabotropic glutamate receptors in the treatment of Parkinson's disease. *Br J Pharmacol* 161(2):271-287.

Duvoisin RM, Zhang C, Pfankuch TF, O'Connor H, Gayet-Primo J, Quraishi S and Raber J (2005) Increased measures of anxiety and weight gain in mice lacking the group III metabotropic glutamate receptor mGluR8. *Eur J Neurosci* 22(2):425-436.

Engin E and Treit D (2008) The effects of intra-cerebral drug infusions on animals' unconditioned fear reactions: a systematic review. *Prog Neuropsychopharmacol Biol Psychiatry* 32(6):1399-1419.

Fairfax BP, Pitcher JA, Scott MG, Calver AR, Pangalos MN, Moss SJ and Couve A (2004) Phosphorylation and chronic agonist treatment atypically modulate GABAB receptor cell surface stability. *J Biol Chem* 279(13):12565-12573.

Fell MJ, Svensson KA, Johnson BG and Schoepp DD (2008) Evidence for the role of metabotropic glutamate (mGlu)2 not mGlu3 receptors in the preclinical antipsychotic pharmacology of the mGlu2/3 receptor agonist (-)-(1R,4S,5S,6S)-4-amino-2-sulfonylbicyclo[3.1.0]hexane-4,6-dicarboxylic acid (LY404039). *J Pharmacol Exp Ther* 326(1):209-217.

Felts AS, Lindsley SR, Lamb JP, Rodriguez AL, Menon UN, Jadhav S, Jones CK, Conn PJ, Lindsley CW and Emmitte KA (2010) 3-Cyano-5-fluoro-N-arylbenzamides as negative allosteric modulators of mGlu(5): Identification of easily prepared tool compounds with CNS exposure in rats. *Bioorg Med Chem Lett* 20(15):4390-4394.

Ferraguti F and Shigemoto R (2006) Metabotropic glutamate receptors. *Cell Tissue Res* 326(2):483-504.

Ferre S, Ciruela F, Quiroz C, Lujan R, Popoli P, Cunha RA, Agnati LF, Fuxe K, Woods AS, Lluis C and Franco R (2007) Adenosine receptor heteromers and their integrative role in striatal function. *ScientificWorldJournal* 7:74-85.

Ferre S, Karcz-Kubicha M, Hope BT, Popoli P, Burgueno J, Gutierrez MA, Casado V, Fuxe K, Goldberg SR, Lluis C, Franco R and Ciruela F (2002) Synergistic interaction between adenosine A2A and glutamate mGlu5 receptors: implications for striatal neuronal function. *Proc Natl Acad Sci U S A* 99(18):11940-11945.

Feyissa AM, Chandran A, Stockmeier CA and Karolewicz B (2009) Reduced levels of NR2A and NR2B subunits of NMDA receptor and PSD-95 in the prefrontal cortex in major depression. *Prog Neuropsychopharmacol Biol Psychiatry* 33(1):70-75.

Flannery BA, Garbutt JC, Cody MW, Renn W, Grace K, Osborne M, Crosby K, Morreale M and Trivette A (2004) Baclofen for alcohol dependence: a preliminary open-label study. *Alcohol Clin Exp Res* 28(10):1517-1523.

Fredriksson R, Lagerstrom MC, Lundin LG and Schioth HB (2003) The G-protein-coupled receptors in the human genome form five main families. Phylogenetic analysis, paralogon groups, and fingerprints. *Mol Pharmacol* 63(6):1256-1272.

Froestl W, Mickel SJ, Hall RG, von Sprecher G, Strub D, Baumann PA, Brugger F, Gentsch C, Jaekel J, Olpe HR and et al. (1995) Phosphinic acid analogues of GABA. 1. New potent and selective GABAB agonists. *J Med Chem* 38(17):3297-3312.

Galandrin S, Oligny-Longpre G and Bouvier M (2007) The evasive nature of drug efficacy: implications for drug discovery. *Trends Pharmacol Sci* 28(8):423-430.

Galici R, Jones CK, Hemstapat K, Nong Y, Echemendia NG, Williams LC, de Paulis T and Conn PJ (2006) Biphenyl-indanone A, a positive allosteric modulator of the metabotropic glutamate receptor subtype 2, has antipsychotic- and anxiolytic-like effects in mice. *J Pharmacol Exp Ther* 318(1):173-185.

Galvez T, Duthey B, Kniazeff J, Blahos J, Rovelli G, Bettler B, Prezeau L and Pin JP (2001) Allosteric interactions between GB1 and GB2 subunits are required for optimal GABA(B) receptor function. *EMBO J* 20(9):2152-2159.

Gasparini F, Lingenhohl K, Stoehr N, Flor PJ, Heinrich M, Vranesic I, Biollaz M, Allgeier H, Heckendorn R, Urwyler S, Varney MA, Johnson EC, Hess SD, Rao SP, Sacaan AI, Santori EM, Velicelebi G and Kuhn R (1999) 2-Methyl-6-(phenylethynyl)-pyridine (MPEP), a potent, selective and systemically active mGlu5 receptor antagonist. *Neuropharmacology* 38(10):1493-1503.

Gerlai R, Roder JC and Hampson DR (1998) Altered spatial learning and memory in mice lacking the mGluR4 subtype of metabotropic glutamate receptor. *Behav Neurosci* 112(3):525-532.

Ghasemzadeh MB, Mueller C and Vasudevan P (2009) Behavioral sensitization to cocaine is associated with increased glutamate receptor trafficking to the postsynaptic density after extended withdrawal period. *Neuroscience* 159(1):414-426.

Gonzalez-Maeso J, Ang RL, Yuen T, Chan P, Weisstaub NV, Lopez-Gimenez JF, Zhou M, Okawa Y, Callado LF, Milligan G, Gingrich JA, Filizola M, Meana JJ and Sealfon SC (2008) Identification of a serotonin/glutamate receptor complex implicated in psychosis. *Nature* 452(7183):93-97.

Gonzalez-Maeso J, Weisstaub NV, Zhou M, Chan P, Ivic L, Ang R, Lira A, Bradley-Moore M, Ge Y, Zhou Q, Sealfon SC and Gingrich JA (2007) Hallucinogens recruit specific cortical 5-HT(2A) receptor-mediated signaling pathways to affect behavior. *Neuron* 53(3):439-452.

Gonzalez-Maeso J, Yuen T, Ebersole BJ, Wurmbach E, Lira A, Zhou M, Weisstaub N, Hen R, Gingrich JA and Sealfon SC (2003) Transcriptome fingerprints distinguish hallucinogenic and nonhallucinogenic 5-hydroxytryptamine 2A receptor agonist effects in mouse somatosensory cortex. *J Neurosci* 23(26):8836-8843.

Goudet C, Gaven F, Kniazeff J, Vol C, Liu J, Cohen-Gonsaud M, Acher F, Prezeau L and Pin JP (2004) Heptahelical domain of metabotropic glutamate receptor 5 behaves like rhodopsin-like receptors. *Proc Natl Acad Sci U S A* 101(1):378-383.

Guetg N, Abdel Aziz S, Holbro N, Turecek R, Rose T, Seddik R, Gassmann M, Moes S, Jenoe P, Oertner TG, Casanova E and Bettler B (2010) NMDA receptor-dependent GABAB receptor internalization via CaMKII phosphorylation of serine 867 in GABAB1. *Proc Natl Acad Sci U S A* 107(31):13924-13929.

Hammond AS, Rodriguez AL, Townsend SD, Niswender CM, Gregory KJ, Lindsley CW and Conn PJ (2010) Discovery of a Novel Chemical Class of mGlu(5) Allosteric Ligands with Distinct Modes of Pharmacology. *ACS Chem Neurosci* 1(10):702-716.

Haney M, Hart CL and Foltin RW (2006) Effects of baclofen on cocaine self-administration: opioid- and nonopioid-dependent volunteers. *Neuropsychopharmacology* 31(8):1814-1821.

Hanyaloglu AC and von Zastrow M (2008) Regulation of GPCRs by endocytic membrane trafficking and its potential implications. *Annu Rev Pharmacol Toxicol* 48:537-568.

Harvey J and Collingridge GL (1993) Signal transduction pathways involved in the acute potentiation of NMDA responses by 1S,3R-ACPD in rat hippocampal slices. *Br J Pharmacol* 109(4):1085-1090.

Hemstapat K, de Paulis T, Chen Y, Brady AE, Grover VK, Alagille D, Tamagnan GD and Conn PJ (2006) A novel class of positive allosteric modulators of metabotropic glutamate receptor subtype 1 interact with a site distinct from that of negative allosteric modulators. *Mol Pharmacol* 70(2):616-626.

Herlitze S, Garcia DE, Mackie K, Hille B, Scheuer T and Catterall WA (1996) Modulation of Ca2+ channels by G-protein beta gamma subunits. *Nature* 380(6571):258-262.

Hirono M, Yoshioka T and Konishi S (2001) GABA(B) receptor activation enhances mGluR-mediated responses at cerebellar excitatory synapses. *Nat Neurosci* 4(12):1207-1216.

Hirsch EC (2000) Nigrostriatal system plasticity in Parkinson's disease: effect of dopaminergic denervation and treatment. *Ann Neurol* 47(4 Suppl 1):S115-120; discussion S120-111.

Hoare SR (2005) Mechanisms of peptide and nonpeptide ligand binding to Class B G-protein-coupled receptors. *Drug Discov Today* 10(6):417-427.

Hu J, Hauache O and Spiegel AM (2000) Human Ca2+ receptor cysteine-rich domain. Analysis of function of mutant and chimeric receptors. *J Biol Chem* 275(21):16382-16389.

Jiang P, Ji Q, Liu Z, Snyder LA, Benard LM, Margolskee RF and Max M (2004) The cysteine-rich region of T1R3 determines responses to intensely sweet proteins. *J Biol Chem* 279(43):45068-45075.

Johnson MP, Baez M, Jagdmann GE, Jr., Britton TC, Large TH, Callagaro DO, Tizzano JP, Monn JA and Schoepp DD (2003) Discovery of allosteric potentiators for the metabotropic glutamate 2 receptor: synthesis and subtype selectivity of N-(4-(2-methoxyphenoxy)phenyl)-N-(2,2,2- trifluoroethylsulfonyl)pyrid-3-ylmethylamine. *J Med Chem* 46(15):3189-3192.

Kachroo A, Orlando LR, Grandy DK, Chen JF, Young AB and Schwarzschild MA (2005) Interactions between metabotropic glutamate 5 and adenosine A2A receptors in normal and parkinsonian mice. *J Neurosci* 25(45):10414-10419.

Kammerer RA, Frank S, Schulthess T, Landwehr R, Lustig A and Engel J (1999) Heterodimerization of a functional GABAB receptor is mediated by parallel coiled-coil alpha-helices. *Biochemistry* 38(40):13263-13269.

Kangrga I, Jiang MC and Randic M (1991) Actions of (-)-baclofen on rat dorsal horn neurons. *Brain Res* 562(2):265-275.

Kaupmann K, Cryan JF, Wellendorph P, Mombereau C, Sansig G, Klebs K, Schmutz M, Froestl W, van der Putten H, Mosbacher J, Brauner-Osborne H, Waldmeier P and Bettler B (2003) Specific gamma-hydroxybutyrate-binding sites but loss of pharmacological effects of gamma-hydroxybutyrate in GABA(B)(1)-deficient mice. *Eur J Neurosci* 18(10):2722-2730.

Kaupmann K, Huggel K, Heid J, Flor PJ, Bischoff S, Mickel SJ, McMaster G, Angst C, Bittiger H, Froestl W and Bettler B (1997) Expression cloning of GABA(B) receptors uncovers similarity to metabotropic glutamate receptors. *Nature* 386(6622):239-246.

Kaupmann K, Malitschek B, Schuler V, Heid J, Froestl W, Beck P, Mosbacher J, Bischoff S, Kulik A, Shigemoto R, Karschin A and Bettler B (1998) GABA(B)-receptor subtypes assemble into functional heteromeric complexes. *Nature* 396(6712):683-687.

Kenny PJ and Markou A (2004) The ups and downs of addiction: role of metabotropic glutamate receptors. *Trends Pharmacol Sci* 25(5):265-272.

Kinney GG, O'Brien JA, Lemaire W, Burno M, Bickel DJ, Clements MK, Chen TB, Wisnoski DD, Lindsley CW, Tiller PR, Smith S, Jacobson MA, Sur C, Duggan ME, Pettibone DJ, Conn PJ and Williams DL, Jr. (2005) A novel selective positive allosteric modulator of metabotropic glutamate receptor subtype 5 has in vivo activity and antipsychotic-like effects in rat behavioral models. *J Pharmacol Exp Ther* 313(1):199-206.

Kleinschmidt S, Grundmann U, Janneck U, Kreienmeyer J, Kulosa R and Larsen R (1997) Total intravenous anaesthesia using propofol, gamma-hydroxybutyrate or midazolam in combination with sufentanil for patients undergoing coronary artery bypass surgery. *Eur J Anaesthesiol* 14(6):590-599.

Klodzinska A, Tatarczynska E, Stachowicz K and Chojnacka-Wojcik E (2004) The anxiolytic-like activity of AIDA (1-aminoindan-1,5-dicarboxylic acid), an mGlu 1 receptor antagonist. *J Physiol Pharmacol* 55(1 Pt 1):113-126.

Kniazeff J, Galvez T, Labesse G and Pin JP (2002) No ligand binding in the GB2 subunit of the GABA(B) receptor is required for activation and allosteric interaction between the subunits. *J Neurosci* 22(17):7352-7361.

Kniazeff J, Prezeau L, Rondard P, Pin JP and Goudet C (2011) Dimers and beyond: The functional puzzles of class C GPCRs. *Pharmacol Ther* 130(1):9-25.

Knoflach F, Mutel V, Jolidon S, Kew JN, Malherbe P, Vieira E, Wichmann J and Kemp JA (2001) Positive allosteric modulators of metabotropic glutamate 1 receptor: characterization, mechanism of action, and binding site. *Proc Natl Acad Sci U S A* 98(23):13402-13407.

Kolber BJ, Montana MC, Carrasquillo Y, Xu J, Heinemann SF, Muglia LJ and Gereau RWt (2010) Activation of metabotropic glutamate receptor 5 in the amygdala modulates pain-like behavior. *J Neurosci* 30(24):8203-8213.

Kulik A, Vida I, Lujan R, Haas CA, Lopez-Bendito G, Shigemoto R and Frotscher M (2003) Subcellular localization of metabotropic GABA(B) receptor subunits GABA(B1a/b) and GABA(B2) in the rat hippocampus. *J Neurosci* 23(35):11026-11035.

Kunishima N, Shimada Y, Tsuji Y, Sato T, Yamamoto M, Kumasaka T, Nakanishi S, Jingami H and Morikawa K (2000) Structural basis of glutamate recognition by a dimeric metabotropic glutamate receptor. *Nature* 407(6807):971-977.

Laborit H, Jouany JM, Gerard J and Fabiani F (1960) [Summary of an experimental and clinical study on a metabolic substrate with inhibitory central action: sodium 4-hydroxybutyrate]. *Presse Med* 68:1867-1869.

Leaney JL and Tinker A (2000) The role of members of the pertussis toxin-sensitive family of G proteins in coupling receptors to the activation of the G protein-gated inwardly rectifying potassium channel. *Proc Natl Acad Sci U S A* 97(10):5651-5656.

Lefkowitz RJ (1998) G protein-coupled receptors. III. New roles for receptor kinases and beta-arrestins in receptor signaling and desensitization. *J Biol Chem* 273(30):18677-18680.

Lehmann A (2008) Novel treatments of GERD: focus on the lower esophageal sphincter. *Eur Rev Med Pharmacol Sci* 12 Suppl 1:103-110.

Linden AM, Shannon H, Baez M, Yu JL, Koester A and Schoepp DD (2005) Anxiolytic-like activity of the mGLU2/3 receptor agonist LY354740 in the elevated plus maze test is disrupted in metabotropic glutamate receptor 2 and 3 knock-out mice. *Psychopharmacology (Berl)* 179(1):284-291.

Litschig S, Gasparini F, Rueegg D, Stoehr N, Flor PJ, Vranesic I, Prezeau L, Pin JP, Thomsen C and Kuhn R (1999) CPCCOEt, a noncompetitive metabotropic glutamate receptor 1 antagonist, inhibits receptor signaling without affecting glutamate binding. *Mol Pharmacol* 55(3):453-461.

Lopez S, Turle-Lorenzo N, Acher F, De Leonibus E, Mele A and Amalric M (2007) Targeting group III metabotropic glutamate receptors produces complex behavioral effects in rodent models of Parkinson's disease. *J Neurosci* 27(25):6701-6711.

Lopez-Bendito G, Shigemoto R, Kulik A, Vida I, Fairen A and Lujan R (2004) Distribution of metabotropic GABA receptor subunits GABAB1a/b and GABAB2 in the rat hippocampus during prenatal and postnatal development. *Hippocampus* 14(7):836-848.

Lu YM, Jia Z, Janus C, Henderson JT, Gerlai R, Wojtowicz JM and Roder JC (1997) Mice lacking metabotropic glutamate receptor 5 show impaired learning and reduced CA1 long-term potentiation (LTP) but normal CA3 LTP. *J Neurosci* 17(13):5196-5205.

Luscher C, Jan LY, Stoffel M, Malenka RC and Nicoll RA (1997) G protein-coupled inwardly rectifying K+ channels (GIRKs) mediate postsynaptic but not presynaptic transmitter actions in hippocampal neurons. *Neuron* 19(3):687-695.

Maj M, Bruno V, Dragic Z, Yamamoto R, Battaglia G, Inderbitzin W, Stoehr N, Stein T, Gasparini F, Vranesic I, Kuhn R, Nicoletti F and Flor PJ (2003) (-)-PHCCC, a positive allosteric modulator of mGluR4: characterization, mechanism of action, and neuroprotection. *Neuropharmacology* 45(7):895-906.

Malcangio M and Bowery NG (1995) Possible therapeutic application of GABAB receptor agonists and antagonists. *Clin Neuropharmacol* 18(4):285-305.

Malcangio M, Ghelardini C, Giotti A, Malmberg-Aiello P and Bartolini A (1991) CGP 35348, a new GABAB antagonist, prevents antinociception and muscle-relaxant effect induced by baclofen. *Br J Pharmacol* 103(2):1303-1308.

Malherbe P, Masciadri R, Norcross RD, Knoflach F, Kratzeisen C, Zenner MT, Kolb Y, Marcuz A, Huwyler J, Nakagawa T, Porter RH, Thomas AW, Wettstein JG, Sleight AJ, Spooren W and Prinssen EP (2008) Characterization of (R,S)-5,7-di-tert-butyl-3-hydroxy-3-trifluoromethyl-3H-benzofuran-2-one as a positive allosteric modulator of GABAB receptors. *Br J Pharmacol* 154(4):797-811.

Margeta-Mitrovic M, Jan YN and Jan LY (2001) Function of GB1 and GB2 subunits in G protein coupling of GABA(B) receptors. *Proc Natl Acad Sci U S A* 98(25):14649-14654.

Martin LJ, Blackstone CD, Huganir RL and Price DL (1992) Cellular localization of a metabotropic glutamate receptor in rat brain. *Neuron* 9(2):259-270.

Marvizon JC, Grady EF, Stefani E, Bunnett NW and Mayer EA (1999) Substance P release in the dorsal horn assessed by receptor internalization: NMDA receptors counteract a tonic inhibition by GABA(B) receptors. *Eur J Neurosci* 11(2):417-426.

Masu M, Iwakabe H, Tagawa Y, Miyoshi T, Yamashita M, Fukuda Y, Sasaki H, Hiroi K, Nakamura Y, Shigemoto R and et al. (1995) Specific deficit of the ON response in visual transmission by targeted disruption of the mGluR6 gene. *Cell* 80(5):757-765.

Maurel D, Comps-Agrar L, Brock C, Rives ML, Bourrier E, Ayoub MA, Bazin H, Tinel N, Durroux T, Prezeau L, Trinquet E and Pin JP (2008) Cell-surface protein-protein interaction analysis with time-resolved FRET and snap-tag technologies: application to GPCR oligomerization. *Nat Methods* 5(6):561-567.

Miedlich SU, Gama L, Seuwen K, Wolf RM and Breitwieser GE (2004) Homology modeling of the transmembrane domain of the human calcium sensing receptor and localization of an allosteric binding site. *J Biol Chem* 279(8):7254-7263.

Misgeld U, Bijak M and Jarolimek W (1995) A physiological role for GABAB receptors and the effects of baclofen in the mammalian central nervous system. *Prog Neurobiol* 46(4):423-462.

Molina-Hernandez M, Tellez-Alcantara NP, Perez-Garcia J, Olivera-Lopez JI and Jaramillo-Jaimes MT (2008) Antidepressant-like actions of minocycline combined with several glutamate antagonists. *Prog Neuropsychopharmacol Biol Psychiatry* 32(2):380-386.

Morishima Y, Miyakawa T, Furuyashiki T, Tanaka Y, Mizuma H and Nakanishi S (2005) Enhanced cocaine responsiveness and impaired motor coordination in metabotropic glutamate receptor subtype 2 knockout mice. *Proc Natl Acad Sci U S A* 102(11):4170-4175.

Moussawi K and Kalivas PW (2010) Group II metabotropic glutamate receptors (mGlu2/3) in drug addiction. *Eur J Pharmacol* 639(1-3):115-122.

Moussawi K, Pacchioni A, Moran M, Olive MF, Gass JT, Lavin A and Kalivas PW (2009) N-Acetylcysteine reverses cocaine-induced metaplasticity. *Nat Neurosci* 12(2):182-189.

Muto T, Tsuchiya D, Morikawa K and Jingami H (2007) Expression, purification, crystallization and preliminary X-ray analysis of the ligand-binding domain of metabotropic glutamate receptor 7. *Acta Crystallogr Sect F Struct Biol Cryst Commun* 63(Pt 7):627-630.

Nakajima Y, Iwakabe H, Akazawa C, Nawa H, Shigemoto R, Mizuno N and Nakanishi S (1993) Molecular characterization of a novel retinal metabotropic glutamate receptor mGluR6 with a high agonist selectivity for L-2-amino-4-phosphonobutyrate. *J Biol Chem* 268(16):11868-11873.

Nelson G, Hoon MA, Chandrashekar J, Zhang Y, Ryba NJ and Zuker CS (2001) Mammalian sweet taste receptors. *Cell* 106(3):381-390.

Neugebauer V, Zinebi F, Russell R, Gallagher JP and Shinnick-Gallagher P (2000) Cocaine and kindling alter the sensitivity of group II and III metabotropic glutamate receptors in the central amygdala. *J Neurophysiol* 84(2):759-770.

Nicoletti F, Bockaert J, Collingridge GL, Conn PJ, Ferraguti F, Schoepp DD, Wroblewski JT and Pin JP (2011) Metabotropic glutamate receptors: from the workbench to the bedside. *Neuropharmacology* 60(7-8):1017-1041.

Nishikawa M, Hirouchi M and Kuriyama K (1997) Functional coupling of Gi subtype with GABAB receptor/adenylyl cyclase system: analysis using a reconstituted system with purified GTP-binding protein from bovine cerebral cortex. *Neurochem Int* 31(1):21-25.

Niswender CM and Conn PJ (2010) Metabotropic glutamate receptors: physiology, pharmacology, and disease. *Annu Rev Pharmacol Toxicol* 50:295-322.

Niswender CM, Johnson KA, Miller NR, Ayala JE, Luo Q, Williams R, Saleh S, Orton D, Weaver CD and Conn PJ (2010) Context-dependent pharmacology exhibited by negative allosteric modulators of metabotropic glutamate receptor 7. *Mol Pharmacol* 77(3):459-468.

Niswender CM, Johnson KA, Weaver CD, Jones CK, Xiang Z, Luo Q, Rodriguez AL, Marlo JE, de Paulis T, Thompson AD, Days EL, Nalywajko T, Austin CA, Williams MB, Ayala JE, Williams R, Lindsley CW and Conn PJ (2008) Discovery, characterization, and antiparkinsonian effect of novel positive allosteric modulators of metabotropic glutamate receptor 4. *Mol Pharmacol* 74(5):1345-1358.

O'Hara PJ, Sheppard PO, Thogersen H, Venezia D, Haldeman BA, McGrane V, Houamed KM, Thomsen C, Gilbert TL and Mulvihill ER (1993) The ligand-binding domain in metabotropic glutamate receptors is related to bacterial periplasmic binding proteins. *Neuron* 11(1):41-52.

Ohishi H, Neki A and Mizuno N (1998) Distribution of a metabotropic glutamate receptor, mGluR2, in the central nervous system of the rat and mouse: an immunohistochemical study with a monoclonal antibody. *Neurosci Res* 30(1):65-82.

Ohishi H, Ogawa-Meguro R, Shigemoto R, Kaneko T, Nakanishi S and Mizuno N (1994) Immunohistochemical localization of metabotropic glutamate receptors, mGluR2 and mGluR3, in rat cerebellar cortex. *Neuron* 13(1):55-66.

Oliet SH, Malenka RC and Nicoll RA (1997) Two distinct forms of long-term depression coexist in CA1 hippocampal pyramidal cells. *Neuron* 18(6):969-982.

Ossowska K, Pietraszek M, Wardas J and Wolfarth S (2004) Potential antipsychotic and extrapyramidal effects of (R,S)-3,4-dicarboxyphenylglycine [(R,S)-3,4-DCPG], a mixed AMPA antagonist/mGluR8 agonist. *Pol J Pharmacol* 56(3):295-304.

Overington JP, Al-Lazikani B and Hopkins AL (2006) How many drug targets are there? *Nat Rev Drug Discov* 5(12):993-996.

Pagano A, Ruegg D, Litschig S, Stoehr N, Stierlin C, Heinrich M, Floersheim P, Prezeau L, Carroll F, Pin JP, Cambria A, Vranesic I, Flor PJ, Gasparini F and Kuhn R (2000) The non-competitive antagonists 2-methyl-6-(phenylethynyl)pyridine and 7-hydroxyiminocyclopropan[b]chromen-1a-carboxylic acid ethyl ester interact with overlapping binding pockets in the transmembrane region of group I metabotropic glutamate receptors. *J Biol Chem* 275(43):33750-33758.

Palucha A and Pilc A (2005) The involvement of glutamate in the pathophysiology of depression. *Drug News Perspect* 18(4):262-268.

Pardi D and Black J (2006) gamma-Hydroxybutyrate/sodium oxybate: neurobiology, and impact on sleep and wakefulness. *CNS Drugs* 20(12):993-1018.

Patil ST, Zhang L, Martenyi F, Lowe SL, Jackson KA, Andreev BV, Avedisova AS, Bardenstein LM, Gurovich IY, Morozova MA, Mosolov SN, Neznanov NG, Reznik AM, Smulevich AB, Tochilov VA, Johnson BG, Monn JA and Schoepp DD (2007) Activation of mGlu2/3 receptors as a new approach to treat schizophrenia: a randomized Phase 2 clinical trial. *Nat Med* 13(9):1102-1107.

Paul IA and Skolnick P (2003) Glutamate and depression: clinical and preclinical studies. *Ann N Y Acad Sci* 1003:250-272.

Pekhletski R, Gerlai R, Overstreet LS, Huang XP, Agopyan N, Slater NT, Abramow-Newerly W, Roder JC and Hampson DR (1996) Impaired cerebellar synaptic plasticity and motor performance in mice lacking the mGluR4 subtype of metabotropic glutamate receptor. *J Neurosci* 16(20):6364-6373.

Peleg S, Varon D, Ivanina T, Dessauer CW and Dascal N (2002) G(alpha)(i) controls the gating of the G protein-activated K(+) channel, GIRK. *Neuron* 33(1):87-99.

Perroy J, Adam L, Qanbar R, Chenier S and Bouvier M (2003) Phosphorylation-independent desensitization of GABA(B) receptor by GRK4. *EMBO J* 22(15):3816-3824.

Perroy J, Raynaud F, Homburger V, Rousset MC, Telley L, Bockaert J and Fagni L (2008) Direct interaction enables cross-talk between ionotropic and group I metabotropic glutamate receptors. *J Biol Chem* 283(11):6799-6805.

Petersen EN and Lassen JB (1981) A water lick conflict paradigm using drug experienced rats. *Psychopharmacology (Berl)* 75(3):236-239.

Petrel C, Kessler A, Dauban P, Dodd RH, Rognan D and Ruat M (2004) Positive and negative allosteric modulators of the Ca2+-sensing receptor interact within overlapping but not identical binding sites in the transmembrane domain. *J Biol Chem* 279(18):18990-18997.

Pin JP and Acher F (2002) The metabotropic glutamate receptors: structure, activation mechanism and pharmacology. *Curr Drug Targets CNS Neurol Disord* 1(3):297-317.

Pin JP, Kniazeff J, Goudet C, Bessis AS, Liu J, Galvez T, Acher F, Rondard P and Prezeau L (2004) The activation mechanism of class-C G-protein coupled receptors. *Biol Cell* 96(5):335-342.

Pin JP and Prezeau L (2007) Allosteric modulators of GABA(B) receptors: mechanism of action and therapeutic perspective. *Curr Neuropharmacol* 5(3):195-201.

Pisani A, Bonsi P, Centonze D, Gubellini P, Bernardi G and Calabresi P (2003) Targeting striatal cholinergic interneurons in Parkinson's disease: focus on metabotropic glutamate receptors. *Neuropharmacology* 45(1):45-56.

Pontier SM, Lahaie N, Ginham R, St-Gelais F, Bonin H, Bell DJ, Flynn H, Trudeau LE, McIlhinney J, White JH and Bouvier M (2006) Coordinated action of NSF and PKC regulates GABAB receptor signaling efficacy. *EMBO J* 25(12):2698-2709.

Price DD, Rafii A, Watkins LR and Buckingham B (1984) A psychophysical analysis of acupuncture analgesia. *Pain* 19(1):27-42.

Puckerin A, Liu L, Permaul N, Carman P, Lee J and Diverse-Pierluissi MA (2006) Arrestin is required for agonist-induced trafficking of voltage-dependent calcium channels. *J Biol Chem* 281(41):31131-31141.

Rondard P, Liu J, Huang S, Malhaire F, Vol C, Pinault A, Labesse G and Pin JP (2006) Coupling of agonist binding to effector domain activation in metabotropic glutamate-like receptors. *J Biol Chem* 281(34):24653-24661.

Sansig G, Bushell TJ, Clarke VR, Rozov A, Burnashev N, Portet C, Gasparini F, Schmutz M, Klebs K, Shigemoto R, Flor PJ, Kuhn R, Knoepfel T, Schroeder M, Hampson DR, Collett VJ, Zhang C, Duvoisin RM, Collingridge GL and van Der Putten H (2001) Increased seizure susceptibility in mice lacking metabotropic glutamate receptor 7. *J Neurosci* 21(22):8734-8745.

Sato M, Horinouchi T, Hutchinson DS, Evans BA and Summers RJ (2007) Ligand-directed signaling at the beta3-adrenoceptor produced by 3-(2-Ethylphenoxy)-1-[(1,S)-1,2,3,4-tetrahydronapth-1-ylamino]-2S-2-propan ol oxalate (SR59230A) relative to receptor agonists. *Mol Pharmacol* 72(5):1359-1368.

Sawynok J (1984) GABAergic mechanisms in antinociception. *Prog Neuropsychopharmacol Biol Psychiatry* 8(4-6):581-586.

Schaffhauser H, Knoflach F, Pink JR, Bleuel Z, Cartmell J, Goepfert F, Kemp JA, Richards JG, Adam G and Mutel V (1998) Multiple pathways for regulation of the KCl-induced [3H]-GABA release by metabotropic glutamate receptors, in primary rat cortical cultures. *Brain Res* 782(1-2):91-104.

Schann S, Menet C, Arvault P, Mercier G, Frauli M, Mayer S, Hubert N, Triballeau N, Bertrand HO, Acher F and Neuville P (2006) Design and synthesis of APTCs (aminopyrrolidinetricarboxylic acids): identification of a new group III metabotropic glutamate receptor selective agonist. *Bioorg Med Chem Lett* 16(18):4856-4860.

Scholten D, Canals M, Maussang D, Roumen L, Smit M, Wijtmans M, de Graaf C, Vischer H and Leurs R (2011) Pharmacological Modulation of Chemokine Receptor Function. *Br J Pharmacol.*

Schweitzer C, Kratzeisen C, Adam G, Lundstrom K, Malherbe P, Ohresser S, Stadler H, Wichmann J, Woltering T and Mutel V (2000) Characterization of [(3)H]-LY354740 binding to rat mGlu2 and mGlu3 receptors expressed in CHO cells using semliki forest virus vectors. *Neuropharmacology* 39(10):1700-1706.

Scrima L, Hartman PG, Johnson FH, Jr., Thomas EE and Hiller FC (1990) The effects of gamma-hydroxybutyrate on the sleep of narcolepsy patients: a double-blind study. *Sleep* 13(6):479-490.

Selvam C, Oueslati N, Lemasson IA, Brabet I, Rigault D, Courtiol T, Cesarini S, Triballeau N, Bertrand HO, Goudet C, Pin JP and Acher FC (2010) A virtual screening hit reveals new possibilities for developing group III metabotropic glutamate receptor agonists. *J Med Chem* 53(7):2797-2813.

Sexton PM, Morfis M, Tilakaratne N, Hay DL, Udawela M, Christopoulos G and Christopoulos A (2006) Complexing receptor pharmacology: modulation of family B G protein-coupled receptor function by RAMPs. *Ann N Y Acad Sci* 1070:90-104.

Shenoy SK and Lefkowitz RJ (2005) Receptor regulation: beta-arrestin moves up a notch. *Nat Cell Biol* 7(12):1159-1161.

Shimazaki T, Iijima M and Chaki S (2004) Anxiolytic-like activity of MGS0039, a potent group II metabotropic glutamate receptor antagonist, in a marble-burying behavior test. *Eur J Pharmacol* 501(1-3):121-125.

Smith GD, Harrison SM, Birch PJ, Elliott PJ, Malcangio M and Bowery NG (1994) Increased sensitivity to the antinociceptive activity of (+/-)-baclofen in an animal model of chronic neuropathic, but not chronic inflammatory hyperalgesia. *Neuropharmacology* 33(9):1103-1108.

Steckler T, Lavreysen H, Oliveira AM, Aerts N, Van Craenendonck H, Prickaerts J, Megens A and Lesage AS (2005) Effects of mGlu1 receptor blockade on anxiety-related behaviour in the rat lick suppression test. *Psychopharmacology (Berl)* 179(1):198-206.

Sudo S, Kumagai J, Nishi S, Layfield S, Ferraro T, Bathgate RA and Hsueh AJ (2003) H3 relaxin is a specific ligand for LGR7 and activates the receptor by interacting with both the ectodomain and the exoloop 2. *J Biol Chem* 278(10):7855-7862.

Sung KW, Choi S and Lovinger DM (2001) Activation of group I mGluRs is necessary for induction of long-term depression at striatal synapses. *J Neurophysiol* 86(5):2405-2412.

Suzuki G, Kimura T, Satow A, Kaneko N, Fukuda J, Hikichi H, Sakai N, Maehara S, Kawagoe-Takaki H, Hata M, Azuma T, Ito S, Kawamoto H and Ohta H (2007) Pharmacological characterization of a new, orally active and potent allosteric metabotropic glutamate receptor 1 antagonist, 4-[1-(2-fluoropyridin-3-yl)-5-methyl-1H-1,2,3-triazol-4-yl]-N-isopropyl-N-methyl-3,6-dihydropyridine-1(2H)-carboxamide (FTIDC). *J Pharmacol Exp Ther* 321(3):1144-1153.

Tamaru Y, Nomura S, Mizuno N and Shigemoto R (2001) Distribution of metabotropic glutamate receptor mGluR3 in the mouse CNS: differential location relative to pre- and postsynaptic sites. *Neuroscience* 106(3):481-503.

Tebano MT, Martire A, Pepponi R, Domenici MR and Popoli P (2006) Is the functional interaction between adenosine A(2A) receptors and metabotropic glutamate 5 receptors a general mechanism in the brain? Differences and similarities between the striatum and the hippocampus. *Purinergic Signal* 2(4):619-625.

Terunuma M, Vargas KJ, Wilkins ME, Ramirez OA, Jaureguiberry-Bravo M, Pangalos MN, Smart TG, Moss SJ and Couve A (2010) Prolonged activation of NMDA receptors promotes dephosphorylation and alters postendocytic sorting of GABAB receptors. *Proc Natl Acad Sci U S A* 107(31):13918-13923.

Thompson SM, Capogna M and Scanziani M (1993) Presynaptic inhibition in the hippocampus. *Trends Neurosci* 16(6):222-227.

Toms NJ and Roberts PJ (1999) Group 1 mGlu receptors elevate [Ca2+]i in rat cultured cortical type 2 astrocytes: [Ca2+]i synergy with adenosine A1 receptors. *Neuropharmacology* 38(10):1511-1517.

Trullas R and Skolnick P (1990) Functional antagonists at the NMDA receptor complex exhibit antidepressant actions. *Eur J Pharmacol* 185(1):1-10.

Tsuchiya D, Kunishima N, Kamiya N, Jingami H and Morikawa K (2002) Structural views of the ligand-binding cores of a metabotropic glutamate receptor complexed with an antagonist and both glutamate and Gd3+. *Proc Natl Acad Sci U S A* 99(5):2660-2665.

Tyacke RJ, Lingford-Hughes A, Reed LJ and Nutt DJ (2010) GABAB receptors in addiction and its treatment. *Adv Pharmacol* 58:373-396.

Ulrich D and Bettler B (2007) GABA(B) receptors: synaptic functions and mechanisms of diversity. *Curr Opin Neurobiol* 17(3):298-303.

Urizar E, Yano H, Kolster R, Gales C, Lambert N and Javitch JA (2011) CODA-RET reveals functional selectivity as a result of GPCR heteromerization. *Nat Chem Biol* 7(9):624-630.

Urwyler S, Mosbacher J, Lingenhoehl K, Heid J, Hofstetter K, Froestl W, Bettler B and Kaupmann K (2001) Positive allosteric modulation of native and recombinant gamma-aminobutyric acid(B) receptors by 2,6-Di-tert-butyl-4-(3-hydroxy-2,2-dimethyl-propyl)-phenol (CGP7930) and its aldehyde analog CGP13501. *Mol Pharmacol* 60(5):963-971.

Valant C, Gregory KJ, Hall NE, Scammells PJ, Lew MJ, Sexton PM and Christopoulos A (2008) A novel mechanism of G protein-coupled receptor functional selectivity. Muscarinic partial agonist McN-A-343 as a bitopic orthosteric/allosteric ligand. *J Biol Chem* 283(43):29312-29321.

Valant C, Sexton PM and Christopoulos A (2009) Orthosteric/allosteric bitopic ligands: going hybrid at GPCRs. *Mol Interv* 9(3):125-135.

Valenti O, Marino MJ, Wittmann M, Lis E, DiLella AG, Kinney GG and Conn PJ (2003) Group III metabotropic glutamate receptor-mediated modulation of the striatopallidal synapse. *J Neurosci* 23(18):7218-7226.

Vienne J, Bettler B, Franken P and Tafti M (2010) Differential effects of GABAB receptor subtypes, {gamma}-hydroxybutyric Acid, and Baclofen on EEG activity and sleep regulation. *J Neurosci* 30(42):14194-14204.

Wettschureck N and Offermanns S (2005) Mammalian G proteins and their cell type specific functions. *Physiol Rev* 85(4):1159-1204.

White JH, Wise A, Main MJ, Green A, Fraser NJ, Disney GH, Barnes AA, Emson P, Foord SM and Marshall FH (1998) Heterodimerization is required for the formation of a functional GABA(B) receptor. *Nature* 396(6712):679-682.

Woolley ML, Pemberton DJ, Bate S, Corti C and Jones DN (2008) The mGlu2 but not the mGlu3 receptor mediates the actions of the mGluR2/3 agonist, LY379268, in mouse models predictive of antipsychotic activity. *Psychopharmacology (Berl)* 196(3):431-440.

Wright RA, Arnold MB, Wheeler WJ, Ornstein PL and Schoepp DD (2000) Binding of [3H](2S,1'S,2'S)-2-(9-xanthylmethyl)-2-(2'-carboxycyclopropyl) glycine ([3H]LY341495) to cell membranes expressing recombinant human group III metabotropic glutamate receptor subtypes. *Naunyn Schmiedebergs Arch Pharmacol* 362(6):546-554.

Yamaguchi S and Ninomiya K (2000) Umami and food palatability. *J Nutr* 130(4S Suppl):921S-926S.

Zhang F, Klebansky B, Fine RM, Xu H, Pronin A, Liu H, Tachdjian C and Li X (2008) Molecular mechanism for the umami taste synergism. *Proc Natl Acad Sci U S A* 105(52):20930-20934.

2

Opioid Kappa Receptor Selective Agonist TRK-820 (Nalfurafine Hydrochloride)

Hideaki Fujii, Shigeto Hirayama and Hiroshi Nagase
School of Pharmacy, Kitasato University
Japan

1. Introduction

TRK-820 (nalfurafine hydrochloride) is a selective opioid κ receptor agonist (Fig. 1) that was launched as an antipruritic for hemodialysis patients in Japan in 2009. In general, clinically used opioids, such as morphine, exhibit potent antinociceptive effects and simultaneous severe adverse effects, including drug dependence, derived from the opioid μ receptor. To develop analgesics without drug dependence, κ receptor agonists are investigated. However, conventional κ agonists, arylacetamide derivatives, showed aversive effects like psychotomimetic effects, and have not yet been used clinically. On the other hand, the novel κ agonist TRK-820 has no dependent or aversive properties. TRK-820, which has a structure different from arylacetamides, was first developed as an analgesic for postoperative pain, but the indication was changed to pruritus (Nakao & Mochizuki, 2009; Nagase & Fujii, 2011). The rational drug design and synthesis of the compound have been reported (Kawai et al., 2008; Nagase et al., 1998; Nagase & Fujii, 2011); therefore, in this chapter, we will focus on its pharmacological properties.

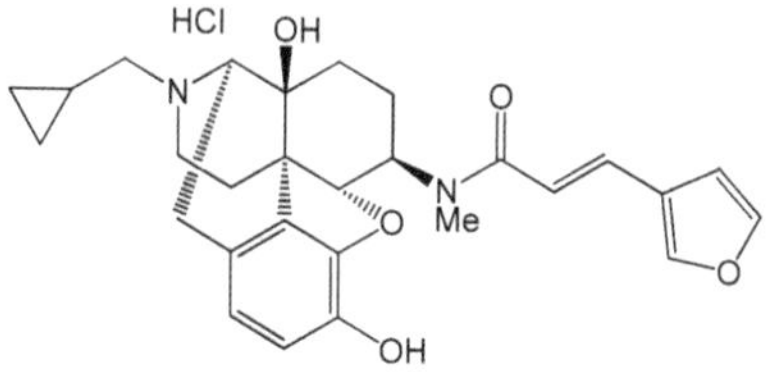

Fig. 1. Structure of nalfurafine hydrochloride (TRK-820)

2. Opioid receptor type selectivity (*In vitro*)

The binding affinities of TRK-820 were evaluated using various tritiated ligands and opioid receptors derived from various species (Table 1). The κ selectivity over the δ receptor (K_i ratio δ/κ) tended to be higher than over the μ receptor (K_i ratio μ/κ). Binding affinities for the L-type Ca^{2+} channel and 45 receptors, except the opioid receptors, were examined (Nakao & Mochizuki, 2009). Among the tested receptors, TRK-820 showed the strongest affinity for the muscarine M_1 receptor, but its K_i value was 1,700 nmol/L and approximately 7,000 times higher than that of the κ receptor. A comparison of the binding properties of TRK-820 and a conventional κ agonist, U-69,593, was noteworthy. In a competitive binding

K_i (nM)			K_i ratio		References
μ	δ	κ	μ/κ	δ/κ	
53	1200	3.5	15	343	Seki et al., 1999
5.2	161	0.075	69	2147	Wang, Y et al., 2005
0.71	49.9	0.36	2.0	139	Vanderah et al., 2008
2.21	484	0.244	9.1	1984	Nakao & Mochizuki, 2009
0.582	96.5	0.225	2.6	429	Nagase et al., 2010

Table 1. Binding affinities (K_i values) and selectivities (K_i ratios) of TRK-820 for the opioid receptors. Seki et al. used [3H]bremazocine and the recombinant rat opioid receptors. Wang, Y et al. used [3H]diprenorphine and recombinant rat μ, recombinant mouse δ, and recombinant human κ receptors. Vanderah et al. used [3H]DAMDO, [3H]pCl-DPDPE, and [3H]U-69,593 for the recombinant human μ, δ, and κ receptors, respectively. Nakao et al. used [3H]diprenorphine and the recombinant human receptors. Nagase et al. used [3H]DAMDO, [3H]NTI, and [3H]U-69,593 for the μ, δ, and κ receptors, respectively. Guinea pig forebrain or guinea pig cerebellum was used to assay the μ and δ receptor or κ receptor, respectively.

Assay	Selectivity		References
	μ/κ	δ/κ	
MVD	980	NC	Kawai et al., 2008
GPI	78.6	–	Kawai et al., 2008
cAMP (Sato et al.)	55	>6,667	Seki et al., 1999
cAMP (Nakao et al.)	203	2,610	Nakao & Mochizuki, 2009
[35S]GTPγS	128	11,560	Wang, Y et al., 2005

Table 2. Selectivities of TRK-820 in various functional assays. Selectivity in MVD and GPI assays was obtained by Ke ratios. The selectivity for the κ receptor over the δ receptor in the MVD assay was not calculated (NC) due to a lack of agonist activity for the δ receptor. The selectivity for the κ receptor over the δ receptor in the GPI assay was not obtained because GPI preparation contained only the μ and κ receptors. Seki et al. and Nakao et al. used the recombinant rat and human receptors in their assays, respectively. In the [35S]GTPγS binding assay, recombinant rat μ, recombinant mouse δ, or recombinant human κ receptors were used.

assay using [3H]TRK-820, TRK-820 completely replaced [3H]TRK-820 binding, whereas U-69,593 did not replace it completely, with roughly 20% of [3H]TRK-820 binding remaining. Moreover, Scatchard analysis of [3H]TRK-820 and [3H]U-69,593 binding using guinea pig cerebellum showed that TRK-820 had stronger binding affinity than U-69,593 (K_d values: 0.46±0.03 nM for [3H]TRK-820, 1.17±0.14 nM for [3H]U-69,593) and that the B_{max} value for [3H]TRK-820 (284±43.3 fmol/mg protein) was significantly higher than the value for [3H]U-69,593 (83.7±7.86 fmol/mg protein). Even in the presence of μ agonist DAMDO (100 nM) and δ agonist DPDPE (200 nM), the K_d and B_{max} values for [3H]TRK-820 did not change (K_d = 0.51±0.03 nM, B_{max} = 265±27.2 fmol/mg protein) (Endoh et al., 2000). These results suggest that TRK-820 was selective ligand for the κ receptor and that its binding property for the κ receptor was different from that of the conventional κ agonist U-69,593. Many binding assays are carried out using [³H]U-69,593 because it is commercially available. However, the binding property of TRK-820 is difficult to be definitively evaluated because [³H]TRK-820 is not available now.

TRK-820 was selective for the κ receptor, but the selectivity over the μ receptor was apparently not as high in the binding assays. Contrarily TRK-820 showed more selectivities for the κ receptor in functional assays: MVD (mouse vas deference) and GPI (guinea pig ileum) assay (Nagase et al., 1998), cAPM assay (Nakao & Mochizuki, 2009; Seki et al., 1999), and [³⁵S]GTPγS binding assay (Wang, Y et al., 2005) (Table 2). The results of the cAMP assay (IC_{50} (μ) = 8.3±1.4 nM, I_{max} (μ) = 69±3%, IC_{50} (δ) > 1,000 nM, I_{max} (δ) not determined, IC_{50} (κ) = 0.15±0.07 nM, I_{max} (κ) = 81±3% by Seki et al.; IC_{50} (μ) = 1.66±0.09 nM, I_{max} (μ) = 53.2±1.3%, IC_{50} (δ) = 21.3±1.0 nM, I_{max} (δ) = 77.9±1.6%, IC_{50} (κ) = 0.00816±0.00138 nM, I_{max} (κ) = 91.3±0.5% by Nakao et al.) indicated that TRK-820 was a selective and potent full agonist for the κ receptor and partial agonist for the μ and δ receptors. The potency for the δ receptor was very low (Nakao & Mochizuki, 2009; Seki et al., 1999). The [³⁵S]GTPγS binding assay provided similar results (EC_{50} (μ) = 3.2±1.3 nM, E_{max} (μ) = 54±7%, EC_{50} (δ) = 289±60 nM, E_{max} (δ) = 51±6%, EC_{50} (κ) = 0.025±0.003 nM, E_{max} (κ) = 93±5%) (Wang, Y et al., 2005). Mizoguchi et al. exhibited partial agonist activity of TRK-820 for the μ receptor in both *in vitro* and *in vivo* assays (Mizoguchi et al., 2003). TRK-820 concentration- or dose-dependently attenuated [³⁵S]GTPγS binding by DAMGO or antinociception induced by intracerebroventricular (i.c.v.) administration of DAMGO. On the other hand, the effects of morphine alone or a mixture with TRK-820 were investigated using a mouse acetic acid-induced writhing test or warm water (50 °C) tail-withdrawal assay in rhesus monkeys (Ko & Husbands, 2009; Nagase, 2010). Isobologram analysis of the results showed that additive or synergetic effects for TRK-820 in combination with morphine in the antinociceptive effect were observed, indicating that TRK-820 had no μ antagonist activity, at least no antagonism against analgesic activity induced by morphine. Why the effects of TRK-820 against DAMGO differed from those against morphine is not clear.

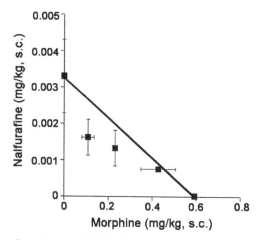

Fig. 2. Isobologram for the mixture of TRK-820- and morphine-induced antinociception in the mouse acetic acid-induced writhing test. Reprinted with permission from Nagase, 2010.

3. Analgesic effects

TRK-820 showed potent analgesic effects in some species (rodents and primates) with various stimuli: chemical, thermal, or mechanical stimuli and inflammatory, diabetic, herpetic, and postherpetic pain models. The antinociceptive effects of TRK-820 are summarized in Tables 3-7. Subcutaneous (s.c.) administration of TRK-820 produced dose-dependent and profound antinociceptive effects in the low temperature hot plate, tail flick, tail pressure, and tail pinch tests. However, TRK-820 was not as effective in high temperature hot plate tests (Table 3) (Endoh et al., 1999).

In a rat paw pressure test, TRK-820 given s.c. or intramuscularly (i.m.) induced dose-dependent and sufficient analgesic effects, which were suppressed by pre-treatment with selective κ antagonist nor-BNI (Table 3). The antinociceptive effect by TRK-820 (ED_{50} = 0.064 mg/kg, s.c.) was 170, 2, 20, and 78-fold more potent than U-50,488H, CI-977, morphine, and pentazocine, respectively (ED_{50} values : 11.0, 0.15, 1.3, and 5.0 mg/kg) (Endoh et al., 2000).

Compound	High temperture hot plate (55 °C)	Low temperature hot plate (51 °C)	Tail flick	Tail pressure	Tail pinch
TRK-820	32.0 % at 0.2	0.129	0.062	0.009	0.035
U-50,488H	63.8 % at 20	8.71	5.18	1.0	11.5
ICI-199,441	n.t.	0.065	0.042	0.024	0.051
U-69,593	n.t.	1.33	n.t.	0.48	2.8
CI-977	n.t.	n.t.	n.t.	n.t.	n.t.
PD-117302	n.t.	n.t.	n.t.	n.t.	n.t.
Pentazocine	44.6 % at 40	52.2	n.t.	n.t.	n.t.
Morphine	3.65	5.30	5.26	1.5	12.2

Compound	Paw pressure	Formalin test	Acetic acid-induced writhing test
TRK-820	0.064	0.0096	0.0033
U-50,488H	11.0	n.t.	1.16
ICI-199,441	0.074	0.0095	0.0071
CI-977	0.15	n.t.	0.0069
PD-117302	n.t.	n.t.	1.22
Pentazocine	5.0	n.t.	n.t.
Morphine	1.3	0.975	0.58

Table 3. ED_{50} values (mg/kg, s.c.) of the antinociceptive effects of some opioid agonists in various tests. U-50,488H, U-69,593, ICI-199,441, CI-977, and PD-117302 are conventional κ agonists. n.t. : not tested. Hot plate, tail flick, tail pressure, tail pinch, and acetic acid-induced writhing tests were performed in mice (Endoh et al., 1999). Paw pressure and formalin tests were performed in rats (Endoh et al., 2000).

In the formalin test, s.c. TRK-820 given 15 min prior to the formalin injection markedly inhibited the second phase of the nociceptive response induced by formalin in a dose-dependent manner. However, the analgesic effect of TRK-820 was low for the first phase of the formalin response. Similarly, a conventional κ agonist, ICI-199,441, also markedly inhibited the second phase. On the other hand, a μ agonist, morphine inhibited both phases in a dose-dependent manner. The antinociceptive potencies of TRK-820 and ICI-199,441 were almost equivalent (Table 3) (Endoh et al., 2000). A potent and dose-dependent antinociceptive effect of TRK-820 (i.m.) was also observed in cynomolgus monkeys. The analgesic effect of TRK-820 was 295 and 492-fold more potent than that of morphine in the 50 °C and 55 °C hot water tests, respectively, and 40 and 1000-fold more potent than that of U-50,488H and pentazocine in the 50 °C hot water test, respectively (Table 4) (Endoh et al., 2001).

Furthermore, the antinociceptive effects of TRK-820 administered s.c. and perorally (p.o.) were compared. The dose-dependent antinociception of TRK-820 (ED_{50} = 0.0033 mg/kg, s.c. and 0.032 mg/kg, p.o.) in the acetic acid-induced writhing test were inhibited by pre-treatment with nor-BNI. The antinociceptive effects induced by s.c. or p.o. administration of TRK-820 were 351 and 796-fold more potent than those induced by U-50,488H, respectively, and 175 and 187-fold more potent than those induced by morphine, respectively. Because the ED_{50} p.o./s.c. ratio for TRK-820 was the least among the tested compounds, TRK-820 was expected to be the most effective agent when administered p.o. (Table 5) (Endoh et al., 1999). Intravenous administration of TRK-820 was also reported to be effective in the same test (Vanderh et al., 2008).

The effect of repeated administration of some κ agonists and morphine on antinociceptive tolerance was examined by the acetic acid-induced writhing test in mice. After five

Compound	50 °C hot water	55 °C hot water
TRK-820	0.0078	0.012
Morphine	2.3	5.9
U-50,488H	0.31	n.t.
Pentazocine	> 10	n.t.

Table 4. ED_{50} values (mg/kg, i.m.) of antinociceptive effects induced by some opioid agonists in the hot water tail withdrawal test in cynomolgus monkeys. n.t. : not tested.

Compound	s.c.	p.o.	ED_{50} p.o./s.c. ratio
TRK-820	0.0033	0.032	9.7
U-50,488H	1.16	25.5	22.0
CI-977	0.0069	> 1.0	> 145
ICI-199441	0.0071	0.3	42.3
PD-117302	1.22	33.0	27.0
Morphine	0.58	6.01	10.4

Table 5. ED_{50} values (mg/kg, s.c. or p.o.) for antinociceptive effects induced by some opioid agonists in the acetic acid-induced writhing test in mice.

administrations of TRK-820 (0.1-0.8 mg/kg, s.c.), U-50,488H (10-80 mg/kg, s.c.), ICI-199,441 (0.025-0.2 mg/kg, s.c.), or morphine (1.25-10 mg/kg, s.c.) over three days, the development of tolerance to the antinociception induced by each compound at a fixed dose was assessed and tolerance ED_{50} was calculated. Comparing the ratio of tolerance ED_{50} to acute antinociceptive ED_{50} of each compound, TRK-820 was found to develop the least tolerance to antinociception (Table 6) (Suzuki et al., 2004).

An analgesic effect of TRK-820 (i.m.) was also examined using rats with arthritis induced by adjuvant. TRK-820 dose-dependently produced potent and equivalent antinociceptive activity in both arthritic and normal rats in the paw pressure test. Similar results were obtained when morphine was injected i.m. However, the analgesic effect of a conventional κ agonist, ICI-199,441, in the arthritic rats was less potent than in normal rats (Table 7) (Endoh et al., 2000).

Compound	Tolerance ED_{50}	Acute antinociceptive ED_{50}	Ratio of tolerance ED_{50}/acute antinociceptive ED_{50}
TRK-820	0.54	0.0033	163.6
U-50,488H	30.7	1.16	26.5
ICI-199,441	0.078	0.0071	11.0
Morphine	5.72	0.58	9.9

Table 6. ED_{50} values (mg/kg, s.c.) for tolerance and antinociceptive effects induced by some opioid agonists in the acetic acid-induced writhing test.

Compound	Normal rat	Arthritic rat	ED50 ratio of arthritic rat/ normal rat
TRK-820	0.055	0.095	1.7
ICI-199,441	0.047	0.24	5.1
Morphine	1.1	1.1	1.0

Table 7. ED_{50} values (mg/kg, i.m.) for antinociceptive effects induced by some opioid agonists in the paw pressure test in normal and arthritic rats.

In streptozotocin-induced diabetic mice, the antinociceptive effects induced by several κ agonists, including TRK-820, were compared in the tail flick test. Intrathecal (i.t.) and i.c.v. administration of TRK-820 produced dose-dependent antinociceptive effects in both diabetic and non-diabetic mice. However, antinociception induced by TRK-820 administered i.t. or i.c.v. in diabetic mice were less potent than antinociception in non-diabetic mice. However, the antinociceptive effects of CI-977 administered i.t., but not i.c.v., in diabetic mice were less potent than those in non-diabetic mice. On the other hand, the antinociceptive effects of ICI-199,441 and R-84760 injected i.c.v., but not i.t., in diabetic mice were less potent than those in non-diabetic mice. These results indicate that the antinociceptive effects of κ agonists in diabetic mice are altered in a region-specific manner in the central nervous system and by chemotypes of κ agonists (Ohsawa et al., 2005).

In acute herpetic and postherpetic pain models induced by herpes simplex virus type-1 infection in mice, TRK-820 dose-dependently and remarkably inhibited the allodynia and hyperalgesia stimulated by von Frey filaments (Takasaki et al., 2004, 2006). The effects of TRK-820, but not morphine, were not significantly different between herpetic and postherpetic pain (Takasaki et al., 2006). TRK-820 (0.1 mg/kg, s.c.) almost completely relieved both allodynia and hyperalgesia in herpetic pain, whereas a high dose of morphine (20 mg/kg, s.c.) did not produce complete inhibition. However, TRK-820 (0.01-0.1 mg/kg, s.c.) did not affect the spontaneous locomotor activity of normal mice (Takasaki et al., 2004). Moreover, repeated administration of TRK-820 (0.1 mg/kg, p.o., twice daily) produced constant inhibition of allodynia and hyperalgesia in herpetic pain. The effects of the fourth administration with TRK-820 were not significantly different from those of the first administration. On the other hand, the effects of morphine rapidly decreased after repeated administration (20 mg/kg, p.o., twice daily). The effects of the third and fourth administration of morphine were significantly weaker than those of the first administration. Pre-treatment with morphine (20 mg/kg, p.o., three times) did not affect the antinociceptive effect of TRK-820 (0.1 mg/kg, p.o.), whereas the effect of morphine (20 mg/kg, p.o.) was significantly reduced (Takasaki et al., 2006). These results indicate that TRK-820 is effective on both herpetic and postherpetic pain in mice. In addition, the analgesic dose of TRK-820 did not develop acute tolerance and induced cross-tolerance to morphine in herpetic pain.

4. Antipruritic effects

4.1 Preclinical studies

The p.o. administration of TRK-820 dose-dependently inhibited scratching behavior induced by histamine in mice, which is one of the representative pruritogenic substances, without obvious suppression of spontaneous locomotor activity. The antiscratching activity of TRK-820 with ED_{50} 7.3 µg/kg was antagonized by nor-BNI (Togashi et al., 2002). TRK-820 was effective in scratching induced by the other pruritogenic substances: substance P (Togashi et al., 2002; Umeuchi et al., 2003; Utsumi et al., 2004), chloroquine (Inan & Cowan, 2004), compound 48/80 (Wang, Y et al., 2005), agmatin (Inan & Cowan, 2006a), and 5'-GNTI (Inan et al., 2009a, 2011) (Table 8). 5'-GNTI-induced scratching was suppressed by both pre-treatment and post-treatment with TRK-820. Tolerance did not develop to the antiscratching effect of TRK-820 in the subchronic study (Inan et al., 2009a).

Pruritogenic substance	Antipruritic effect	References
Histamine	ED_{50} = 7.3 µg/kg, p.o.	Togashi et al., 2002
Substance P	ED_{50} = 19.6 µg/kg, p.o.	Togashi et al., 2002
Chloroquine	TRK-820 (120 µg/kg, p.o.) suppressed the scratching almost completely	Inan & Cowan, 2004
Compound 48/80	ED_{50} = 6.64 µg/kg, s.c.	Wang, Y et al., 2005
Agmatin	TRK-820 (0.02 mg/kg, s.c.) was effective	Inan & Cowan, 2006a
5'-GNTI	TRK-820 (20 µg/kg, s.c.) suppressed the scratching almost completely	Inan et al., 2009a

Table 8. The antipruritic effects of TRK-820 against itching behaviors induced by various pruritogenic substances.

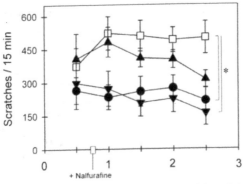

Fig. 3. Effects of TRK-820 on scratching induced by i.t. administration of morphine in rhesus monkeys. TRK-820 (0 (□), 0.1 (▲), 0.3 (●), and 1 (▼) μg/kg, i.m.) was given 45 min after the administration of morphine (0.03 mg, i.t.). * $p < 0.05$ between vehicle and time points 1 and 2.5 h. Reprinted with permission from Ko & Husbands, 2009.

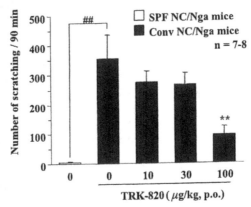

Fig. 4. Effects of TRK-820 on scratching behaviors observed in NC/Nag mice maintained in a conventional environment. ## $p < 0.01$, Welch test. ** $p < 0.01$ compared to NC/Nag mice not treated with TRK-820, parametric Dunnett multiple comparison test. Reprinted with permission from Nakao et al., 2008.

Although epidural or i.t. administration of a μ agonist like morphine is an important method for pain management, an itching sensation is the most common side effect (Ballantyne et al., 1988; Cousins & Mather, 1984). The effect of TRK-820 on morphine-induced scratching in mice or primates was also evaluated (Ko & Husbands, 2009; Utsumi et al., 2004; Wakasa et al., 2004). Intramuscular administration of TRK-820 (0.3–1 μg/kg) dose-dependently attenuated scratching induced by morphine (i.t.) in rhesus monkeys without affecting antinociception by morphine (Fig. 3) (Ko & Husbands, 2009).

TRK-820 reportedly exhibited antipruritic effects on spontaneous scratching behavior in aged MRL/*lpr* mice (a possible model for pruritus in autoimmune disease) (Umeuchi et al.,

2005) or NC/Nag mice maintained in a conventional environment (an animal model for atopic dermatitis) (Nakao et al., 2008), and scratching behavior secondary to cholestasis induced chronic ethynylestradiol injections in rats (Inan & Cowan, 2006b). Interestingly, TRK-820 was effective in scratching behaviors observed in conventional NC/Nag mice, which were considered a model of atopic dermatitis (Fig. 4).

4.2 Clinical studies

Wikström et al. (2005) and Kumagai et al. (2010) reported the results of randomized, double-blind, placebo-controlled clinical studies in which TRK-820 was administered to patients undergoing hemodialysis intravenously or orally (Fig. 5). In these studies, TRK-820 exhibited significant antipruritic effects without severe adverse drug reactions. These outcomes suggest that TRK-820 can be considered a safe agent.

TRK-820 is prescribed in Japan as an antipruritic for hemodialysis. Very recently, Kumagai et al. reported that TRK-820 has been prescribed for approximately 18,000 hemodialysis patients and effective in 70 to 80% (Kumagai et al., 2011).

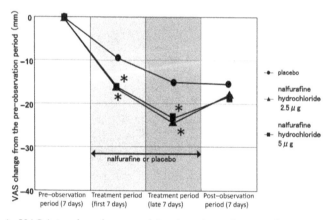

Fig. 5. Changes in VAS (visual analogue scale) values from the pre-observation period. All symbols show the mean values of VAS changes. *$p < 0.025$ compared to placebo, one-sided ANCOVA. Reprinted from Nagase & Fujii, 2011 with permission from Springer Science+Business Media. The VAS test consisted of a 100-mm horizontal line without scale markings. The patients were asked to mark the intensity of itching on the scale, with the right end of the line (100 mm) indicating the strongest possible itching and the left end (0 mm) indicating no itching.

5. Effects of TRK-820 on drug dependence

5.1 Effects of TRK-820 in the conditioned place preference (CPP) test

The μ agonists have a rewarding effect, which accounts for the abuse of morphine by humans. In animal models, the rewarding effects of μ agonists have been evaluated by the conditioned place preference (CPP) and self-administration paradigms (Di Chiara & North, 1992). In contrast to μ agonists, conventional κ agonists such as U-50,488H and U-69,593 generally lack a rewarding effect (Dykstra et al., 1997). However in the CPP test, animals avoid an environment associated with the administration of the κ agonists, indicating that these drugs have aversive effects (Barr et al., 1994; Funada et al., 1993). In contrast to conventional κ agonists, such as U-50,488H, TRK-820 (3.0-30 μg/kg, s.c.) did not induce significant place aversion in mice at doses producing significant antinociception (Fig. 6) (Nagase, 2010). Notably, TRK-820 exhibited neither preferential nor aversive properties. Recently, the peroral administration of TRK-820 (5.0 μg/day) was reported to show no signs of psychological or physical dependence in an open-labeled clinical trial for one year (Nagase & Fujii, 2011).

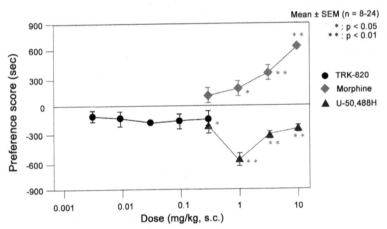

Fig. 6. The effect of TRK-820 in the CPP test. Reprinted with permission from Nagase, 2010.

5.2 The effects of TRK-820 on morphine and cocaine-induced rewarding effects

The mechanism of μ agonist-induced rewarding effects is outlined below. The activation of the μ receptor on γ-aminobutyric acid-containing interneurons is likely to disinhibit ventrotegmental area dopaminergic neurons, thereby increasing dopamine release in their terminal areas, including the nucleus accumbens (N.Acc). On the other hand, the activation of the κ receptor decreases dopamine release in the N.Acc (Di Chiara & Imperato, 1988; Spanagel et al., 1992). Therefore, κ agonists may be useful for treating morphine dependence. Indeed, the pretreatment with U-50,488H attenuated the morphine-induced place preference in mice (Funada et al., 1993). TRK-820 also significantly suppressed the place preference produced by morphine, and the effect of TRK-820 was antagonized by pre-treatment with nor-BNI (3.0 mg/kg, s.c.) in mice (Tsuji et al., 2001). In addition, TRK-820 was effective in reducing the rewarding effect produced by cocaine. TRK-820 (20 and 40 μg/kg, i.p.), at doses producing no aversive or sedative effects, suppressed the rewarding effect of cocaine (4.0 mg/kg, i.p.) in rats (Mori et al., 2002). U-50,488H and U-69,593 exhibited similar effects as TRK-820 (Shippenberg et al., 1996; Suzuki et al., 1992). Drug discrimination procedures provide relevant information about neuropharmacological mechanisms underlying the subjective effects of abused drugs, including cocaine, methamphetamine, and opioids, in animals. Therefore, the procedures are potentially useful for identifying candidate therapeutics for the management of drug abuse (Schuster & Johanson, 1988). Pre-treatment with TRK-820 (10 and 20 μg/kg, s.c.) significantly shifted the dose-response curve for cocaine (10 mg/kg, i.p.) to the right without changing the response rate. This attenuating effect of TRK-820 was completely reversed by pre-treatment with nor-BNI (10 mg/kg, s.c.) (Mori et al., 2002).

5.3 Effects of TRK-820 on the morphine withdrawal response

In humans, withdrawal from the chronic administration of opioids such as morphine results in characteristic behaviors, including anxiety, nausea, insomnia, hot and cold flashes, muscle aches, perspiration, and diarrhea. Such symptoms would pose clinical problems in patients receiving long-term treatment with opioids for pain relief. Rodents that are physically dependent on morphine elicit characteristic signs (jumping, wet dog shakes, rearing, diarrhea, ptosis, and forepaw tremor) when administrated naloxone. The withdrawal signs precipitated by naloxone are used as an index of the physical dependence on morphine. The effects of κ agonists TRK-820 and U-50,488H on the development of physical dependence on morphine were reported. Co-injection of TRK-820 (0.003-0.03 mg/kg, s.c.) during chronic morphine treatment dose-dependently suppressed naloxone-precipitated body weight loss, and the other withdrawal signs in morphine-dependent mice treated with TRK-820 (0.03 mg/kg, s.c.) were significantly fewer than those in untreated mice. In contrast to TRK-820, co-injection of U-50,488H (1.0-10 mg/kg, s.c.) did not inhibit naloxone-precipitated body weight loss and other withdrawal signs (Tsuji et al., 2000).

5.4 The effect of TRK-820 on the nicotine-withdrawal response

Nicotine withdrawal produces characteristic syndromes, including irritability, anxiety, depression, and craving for nicotine. Pre-treatment with TRK-820 (10 and 30 µg/kg, s.c.) or U-50,488H (0.01-1.0 mg/kg, s.c.) has been reported to decrease dose-dependently mecamylamine-precipitated nicotine-withdrawal aversion in nicotine-dependent rats (Ise et al., 2002).

6. Comparison of pharmacological properties between TRK-820 and conventional κ agonists

We described in the previous sections some pharmacological properties of TRK-820 that are different from conventional κ agonists, arylacetamides such as U-50,488H and U-69,593: binding properties (section 2) and exhibition of no preferential and no aversive effect in the CPP paradigm (section 5). As described below, drug discrimination procedures indicate conclusive difference between TRK-820 and arylacetamides.

6.1 Discriminative tests

Drug discrimination procedures have shown that the properties of TRK-820 differ from those of conventional κ agonists, such as U-50,488H. In the cross-substitution tests using rats, U-50,488H (1.0-3.0 mg/kg) substituted for the discriminative stimulus effects of TRK-820 (40 µg/kg, i.p.), whereas TRK-820 (10-76 µg/kg) did not completely substitute for those of U-50,488H (3.0 mg/kg, i.p.). E-2078 (0.3-3.0 mg/kg), but not R-84760 (0.01-0.3 mg/kg), substituted for the discriminative stimulus effects of both TRK-820 and U-50,488H. KT-90 (0.03-3.0 mg/kg), CI-977 (1-30 mg/kg), or ICI-199441 (3.0-56 mg/kg) substituted for the discriminative stimulus effects of U-50,488H, but not for those of TRK-820 (Mori et al., 2004).

In this study, cross-substitution between the discriminative effects of U-50,488H and TRK-820 was not observed. The κ agonists tested in this study, except E-2078, tended to substitute for the discriminative stimulus effects of U-50,488H rather than those of TRK-820. These results suggest that U-50,488H and TRK-820 have differential properties. Furthermore, non-competitive NMDA antagonists phencyclidine (PCP, 0.5-2.0 mg/kg) and MK-801 (10-80 µg/kg) dose-dependently generalized to the discriminative stimulus effects of U-50,488H (3.0 mg/kg, i.p.) in the cross-substitution tests. On the other hand, PCP and MK-801 at doses that generalized to the discriminative stimulus effects of U-50,488H did not generalize to those of TRK-820 (40 µg/kg, i.p.) (Mori et al., 2006). The outcomes clearly indicate different properties between TRK-820 and U-50,488H.

7. Other pharmacological effects

7.1 The effect of TRK-820 on a rat model of schizophrenia

The effects of TRK-820 on hyperlocomotion and stereotyped behaviors (head-weaving, sniffing, and turning) induced by PCP were evaluated. These behaviors are thought to resemble the schizophrenia-like effects in humans. TRK-820 (10–100 µg/kg, s.c.) dose-dependently inhibited PCP (10 mg/kg, i.p.)-induced hyperlocomotion, and this effect was antagonized with nor-BNI (20 mg/kg, s.c.). PCP-induced stereotyped behaviors were also inhibited by treatment with TRK-820 in a dose-dependent manner. These findings that TRK-820 potentially ameliorates abnormal behaviors induced by PCP suggest its therapeutic potential against the symptoms of schizophrenia (Yoshikawa et al., 2009).

7.2 The effect of TRK-820 on dyskinesia symptoms in a parkinsonian rat model

The effects of TRK-820 on rotational behavior were investigated in unilateral 6-hydroxydopamine (6-OHDA)-treated rats (hemi-parkinsonian rats), and on dyskinesia produced by administering L-DOPA to hemi-parkinsonian rats for 3 weeks (dyskinesia rats). TRK-820 significantly ameliorated abnormal behavior in hemi-parkinsonian rats at 30 µg/kg (s.c.), and L-DOPA induced dyskinesia at 10 and 30 µg/kg (s.c.). This effect was antagonized by pretreatment with nor-BNI (20 mg/kg, s.c.). Additionally, co-administration of TRK-820 (3 and 10 µg/kg, s.c.) with L-DOPA for 3 weeks suppressed the development of L-DOPA-induced dyskinesia. TRK-820 may be a suitable drug for the treatment of parkinsonian patients with dyskinesia symptoms (Ikeda et al., 2009).

7.3 The diuretic effect of TRK-820 in rats

Diuresis is a well-recognized effect of conventional κ agonists in animals and humans. A diuretic effect of TRK-820 in rats has also been reported. TRK-820 (0.005-0.02 mg/kg, s.c.) dose-dependently induced a diuretic effect without developing tolerance, and this effect was inhibited by selective κ antagonist 5′-GNTI (Inan et al., 2009b).

7.4 The effects of TRK-820 on endothelial cell differentiation and development of vasculature

The roles of the opioid κ system in vascular development were investigated (Yamamizu et al., 2011). U-50,488H and TRK-820 significantly inhibited endothelial cell differentiation and vascular formation through the inhibition of cAMP/PKA signaling.

8. Conclusion

TRK-820 was a selective κ agonist. However, its pharmacological properties were different from those of conventional arylacetamide κ agonists, including U-50,488H. A noteworthy feature of TRK-820 was that it showed no preferential or aversive properties, whereas U-50,488H produced aversion. This disparity of properties between TRK-820 and arylacetamide κ agonists was reported to stem from the difference in κ receptor subtypes each compound interacted with: arylacetamide κ agonists would interact with κ_1 receptor subtype, whereas TRK-820 may interact with another κ receptor subtype (perhaps κ_3) (Endoh et al., 1999; 2000; 2001; Tsuji et al., 2000a; 2000b). Although opioid receptors have been classified historically into three types (μ, δ, and κ types) and further divided into several subtypes from the pharmacological viewpoint (Dhawan et al., 1996), only the three major types have been cloned (Satoh & Minami, 1995). Much evidence has been compiled indicating that various receptors, including opioid receptors, exist as homo- or hetero dimers of the receptors (George et al., 2000, 2002; Gomes et al., 2000, 2004; Devi, 2001; Levac et al., 2002; Wang, D et al., 2005), and receptor dimerization has been invoked to explain the discrepancy between widely varied pharmacologies and the identification of only three opioid receptor types. Therefore, the disparity of properties between TRK-820 and arylacetamide κ agonists may stem from the difference in receptor dimers each compound interacts with. Both TRK-820 and arylacetamide κ agonists are expected to be useful tools for the investigation of receptor dimerization and/or κ receptor subtype. As mentioned in section 2, a binding assay using [³H]TRK-820 and [³H]U-69,593 is thought to be a facile and useful method for achieving that purpose. However, [³H]TRK-820 is not currently available.

In addition to antipruritic and antinociceptive effects, TRK-820 exhibited various pharmacological effects, such as the treatment of the symptoms of schizophrenia or dyskinesia symptoms of parkisonian patients, or remedy for drug addiction. Moreover, TRK-820 has been already launched in Japan. TRK-820 is expected not only to be developed with the other indication, such as symptoms of schizophrenia or parkinson's disease, but also to be utilized to investigate pharmacology *via* the κ receptor.

9. References

Ballantyne, J.C.; Loach, A. B. & Carr, D. B. (1988). Itching after epidural and spinal opiates, *Pain*, 33, 2, 149-160, ISSN 0304-3959.

Barr, G. A.; Wang, S.; Carden, S. (1994). Aversive properties of the κ opioid agonist U50,488 in the week-old rat pup, *Psychopharmacology*, 113, 3-4, 422-428, ISSN 0033-3158.

Cousins, M.J. & Mather, L.E. (1984). Intrathecal and Epidural Administration of Opioids, *Anesthesiology*, 61, 3, 276-310, ISSN 0003-3022.

Devi, L. A. (2001). Heterodimerization of G-protein-coupled receptors: pharmacology, signaling and trafficking, *Trends Pharmacol. Sci.*, 22, 10, 532-537, ISSN 0165-6147.

Dhawan, B. N.; Cesselin, F.; Raghubir, R.; Reisine, T.; Bradley, P. B.; Portoghese, P. S. & Hamon, M. (1996). International Union of Pharmacology. XII. Classification of Opioid Receptors, *Pharmacol. Rev.*, 48, 4, 567-592, ISSN 0031-6997.

Di Chiara, G.; Imperato, A. (1988). Drugs abused by humans preferentially increase synaptic dopamine concentrations in the mesolimbic system of freely moving rats, *Proc. Natl. Acad. Sci. U. S. A.*, 85, 14, 5274-5278, ISSN 0027-8424.

Di Chiara, G.; North, R. A. (1992). Neurobiology of opiate abuse, *Trends Pharmacol. Sci.*, 13, 5, 185-193, ISSN 0165-6147.

Dykstra, L. A.; Preston, K. L.; Bigelow, G. E. (1997). Discriminative stimulus and subjective effects of opioids with *mu* and *kappa* activity: data from laboratory animals and human subjects, *Psychopharmacology*, 130, 1, 14-27, ISSN 0033-3158.

Endoh, T.; Matsuura, H.; Tajima, A.; Izumimoto, N.; Tajima, C.; Suzuki, T.; Saitoh, A.; Suzuki, T.; Narita, M.; Tseng, L. & Nagase, H. (1999). POTENT ANTINOCICEPTIVE EFFECTS OF TRK-820, A NOVEL κ-OPIOID RECEPTOR AGONIST, *Life Sci.*, 65, 16, 1685-1694, ISSN 0024-3205.

Endoh, T.; Tajima, A.; Suzuki, T.; Kamei, J.; Suzuki, T.; Narita, M.; Tseng, L. & Nagase, H. (2000). Characterization of the antinociceptive effects of TRK-820 in the rat, *Eur. J. Pharmacol.*, 387, 2, 133-140. ISSN 0014-2999.

Endoh, T.; Tajima, A.; Izumimoto, N.; Suzuki, T.; Saitoh, A.; Suzuki, T.; Narita, M.; Kamei, J.; Tseng, L. F.; Mizoguchi, H.; Nagase, H. (2001). TRK-820, a Selective κ-Opioid Agonist, Produces Potent Antinociception in Cynomolgus Monkeys, *Jpn. J. Pharmacol.*, 85, 3, 282-290, ISSN 0021-5198.

Funada, M.; Suzuki, T.; Narita, M.; Misawa, M.; Nagase, H. (1993). Blockade of morphine reward through the activation of κ-opioid receptors in mice, *Neuropharmacology*, 32, 12, 1315-1323, ISSN 0028-3908.

George, S. R.; Fan, T.; Xie, Z.; Tse, R.; Tam, V.; Varghese, G. & O'Dowd, B. F. (2000). Oligomerization of *μ*- and *δ*-Opioid Receptors. GENERATION OF NOVEL FUNCTIONAL PROPERTIES, *J. Biol. Chem.*, 275, 34, 26128-26135, ISSN 0021-9258.

George, S. R.; O'Dowd, B. F. & Lee, S. P. (2002). G-protein-coupled receptor oligomerization and its potential for drug discovery, *Nat. Rev. Drug Discov.*, 1, 10, 808-820, ISSN 1474-1776.

Gomes, I.; Jordan, B. A.; Gupta, A.; Trapaidze, N.; Nagy, V. & Devi, L. A. (2000). Heterodimerization of *μ* and *δ* Opioid Receptors: A Role in Opiate Synergy, *J. Neurosci.*, 20, 22, RC110, ISSN 0270-6474.

Gomes, I.; Gupta, A.; Filipovska, J.; Szeto, H. H.; Pintar, J.E. & Devi, L. A. (2004). A role for heterodimerization of *μ* and *δ* opiate receptors in enhancing morphine analgesia, *Proc. Nat. Acad. U.S.A.*, 101, 14, 5135-5139 ISSN 0027-8424.

Ikeda, K.; Yoshikawa, S.; Kurokawa, T.; Yuzawa, N.; Nakao, K.; Mochizuki, H. (2009). TRK-820, a selective kappa opioid receptor agonist, could effectively ameliorate L-DOPA-induced dyskinesia symptoms in a rat model of Parkinson's disease, *Eur. J. Pharmacol.*, 620, 1-3, 42-48, ISSN 0014-2999.

Inan, S. & Cowan, A. (2004). Kappa opioid agonists suppress chloroquine-induced scratching in mice, *Eur. J. Pharmacol.*, 502, 3, 233-237. ISSN 0014-2999.

Inan, S. & Cowan, A. (2006a). AGMATINE-INDUCED STEREOTYPED SCRATCHING IN MICE IS ANTAGONIZED BY NALFURAFINE, A KAPPA OPIOID AGONIST, *Pharmacologist*, 48, 1, 38, ISSN 0031-7004.

Inan, S. & Cowan, A. (2006b). Nalfurafine, a kappa opioid receptor agonist, inhibits scratching behavior secondary to cholestasis induced by chronic ethynylestradiol injections in rats, *Pharmacol. Biochem. Behav.*, 85, 1, 39-43. ISSN 0091-3057.

Inan, S.; Dun, N. J. & Cowan, A. (2009a). NALFURAFINE PREVENTS 5'-GUANIDINONALTRINDOLE- AND COMPOUND 48/80-INDUCED SPINAL c-fos EXPRESSION AND ATTENUATES 5'-GUANIDINONALTRINDOLE-

ELICITED SCRATCHING BEHAVIOR IN MICE, *Neuroscience*, 163, 1, 23-33, ISSN 0306-4522.

Inan, S.; Lee, D. Y. -W; Liu-Chen, L. Y.; Cowan, A. (2009b). Comparison of the diuretic effects of chemically diverse kappa opioid agonists in rats: nalfurafine, U50,488H, and salvinorin A, *Naunyn Schmiedebergs Arch. Pharmacol.*, 379, 3, 263-270, ISSN 0028-1298.

Inan, S.; Dun, N. J. & Cowan, A. (2011). Investigation of gastrin-releasing peptide as a mediator for 5'-guanidinonaltrindole-induced compulsive scratching in mice, *Peptides*, 32, 2, 286-292, ISSN 0196-9781.

Ise, Y.; Narita, M.; Nagase, H.; Suzuki, T. (2002). Modulation of κ-opioidergic systems on mecamylamine-precipitated nicotine-withdrawal aversion in rats, *Neurosci. Lett.*, 323, 2, 164-166, ISSN 0304-3940.

Kawai, K.; Hayakawa, J.; Miyamoto, T.; Imamura, Y.; Yamane, S.; Wakita, H.; Fujii, H.; Kawamura, K.; Matsuura, H.; Izumimoto, N.; Kobayashi, R.; Endo, T. & Nagase, H. (2008). Design, synthesis, and structure–activity relationship of novel opioid κ-agonists, *Bioorg. Med. Chem.*, 16, 20, 9188-9201. ISSN 0968-0896.

Ko, M. –C. & Husbands, S. M. (2009). Effects of Atypical κ-Opioid Receptor Agonists on Intrathecal Morphine-Induced Itch and Analgesia in Primates, *J. Pharmacol. Exp. Ther.*, 328, 1, 193-200. ISSN 0022-3565.

Kumagai, H.; Ebata, T.; Takamori, K.; Muramatsu, T.; Nakamoto, H. & Suzuki, H. (2010). Effect of a novel kappa-receptor agonist, nalfurafine hydrochloride, on severe itch in 337 haemodialysis patients: a Phase III, randomized, double-blind, placebo-controlled study, *Nephrol. Dial. Transplant.*, 25, 4, 1251-1257, ISSN 0931-0509.

Kumagai, H.; Yamamoto, K.; Kushiyama, T.; Higashi, Y.; Takechi, H. & Suzuki, H. (2011). A novel κ-receptor agonist, nalfurafine, for severe itch in hemodialysis patients, *Kidney and Dialysis*, 70, 4, 651-657, ISSN 0385-2156.

Levac, B. A. R.; O'Dowd, B. F. & George, S. R. (2002). Oligomerization of opioid receptors: generation of novel signaling units, *Curr. Opin. Pharmacol.*, 2, 1, 76-81, ISSN 1471-4892.

Mori, T.; Nomura, M.; Nagase, H.; Narita, M.; Suzuki, T. (2002). Effects of a newly synthesized κ-opioid receptor agonist, TRK-820, on the discriminative stimulus and rewarding effects of cocaine in rats, *Psychopharmacology*, 161, 1, 17-22, ISSN 0033-3158.

Mori, T.; Nomura, M.; Yoshizawa, K.; Nagase, H.; Narita, M.; Suzuki, T. (2004). Differential properties between TRK-820 and U-50,488H on the discriminative stimulus effects in rats, *Life Sci.*, 75, 20, 2473-2482, ISSN 0024-3205.

Mori, T.; Nomura, M.; Yoshizawa, K.; Nagase, H.; Sawaguchi, T.; Narita, M.; Suzuki, T. (2006). Generalization of NMDA-Receptor Antagonists to the Discriminative Stimulus Effects of κ-Opioid Receptor Agonists U-50,488H, but Not TRK-820 in Rats, *J. Pharmacol. Sci.*, 100, 2, 157-161, ISSN 1347-8613.

Nagase, H.; Hayakawa, J.; Kawamura, K.; Kawai, K.; Takezawa, Y.; Matsuura, H.; Tajima, C. & Endo, T. (1998). DISCOVERY OF A STRUCTURALLY NOVEL OPIOID κ-AGONIST DERIVED FROM 4,5-EPOXYMORPHINAN, *Chem. Pharm. Bull.*, 46, 2, 366-369. ISSN 0009-2363.

Nagase, H. (2010). Design and Synthesis of a Novel Antipruritic Drug, Nalfurafine Hydrochloride and Its Pharmacological Feature, *Jpn. J. Pharm. Palliat. Care Sci.* 3, 4, 115-122. ISSN 1882-9783.

Nagase, H.; Watanabe, A.; Nemoto, T.; Yamaotsu, N.; Hayashida, K.; Nakajima, M.; Hasebe, K.; Nakao, K.; Mochizuki, H.; Hirono, S. & Fujii, H. (2010). Drug design and synthesis of a novel κ opioid receptor agonist with an oxabicyclo[2.2.2]octane skeleton and its pharmacology, *Bioorg. Med. Chem. Lett.* 20, 1, 121-124. ISSN 0960-894X.

Nagase, H. & Fujii, H. (2011). Opioids in Preclinical and Clinical Trials, In: *Chemistry of Opioid*, Nagase, H. (Ed.), 29-62, Springer, ISBN 978-3-642-18106-1, Heidelberg.

Nakao, K.; Ikeda, K.; Kurokawa, T.; Togashi, Y.; Umeuchi, H.; Honda, T.; Okano, K. & Mochizuki, H. (2008). Effect of TRK-820, a selective κ opioid receptor agonist, on scratching behavior in an animal model of atopic dermatitis, *Jpn. J. Neuropsychopharmacol.*, 28, 2, 75-83, ISSN 1340-2544.

Nakao, K. & Mochizuki, H. (2009). NALFURAFINE HYDROCHLORIDE: A NEW DRUG FOR THE TREATMENT OF UREMIC PRURITUS IN HEMODIALYSIS PATIENTS, *Drugs Today* 45, 5, 323-329. ISSN 1699-3993.

Ohsawa, M.; Kamei, J. (2005). Modification of κ-Opioid Receptor Agonist-Induced Antinociception by Diabetes in the Mouse Brain and Spinal Cord, *J. Pharmacol. Sci.*, 98, 1, 25-32, ISSN 1347-8613.

Satoh, M. & Minami, M. (1995). MOLECULAR PHARMACOLOGY OF THE OPIOID RECEPTORS, *Pharmacol. Ther.*, 68, 3, 343-364, ISSN 0163-7258.

Schuster, C. R.; Johanson, C. E. (1988). Relationship between the discriminative stimulus properties and subjective effects of drugs, *Psychopharmacol. Ser.* 4, 161–175, ISBN 0931-6795.

Seki, T.; Awamura, S.; Kimura, C.; Ide, S.; Sakano, K.; Minami, M.; Nagase, H. & Satoh, M. (1999). Pharmacological properties of TRK-820 on cloned μ-, δ- and κ-opioid receptors and nociceptin receptor, *Eur. J. Pharmacol.* 376, 1-2, 159-167. ISSN 0014-2999.

Shippenberg, T. S.; LeFevour, A.; Heidbreder, C. (1996). κ-Opioid Rreceptor Agonists Prevent Sensitization to the Conditioned Rewarding Effects of Cocaine, *J. Pharmacol. Exp. Ther.*, 276, 2, 545-554, ISSN 0022-3565.

Spanagel, R.; Herz, A.; Shippenberg, T. S. (1992). Opposing tonically active endogenous opioid systems modulate the mesolimbic dopaminergic pathway, *Proc. Natl. Acad. Sci. U. S. A.*, 89, 6, 2046-2050, ISSN 0027-8424.

Suzuki, T.; Shiozaki, Y.; Masukawa, Y.; Misawa, M.; Nagase, H. (1992). The Role of Mu- and Kappa-Opioid Receptors in Cocaine-Induced Conditioned Place Preference, *Jpn. J. Pharmacol.*, 58, 4, 435-442, ISSN 0021-5198.

Suzuki, T.; Izumimoto, N.; Takezawa, Y.; Fujimura, M.; Togashi, Y.; Nagase, H.; Tanaka, T.; Endoh, T. (2004). Effect of repeated administration of TRK-820, a κ-opioid receptor agonist, on tolerance to its antinociceptive and sedative actions, *Brain Res.*, 995, 2, 167-175, ISSN 0006-8993.

Takasaki, I.; Suzuki, T.; Sasaki, A.; Nakao, K.; Hirakata, M.; Okano, K.; Tanaka, T.; Nagase, H.; Shiraki, K.; Nojima, H.; Kuraishi, Y. (2004). Suppression of Acute Herpetic Pain Related Responses by the κ-Opioid Receptor Agonist (-)-17- Cyclopropylmethyl-3,14β-dihydroxy-4,5α-epoxy-6β-[N-methyl-3-trans-3-(3-furyl)Acrylamido]

Morphinan Hydrochloride (TRK-820) in Mice, *J. Pharmacol. Exp. Ther.*, 309, 1, 36-41, ISSN 0022-3565.

Takasaki, I.; Nojima, H.; Shiraki, K.; Kuraishi, Y. (2006). Specific down-regulation of spinal µ-opioid receptor and reduced analgesic effects of morphine in mice with postherpetic pain, *Eur. J. Pharmacol.*, 550, 1-3, 62-67, ISSN 0014-2999.

Togashi, Y.; Umeuchi, H.; Okano, K.; Ando, N.; Yoshizawa, Y.; Honda, T.; Kawamura, K.; Endoh, T.; Utsumi, J.; Kamei, J.; Tanaka, T. & Nagase, H. (2002). Antipruritic activity of the κ-opioid receptor agonist, TRK-820, *Eur. J. Pharmacol.*, 435, 2-3, 259-264. ISSN 0014-2999.

Tsuji, M.; Yamazaki, M.; Takeda, H.; Matsumiya, T.; Nagase, H.; Tseng, L. F.; Narita, M. & Suzuki, T. (2000a). The novel κ-opioid receptor agonist TRK-820 has no affect on the development of antinociceptive tolerance to morphine in mice, *Eur. J. Pharmacol.*, 394, 1, 91-95. ISSN 0014-2999.

Tsuji, M.; Takeda, H.; Matsumiya, T.; Nagase, H.; Yamazaki, M.; Narita, M. & Suzuki, T. (2000b). A NOVEL κ-OPIOID RECEPTOR AGONIST, TRK-820, BLOCKS THE DEVELOPMENT OF PHYSICAL DEPENDENCE ON MORPHINE IN MICE, *Life Sci.*, 66, 25, PL353-358, ISSN 0024-3205.

Tsuji, M.; Takeda, H.; Matsumiya, T.; Nagase, H.; Narita, M.; Suzuki, T. (2001). The novel κ-opioid receptor agonist TRK-820 suppresses the rewarding and locomotor-enhancing effects of morphine in mice, *Life Sci.*, 68, 15, 1717-1725, ISSN 0024-3205.

Umeuchi, H.; Togashi, Y.; Honda, T.; Nakao, K.; Okano, K.; Tanaka, T. & Nagase, H. (2003). Involvement of central µ-opioid system in the scratching behavior in mice, and the suppression of it by the activation of κ-opioid system, *Eur. J. Pharmacol.*, 477, 1, 29-35. ISSN 0014-2999.

Umeuchi, H.; Kawashima, Y.; Aoki, C. A.; Kurokawa, T.; Nakao, K.; Itoh, M.; Kikuchi, K.; Kato, T.; Okano, K.; Gershwin, M. E. & Miyakawa, H. (2005). Spontaneous scratching behavior in MRL/*lpr* mice, a possible model for pruritus in autoimmune diseases, and antipruritic activity of a novel κ-opioid receptor agonist nalfurafine hydrochloride, *Eur. J. Pharmacol.*, 518, 2-3, 133-139. ISSN 0014-2999.

Utsumi, J.; Togashi, Y.; Umeuchi, H.; Okano, K.; Tanaka, T. & Nagase, H. (2004). Antipruritic Activity of a Novel κ-Opioid Receptor Agonist, TRK-820, In: *Itch: Basic Mechanisms and Therapy* Yosipovitch, G.; Greaves, M. W.; Fleischer A. B. Jr.; McGlone, F. (Ed.) 107-114. ISBN 0-8247-4747-X.

Vanderah, T. W.; Largent-Milnes, T.; Lai, J.; Porreca, F.; Houghten, R. A.; Menzaghi, F.; Wisniewski, K.; Stalewski, J.; Sueiras-Diaz, J.; Galyean, R.; Schteingart, C.; Junien, J. -L.; Trojnar, J.; Riviere, P. J. -M.(2008). Novel D-amino acid tetrapeptides produce potent antinociception by selectively acting at peripheral κ-opioid receptors, *Eur. J. Pharmacol.*, 583, 1, 62-72, ISSN 0014-2999.

Wakasa, Y.; Fujiwara, A.; Umeuchi, H.; Endoh, T.; Okano, K.; Tanaka, T. & Nagase, H. (2004). Inhibitory effects of TRK-820 on systemic skin scratching induced by morphine in rhesus monkeys, *Life Sci.*, 75, 24, 2947-2957, ISSN 0024-3205.

Wang, D.; Sun, X.; Bohn, L. M. & Sadée, W. (2005). Opioid Receptor Homo- and Heterodimerization in Living Cells by Quantitative Bioluminescence Resonance Energy Transfer, *Mol. Pharmacol.*, 67, 6, 2173-2184, ISSN 0026-895X.

Wang, Y.; Tang, K.; Inan, S.; Siebert, D.; Holzgrabe, U.; Lee, D. Y. W.; Huang, P.; Li, J. -G.; Cowan, A. & Liu-Chen, L. -Y. (2005). Comparison of Pharmacological Activities of

Three Distinct κ Ligands (Salvinorin A, TRK-820 and 3FLB) on κ Opioid Receptors in Vitro and Their Antipruritic and Antinociceptive Activities in Vivo, *J. Pharmacol. Exp. Ther.*, 312, 1, 220-230. ISSN 0022-3565.

Wikström, B.; Gellert, R.; Ladefoged, S. D.; Danda, Y.; Akai, M.; Ide, K.; Ogasawara, M.; Kawashima, Y.; Ueno, K.; Mori, A. & Ueno, Y. (2005). κ-Opioid System in Uremic Pruritus: Multicenter, Randomized, Double-Blind, Placebo-Controlled Clinical Studies, *J. Am. Soc. Nephrol.*, 16, 12, 3742-3747, ISSN 1046-6673.

Yamamizu, K.; Furuta, S.; Katayama, S.; Narita, M.; Kuzumaki, N.; Imai, S.; Nagase, H.; Suzuki, T.; Narita, M.; Yamashita, J. K. (2011). The κ opioid system regulates endothelial cell differentiation and pathfinding in vascular development, *Blood*, 118, 3, 775-785, ISSN 0006-4971.

Yoshikawa, S.; Hareyama, N.; Ikeda, K.; Kurokawa, T.; Nakajima, M.; Nakao, K.; Mochizuki, H.; Ichinose, H. (2009). Effects of TRK-820, a selective kappa opioid receptor agonist, on rat schizophrenia models, *Eur. J. Pharmacol.*, 606, 1-3, 102-108, ISSN 0014-2999.

The Cannabinoid 1 Receptor and Progenitor Cells in the Adult Central Nervous System

Alexandra Sideris[1], Thomas Blanck[2] and Esperanza Recio-Pinto[3]
[1]Department of Anesthesiology,
[2]Department of Anesthesiology, Department of Physiology and Neuroscience
[3]Department of Anesthesiology; Department of Pharmacology
New York University Langone Medical Center, New York
USA

1. Introduction

The aims of this chapter are to: (1) examine the key developments leading up to the discovery the cannabinoid 1 receptor (CB1R) and (2) assess the potential therapeutic benefits of cannabinoid drugs with respect to neurogenesis in the adult brain and spinal cord. As one of the most abundant G-protein coupled receptors found in the central nervous system, localization of CB1R and its role in the mature and in the developing brain will be discussed. Pharmacological studies with cannabinergic drugs, and studies utilizing knock-out mice of various endocannabinoid system components will be reviewed in the context of adult brain neurogenesis. The apparent conflicting data reveal the complexity of endocannabinoid signaling in this process. Though many studies have focused on CB1R and neurogenesis in the brain, none have evaluated the potential ability for CB1R to modulate the fate, and specifically neuronal differentiation, of adult spinal cord progenitors. The implications for CB1R modulation of adult neurogenesis are pivotal for understanding the behavioral and cognitive effects of chronic marijuana use, but also for assessing the potential consequences of pharmacotherapeutics with CB1R agonists or antagonists

2. Discovery of an endogenous cannabinoid system

The history leading up to the discovery of the "endocannabinoid (eCB) system" is an interesting one, sprouting from a decades- long quest for the active constituents of the marijuana plant, *Cannabis sativa*. Though the cannabis plant has long been used for a variety of purposes dating back more than 4000 years (O'Shaughnessy 1842; Mechoulam and Hanus 2000), only recently was it found that delta 9- tetrahydrocannabinol (Δ^9-THC) was the ingredient responsible for the psychotropic effects associated and exploited with its use (Mechoulam and Gaoni 1965).

One of the original and most ancient uses of the *Cannabis sativa* plant was to induce a trance-like state, often an essential component to the elaborate religious rites in ancient cultures ranging from the Chinese, to the Ayurvedic Indians, to the Persians and Greeks (O'Shaughnessy 1842; Aldrich 2006). Herodotus referred to the use of the hemp plant by the

Scythians as incense in funeral rites, and also described the use of the hemp plant by the Phoenicians to make 'cordage' for building bridges (Herodotus 1824). The plant was extensively cultivated for its fiber which was used to make fabric for ship sails and clothing, but was also used for food, cooking oil, as a lubricant, and as an analgesic (Grinspoon 1993).

The earliest work to find the active ingredient began in the late 19th century after reports from Dr. O'Shaugnessy during his travels in India. In the true spirit of a responsible clinical researcher, before testing on humans, Dr. O'Shaugnessy described the use of hemp on various animals, a practice not standard for physicians at his time. Based on his findings, he believed that certain patients could benefit from the use of cannabis extracts (O'Shaughnessy 1842). His case studies described the use of the drug in humans for rheumatism, hydrophobia, cholera, tetanus, and infantile convulsions. He cautioned, however, of the "delirium occasioned by continued Hemp inebriation," which continues to be a great -but not insurmountable- obstacle for modern pharmacologists synthesizing drugs targeting the endocannabinoid system. He detailed the effects of cannabis preparations for a variety of ailments in a lecture given to the Medical College of Calcutta in 1839. Based on his work, a renewed interest in active cannabis extracts led to scientific inquiry in Europe and the United States, but an active component was not isolated mostly due to lack of effective techniques available at the time. It was not until 1965 that the major psychoactive constituent Δ^9-THC by Mechoulam's group (Mechoulam and Gaoni 1965). By the 1970s, many phytocannabinoids were characterized, and it was determined that they were lipid derivatives. Because of the lipophilic nature of these compounds, their mechanism of action was thought to be mediated by their ability to adhere to cellular membranes, much like the proposed mechanism of anesthetic action (Paton 1975). The isolation of Δ^9-THC was a key breakthrough in the discovery of an endogenous cannabinoid system because it allowed for the unexpected identification of a highly specific binding site in the body (Devane, Dysarz et al. 1988). This binding site was isolated and cloned in 1990, from both rat and human tissues (Matsuda, Lolait et al. 1990; Gerard, Mollereau et al. 1991) and was named the cannabinoid 1 receptor (CB1R).

Since it did not seem logical that the body would invest energy in the synthesis of receptors that specifically bind the constituents of this one plant, scientists began looking for compounds produced by the body that could also bind to CB1R. Binding studies with known neurotransmitters and hormones proved to be unfruitful, indicating that a unique ligand was utilizing this newly discovered CB1R. By using a highly specific probe for CB1R labeled with tritium (Devane, Breuer et al. 1992), competitive binding studies in pig brain fractions indicated the presence of endogenous compounds with cannabimimetic activity. Chromatography, nuclear magnetic resonance and mass spectrometry were used to identify arachidonoylethanolamide (Devane, Hanus et al. 1992). An amide group in this newly discovered compound and the historically acknowledged effect of cannabis use, led to the witty alternate name for the very first endocannabinoid 'anandamide', deriving from the Sanskrit word for 'bliss' (Devane, Hanus et al. 1992; Mechoulam 2000). Not only did anandamide work like Δ^9-THC in binding assays, it also mimicked its effects on motor functions, sedation and pain relief (Mechoulam 2000).

In 1993, shortly after the discovery of anandamide, another cannabinoid receptor was found and cloned from the periphery (rat spleen), and identified mostly on immune cells (Munro, Thomas et al. 1993). It was referred to as the CB2 receptor (CB2R). Two groups, made the separate discovery of another endocannabinoid, 2-arachidonoyl glycerol (2-AG), that was capable of binding to both the original CB1R, and to this novel CB2R receptor [(Mechoulam, Ben-Shabat et al. 1995; Sugiura, Kondo et al. 1995) and see **Figure 1** for a timeline].

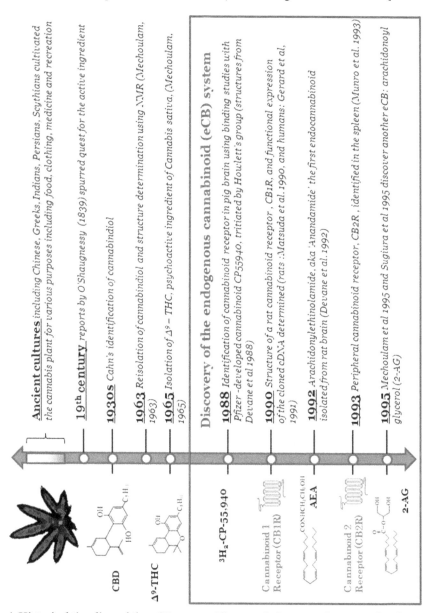

Fig. 1. **A Historical timeline of the eCB system.** Illustrated above are the major developments leading up to the discovery of an endogenous cannabinoid system, with the pivotal discoveries of the cannabinoid receptors, CB1R and CB2R, and the ligands AEA & 2-AG. Partly summarized from (Mechoulam and Hanus 2000). Receptors made with motifolio.com©.

By the end of the 20th century, the basic components of the endocannabinoid system- the receptors, endogenous ligands, and the enzymes responsible for their synthesis and degradation- were identified, paving the way for the groundbreaking discoveries that continually emerge, bringing forth the often surprising and unexpected ways in which this system works in the body.

3. CB1R localization in the central nervous system

With the discovery of the endocannabinoid system came the natural question as to what exactly these ligands and receptors are doing in the body. The location and density of CB1R could not only help explain some of the effects of cannabis use, but also has suggested the potential role of the endocannabinoids in learning, memory, motor function, emesis, reward behaviors and pain.

CB1R is a G-protein coupled receptor encoded by a single gene located on chromosome 4 in the mouse, 5 in the rat and 6 in humans. The mouse and rat display 95% nucleic acid homology, and 99.5% amino acid homology, while the mouse and human display 90% nucleic acid homology, and 97% amino acid homology (Onaivi, Leonard et al. 2002).

This receptor has been identified in both cortical and subcortical areas, the olfactory bulb, the retina, periaqueductal gray area, the cerebellum and the spinal cord (Mackie 2005). Original autoradiography studies revealed that the substantia nigra contains the highest density of CB1R in the central nervous system (CNS) (Herkenham, Lynn et al. 1991). The substantia nigra is a structure in the midbrain that plays an important role in movement, reward and addiction. CB1R is localized to the GABAergic (GABA = Gamma-aminobutyric acid) axons that project to the substantia nigra from the putamen. CB1R is also found in the caudate putamen, and on axons of medium spiny neurons projecting into the globus pallidus, on excitatory glutamatergic axons projecting from the sub-thalamic nucleus into the substantia nigra (Mailleux, Verslijpe et al. 1992; Sanudo-Pena, Tsou et al. 1997; Mackie 2005).

Much attention has been paid to the hippocampus and CB1R expression mainly because of the striking effects of marijuana on cognitive processes like memory. CB1R is widely distributed in the hippocampal structures. For example, high amounts of the receptor are found in the molecular and granule cell layer of the dentate gyrus (Mackie 2005), in the perisomatic region of CA1 indicative of expression that is post-synpaptic to basket cells, and may also be found on glutamatergic terminals of the perforant path (Kirby, Hampson et al. 1995). In the frontal cortex, double-immunocytochemical labeling experiments revealed GABAergic cholecystokinin (CCK) positive interneurons have somatic immunoreactivity for CB1R (Katona, Sperlagh et al. 1999; Tsou, Mackie et al. 1999). In terms of the laminar distribution within the neocortex high expression is found in layer II, upper III, layer IV and VI. Also it was found that the majority of cells in the neocortex which express the CB1R also express GAD65 (glutamic acid decarboxylase), the enzyme which converts L-glutamate to GABA, thus identifying inhibitory neurons in the CNS. In the cerebellum, there is a very high expression of CB1R in the molecular layer where the Purkinje neuron- parallel fiber synapse is found. Also, electrophysiological experiments infer that there are somatic CB1Rs on basket cells within the cerebellum. Therefore, there is strong evidence to suggest the presence of CB1R on GABAergic and glutamatergic neurons within the cerebellum (Mackie 2005).

Since it is believed that cannabis can be habit forming, evidence suggests that the brain area that processes addictive and reinforcing behaviors, the ventral tegmental area (VTA), contain GABAergic and glutamatergic terminals that express CB1R (Melis, Pistis et al. 2004). A potential, but yet unsubstantiated, role of CB1R in this area may be to facilitate other addictive behaviors such as alcoholism or illicit drug use (Mackie 2005). Cannabis and cannabinoid compounds have also been used as anti-emetics (Darmani 2001). Studies have illustrated that indeed the brain area responsible for emesis, the medullary nuclei of the brainstem (i.e. area postrema) contain high levels of the CB1R predominantly located on axon terminals. It is strongly believed that this anti-emesis may be attributed to CB1R activation in this area (Van Sickle, Oland et al. 2001; Van Sickle, Oland et al. 2003; Martin and Wiley 2004; Mackie 2005).

In the spinal cord, several studies have been published demonstrating that CB1R is found throughout the gray matter, but at higher densities in the dorsal areas relative to the ventral areas (Herkenham, Lynn et al. 1991; Tsou, Brown et al. 1998; Ong and Mackie 1999; Farquhar-Smith, Egertova et al. 2000; Mackie 2005; Hegyi, Kis et al. 2009). Many of our essential functions depend on an intact and healthy spinal cord, such as sensation (modulated primarily by the dorsal spinal cord) and locomotion (modulated primarily by the ventral spinal cord). This is evident particularly is diseases of the spinal cord or after traumatic injury, in which the most severe cases render the individual incapable of feeling or moving, or even death. At the spinal cord level, endocannabinoid tone and receptor expression appear to play a role in modulating movement (El Manira, Kyriakatos et al. 2008; El Manira and Kyriakatos 2010), but also nociception (Pernia-Andrade, Kato et al. 2009). Therefore, understanding the role of the eCB system in the adult spinal cord is clinically relevant, and deserves as much attention as other areas of the CNS.

Though strong evidence exists for neuronal CB1R expression, evidence also exists for its expression on astrocytes in the rat striatum (Rodriguez, Mackie et al. 2001), hippocampus (Navarrete and Araque 2008), and spinal cord (Salio, Doly et al. 2002). In addition, microglia derived from neonatal rat brains, were also found to be immunoreactive for CB1R (Waksman, Olson et al. 1999). RIP-positive or APC-positive oligodendrocytes in healthy adult rat brains and spinal cords, respectively, constitutively express CB1R (Molina-Holgado, Vela et al. 2002).

4. Role of CB1R activation in adult neurons

CB1R is included among the most abundant receptors in the brain, with picomolar ranges per milligram of tissue (as determined from rat brain (Herkenham, Lynn et al. 1991; Pazos, Nunez et al. 2005). Interestingly, compared to the abundance of CB1R, under physiological conditions, the amounts of eCBs (AEA and 2-AG) reach only into the low femtomolar range (Bisogno, Berrendero et al. 1999; Pazos, Nunez et al. 2005). This discrepancy - higher amounts of receptor and lower amounts of endogenous ligands- can be reconciled by understanding the function of the endocannabinoid system as an elegant and efficient negative feedback mechanism to control the levels of neurotransmitters released into the synaptic cleft.

Neurotransmitters are synthesized in the pre-synaptic neuron, and stored in vesicles ready to be released into the synaptic cleft after depolarization leads to an influx of calcium through voltage-dependent calcium channels. In contrast, eCBs are synthesized on demand in the post-synaptic neuron using lipid precursors from cell membranes (Di Marzo, Bifulco et al. 2004) - **Figure 2**.

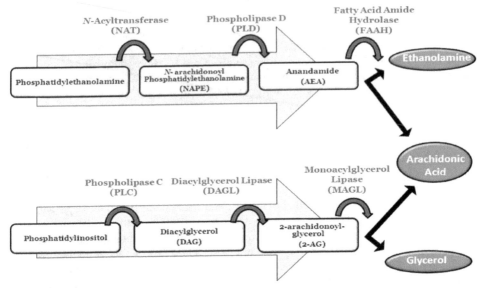

Fig. 2. The enzymes responsible for the synthesis and degradation of the two major eCBs, AEA and 2-AG. They are made on-demand from membrane lipid precursors in the post-synaptic neuron. The endocannabinoid membrane transporter (EMT) facilitates their re-uptake into either the post-synaptic (2-AG) or pre-synaptic (AEA) neuron for degradation by MAGL, or FAAH, respectively (Di Marzo, Bifulco et al. 2004; El Manira and Kyriakatos 2010)

Endocannabinoids readily pass through the post-synaptic membrane, travel retrogradely into the synaptic cleft, and bind to pre-synaptically located CB1Rs (Wilson and Nicoll 2002). As a G-protein coupled receptor, activation of CB1R by the endocannabinoids results in various cellular consequences, two of which are the ability to inhibit voltage-dependent calcium channels, or activate inwardly rectifying potassium channels. These processes affect the pre-synaptic neuron by ultimately decreasing the probability of neurotransmitter release (**Figure 3**).

The magnitude and duration of CB1R activation affects the machinery responsible for the release of several neurotransmitters such as glutamate, GABA, glycine, acetylcholine, noradrenaline and serotonin (Szabo and Schlicker 2005). Therefore, within a neuronal circuit, cells are able to regulate the strength of their synaptic inputs by on-demand release of eCBs which can then bind to CB1R (Freund, Katona et al. 2003). The high abundance of CB1Rs coupled with the relatively low-levels of detectable eCBs can be attributed to the fact that released ligand does not accumulate, but rather acts rapidly and transiently to mediate synaptic plasticity (Pazos, Nunez et al. 2005). In order to achieve such a highly efficient modulation of activity without accumulation of ligand, there must be a high density of receptors. This is precisely the state of the endocannabinoid system under physiological conditions.

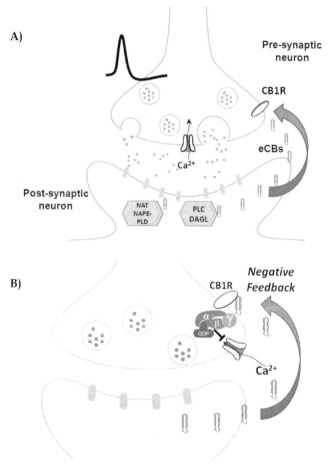

Fig. 3. **Endocannabinoids act as retrograde messengers in the CNS. (A)** Neurotransmitters bind to their postsynaptic receptors causing the synthesis of AEA or 2-AG via their synthetic enzymes, NAT/NAPE-PLD and PLC DAGL, respectively, before traveling retrogradely to bind to CB1Rs. **(B)** Inhibition of voltage-dependent calcium channels is one way by which neurotransmitter release probability is decreased. Binding of ligand to CB1R can result in the inactivation of N and P/Q- type, but not L-type calcium (Ca^{2+}) channels (Caulfield and Brown 1992; Mackie and Hille 1992; Mackie, Devane et al. 1993; Pertwee 1997). The particular channel involved is related to the brain region: in rat striatum, CB1Rs modulate N-type Ca^{2+} channels (Huang, Lo et al. 2001; Schlicker and Kathmann 2001) and not L, P or Q-type Ca^{2+} channels. In cultured rat hippocampal neurons, the CB1R modulates N- and Q-, but not P-type calcium channels (Sullivan 1999; Schlicker and Kathmann 2001). However, CB1R does not modulate any of the voltage- dependent Ca^{2+} channels found in the nucleus accumbens (Robbe, Alonso et al. 2001; Schlicker and Kathmann 2001). In contrast, newer evidence suggests that CB1R activation modulates all of the voltage-dependent Ca^{2+} channels found at the granule cell-Purkinje cell synapse of the cerebellum: the N-, P/Q- and R-type Ca^{2+} channels (Brown, Safo et al. 2004).

Furthermore, CB1R activation causes cAMP levels to drop because CB1R is negatively coupled to adenylate cyclase (AC) through heterotrimeric $G_{i/o}$ proteins, (Matsuda, Lolait et al. 1990; Munro, Thomas et al. 1993; Guzman, Sanchez et al. 2002). CB1R activation is also associated with activation of extracellular signal-related kinase (ERK) (Bouaboula, Poinot-Chazel et al. 1995; Wartmann, Campbell et al. 1995) c-Jun N-terminal kinase (Jnk) p38 mitogen activated-protein kinase (p38) (Rueda, Navarro et al. 2002), protein kinase B (Gomez del Pulgar, Velasco et al. 2000), and increased levels of the second messenger ceramide (Sanchez, Galve-Roperh et al. 1998; Guzman, Sanchez et al. 2002) (**Figure 4**). These pathways have been shown to modulate various cellular functions including cell fate, apoptosis and survival in different cell types (Guzman, Sanchez et al. 2001).

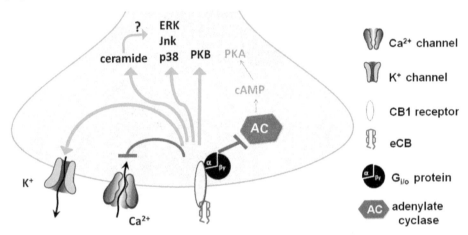

Fig. 4. **The effects of pre-synaptic CB1 receptor activation**. CB1R activation on pre-synaptic neurons inhibits voltage dependent calcium channels, and adenylate cyclase, but can also activate inwardly rectifying potassium channels, and the MAPK pathway. (Image adapted from DiMarzo et al. 2004, and Guzman et al. 2002. and created with motifolio.com©)

5. Role of cannabinoid receptors during pathological states

Because of the ubiquitous expression of the receptor throughout the CNS, several pre-clinical and clinical studies have addressed the potential therapeutic value in modulating the endocannabinoid system for analgesia, weight loss, appetite stimulation, neuroprotection after ischemic injuries, and for anti-emetic, anti-epileptic and anti-spasmodic purposes (Nogueiras, Diaz-Arteaga et al. 2009; Bisogno and Di Marzo 2010; Karst, Wippermann et al. 2010; Scotter, Abood et al. 2010). The premise of many of these therapeutic approaches lies in the neuromodulatory function of CB1R, or in the anti-inflammatory effects on CB2R activation.

During disease or following injury, cannabinoid receptor expression and levels of eCBs are altered. For example, after rat spinal cord injury, cannabinoid receptor expression is altered at the spinal level, but also in brain areas: in the spinal cord, CB1R becomes expressed in reactive astrocytes, and CB2R becomes strongly upregulated in microglia, astrocytes and macrophages. In the brain, CB1R is upregulated in thalamic and hippocampal areas, while downregulated in the amygdala and Periaqueductal Gray Area (Garcia-Ovejero, Arevalo-Martin et al. 2009; Knerlich-Lukoschus, Noack et al. 2011). In healthy spinal cords, several studies indicate that there are very low levels of CB2R, but peripheral nerve injury, for example, leads to significant upregulation of this receptor, corresponding to significant microglial activation in the spinal cord (Zhang, Hoffert et al. 2003; Romero-Sandoval, Nutile-McMenemy et al. 2008). Microglial cells contribute to the inflammatory response by producing and secreting the pro-inflammatory cytokines that contribute to excitotoxic damage in the CNS, but also to the differentiation of pathogenic lymphocytes entering the CNS (Arevalo-Martin, Garcia-Ovejero et al. 2008). Activation of CB2R in cultured microglial cells inhibits these inflammatory cytokines, making CB2R activation an anti-inflammatory target. However, the potential role of CB2R in microglial cells following injury is not clear. Cultured rat microglial cells can produce the eCBs 2-AG and AEA, which in turn auto-stimulate their CB2Rs to induce proliferation (Carrier, Kearn et al. 2004).

Whether these changes reflect an adaptive defense mechanism or contribute to pathology is still a matter of debate. These studies implicate CB1R and CB2R as double edged swords for CNS insult, and whether their activation promotes protection or contributes to damage likely depends on the etiology and progression of the disease or injury, but also in the localization of each receptor on specific cell types.

6. Adult CNS progenitor cells and CB1R

Progenitor cells in the adult CNS are promising targets as endogenous repair mechanisms following insult, and their proliferation and differentiation may provide an avenue to do so. The functional significance of constitutive or pathologically-induced neurogenesis in the adult brain has been associated with wide ranging processes such as memory formation and consolidation, depression, anxiety, and seizure- like activity (Ming and Song 2011). Endocannabinoid system elements have recently been discovered in adult brain progenitor cells (Aguado, Monory et al. 2005; Aguado, Palazuelos et al. 2006; Palazuelos, Aguado et al. 2006). There is an emerging and critical role for the eCB system and specifically, CB1R in adult brain progenitor cells, revealing a novel strategy to help the brain repair itself (Galve-Roperh, Aguado et al. 2007).

In the adult brain, the subgranular zone (SGZ) of the hippocampus, and the subventricular zone (SVZ) contain two different populations of progenitor cells. The first population is referred to as the type 1 or type B cells (SGZ and SVZ, respectively). These cells resemble their developmental counterparts; the radial glia. They are characterized by their slow proliferation kinetics, their morphological hallmarks (tiny processes extending from their somata in the SVZ), and these cells express both Nestin and Glial Fibrillary Acidic Protein (GFAP). The type 2 or C cells (SGZ and SVZ, respectively) are actively dividing, non-radial cells that maintain their Nestin expression, but do not express GFAP. They are occasionally positive for the immature neuronal marker Doublecortin (DCX). Ablation studies indicate that these two different populations are distinct in their characteristics, but they are developmentally connected to one another. The type 1, B cells give rise to the type 2, C cells, and if the latter are destroyed, they can eventually be replenished by the former (Suh, Deng et al. 2009). These progenitor cells give birth to new neurons continually throughout adulthood, in a process known as adult neurogenesis.

It is imperative to distinguish these progenitor populations when assessing the role of the various eCB components in the neurogenic process. This distinction is rarely made in the literature, and yet it is very plausible that the various eCB system components affect these progenitor populations differently. The results from the following studies indicate that the distinct processes involved in adult brain neurogenesis cannot be grouped together with regards to endocannabinoid modulation.

The role of the eCB system, and in particular CB1R, on adult brain neurogenesis is not clear, partly because the separation between effects on progenitor proliferation and neuronal differentiation have not always been made. A study published in 2004 concluded that that there is defective neurogenesis in the CB1R knockout (KO) mouse (Jin, Xie et al. 2004). A major limitation to this study is that the authors equated changes in BrdU (thymidine analog) incorporation with changes in neurogenesis. Their data strongly support the view that CB1R is critical in progenitor proliferation in the hippocampus, but nothing more can be deduced with regards to which progenitor population is affected, nor about neuronal differentiation and maturation of the remaining progenitor cells.

Pharmacological studies in wild-type mice support the conclusions from CB1R KO mice. Treatment with CB1R agonists (either with the endocannabinoid anandamide, the synthetic agonists WIN 55, 212-2 or HU-210) increased the number of BrdU positive(+)/NeuN negative(-) hippocampal cells, but decreased the number of co-labeled, newly generated BrdU(+)/NeuN(+) neurons *in vivo* (Rueda, Navarro et al. 2002; Aguado, Palazuelos et al. 2006; Galve-Roperh, Aguado et al. 2006). Furthermore, these studies showed that a CB1R antagonist, SR141716, reversed the agonist actions- the number of co-labeled cells increased, while BrdU(+)/NeuN(-) cells decreased. Similarly, in a study by Jiang et al, 2005, CB1R activation resulted in increased BrdU(+) cells, which was interpreted as enhanced neurogenesis by cannabinoids; however, the authors themselves never show increases in co-labeled cells, and also point out that relative to no treatment, CB1R agonists do not change the percentage of cells expressing immature neuronal markers (Jiang, Zhang et al. 2005).

Adult hippocampal progenitor cells from mouse brains express CB1R *in vitro* and *in vivo* (Aguado, Monory et al. 2005; Aguado, Palazuelos et al. 2006). CB1R activation induced proliferation of these progenitors assessed by quantifying the amount of cells expressing Nestin and incorporating the thymidine analog BrdU. Interestingly, these studies showed CB1R and FAAH are selectively enriched in type 1 (Nestin(+)/GFAP(+)) progenitors *in vivo* compared to type 2 (Nestin(+)/ GFAP(-)) (Aguado, Palazuelos et al. 2006). Utilizing various markers for immature neurons and glia, CB1R activation appears to promote astroglial differentiation, while inhibition of the receptor appears to promote neuronal differentiation (Aguado, Palazuelos et al. 2006). In contrast, a recent study indicated that CB1R was preferentially expressed on type 2b/3 cells that are also expressing DCX, suggesting that CB1Rs have a role in later stages of neuronal differentiation, and migration of the nascent neuron (Wolf, Bick-Sander et al. 2010). This study examined the levels of DCX expressing cells in the hippocampi of CB1R KO mice, and also in Nestin-GFP reporter mice treated with the CB1R antagonist AM251. According to the authors, genetic deletion of CB1R resulted in increased proliferation but decreased net neurogenesis relative to wild-type mice. But, administration of the CB1R specific antagonist AM251 to wild-type mice promoted proliferation of type 2b/3 DCX(+) cells 7 days after BrdU administration (**Figure 5**).

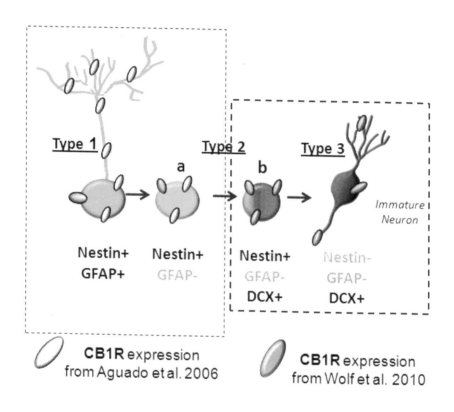

Fig. 5. CB1R is expressed throughout neuronal development (Harkany, Guzman et al. 2007; Harkany, Keimpema et al. 2008), and also at all stages of adult hippocampal neurogenesis. It is not clear whether CB1R is enriched in certain progenitor populations, and if so, how endogenous cannabinoids differentially affect these populations. Equally compelling is how exogenous CB1R agonists or antagonists may affect these different populations, and what the functional outcomes of such interventions may be. Image created with motifolio.com©.

Clarification through additional studies must be made to reconcile these seemingly disparate results. Species, sex and strain of the animals used, chronic versus acute treatment with cannabinergic drugs, specificity, dose/concentration of cannabinergic drugs, BrdU injection protocol and immunohistochemical markers must all be considered when interpreting the many studies published on CB1R's role on adult hippocampal neurogenesis. Table 1 summarizes several knock-out mice that have been developed that target endocannabinoid system components, and the consequences on progenitor proliferation, neuronal differentiation and glial differentiation.

✓ = successful induction ✖ = impaired induction nc = no change N.D. = Not determined		CB1 -/- (Cannabinoid 1 Receptor)	CB2 -/- (Cannabinoid 2 Receptor)	FAAH -/- (Fatty Acid Amide Hydrolase)	DAGLαβ -/- [d] (Diacyl-glycerol Lipase)	
					in vivo, SVZ	in vivo, Hippocampus
Neural Progenitor Proliferation	Embryonic/ Postnatal	✖ *in vivo* P2 hippocampus[a]	✖ *in vitro,*[c]	N.D.	N.D.	
	Adult	✖ *in vivo* 3 months old hippocampus[a]	✖ *in vitro* & *in vivo*[c]	✓ *in vivo,* 3 months old hippocampus[a]	α-/- ✖ β-/- nc	✖ ✖
Glial differentiation or Gliogenesis	Embryonic/ Postnatal	✖ *in vivo* P2 hippocampus[a]	N.D.	N.D.	N.D.	
	Adult	✖ *in vivo,* 3 months old hippocampus[a]	N.D.	✓ *in vivo,* 3months old hippocampus[a]	N.D.	
Neuronal Differentiation or Neurogenesis	Embryonic/ Postnatal	✓ *in vivo,* P2 hippocampus[a]	N.D	N.D.	N.D.	
	Adult	✓ *in vivo* 3 months old hippocampus[a]	N.D	✖ *in vivo,* 3 months old hippocampus[a]	α-/- ✖	✖
		✖ *in vivo* hippocampus[b]			β-/- N.D.	N.D.

Table 1. **eCB Knock-out mice and adult CNS progenitor cells.** [a] (Aguado, Palazuelos et al. 2006); [b](Jin, Xie et al. 2004); [c](Palazuelos, Aguado et al. 2006); [d](Gao, Vasilyev et al. 2010); KO= Knockout; SVZ = subventricular zone. The apparent conflicting results in the adult CB1 -/- brains may be attributed to the interpretation of 'neurogenesis'(see Section 6).

7. Neurogenesis in the adult spinal cord

Compared to the brain, even though progenitor cells also exist in the adult spinal cord, the spinal cord environment does not seem to support robust constitutive neurogenesis, nor does it seem to support neurogenesis following region specific injury or disease. Though injury results in different functional consequences for the brain and spinal cord, it is not clear why one region of the CNS is capable of generating new neurons, while another area is not. There are several clinical examples where new neuron formation in the adult spinal cord could potentially ameliorate disease symptoms or progression, or replace damaged neurons following trauma. Replacement of dead or damaged neurons in the compromised spinal cord may be able to promote functional motor recovery, but also reduce pain (Hofstetter, Holmstrom et al. 2005; Scholz, Broom et al. 2005; Ohori, Yamamoto et al. 2006; Meisner, Marsh et al. 2010). Manipulating the spinal cord environment to coerce neurogenesis from endogenous progenitors is a promising therapeutic intervention, which may bypass the many obstacles inherent to transplantation of exogenous stem/progenitor cells (Obermair, Schroter et al. 2008).

Several models propose distinct locations for the endogenous spinal cord progenitors, and how they respond to physiological and pathological stimuli (Namiki and Tator 1999; Horner, Power et al. 2000; Horky, Galimi et al. 2006; Meletis, Barnabe-Heider et al. 2008; Hamilton, Truong et al. 2009; Barnabe-Heider, Goritz et al. 2010; Hugnot and Franzen 2011). The overwhelming majority of progenitor cells do not differentiate into neurons *in vivo*. Nevertheless, these progenitors have neurogenic potential revealed from *in vitro* studies, but also from *in vivo* transplantation studies. Progenitors isolated from all levels and areas of the adult spinal cord can give rise to neurons in culture (Weiss, Dunne et al. 1996; Yamamoto, Yamamoto et al. 2001). When spinal cord progenitors were transplanted into the hippocampus- a pro-neurogenic environment, they readily formed neurons (Shihabuddin, Horner et al. 2000). These studies imply that the spinal cord environment is restricting the neurogenic potential of the endogenous progenitors, and astrocytes may be one of the culprits (Song, Stevens et al. 2002).

New evidence is emerging to challenge the idea that new neurons cannot be generated in the adult spinal cord. Direct injury to the spinal cord results in massive progenitor proliferation leading to astrocyte differentiation, and a massive inflammatory response which contributes to glial scar formation (Barnabe-Heider, Goritz et al. 2010; Wang, Cheng et al. 2011). This injured environment has been demonstrated as non-neurogenic (Yamamoto, Nagao et al. 2001; Hannila, Siddiq et al. 2007); however, there are instances in which an environment filled with inflammatory cytokines can still elicit neurogenesis in the adult spinal cord. For example, in an experimental rat model of multiple sclerosis (experimental autoimmune encephalomyelitis), newly generated neurons migrated towards the neuroinflammatory lesion (Danilov, Covacu et al. 2006). Also there are instances of indirect injury to the adult spinal cord, such as dorsal rhizotomy (cutting of the dorsal root at the cervical spinal level) in which neurogenesis is observed in the dorsal horn at the corresponding spinal level (Vessal, Aycock et al. 2007). Recent papers showed that in non-injured, intact adult spinal cords, immature neurons can be found in the area surrounding the central canal (Shechter, Ziv et al. 2007; Marichal, Garcia et al. 2009), but also throughout the spinal cord, with a preferential dorsal gray matter localization and exclusive GABAergic phenotype (Shechter, Ziv et al. 2007; Shechter, Baruch et al. 2011). The exact roles of these immature neurons in the healthy spinal cord have not been determined, but may indicate physiological roles for new GABAergic neurons in nociception (Shechter, Baruch et al. 2011), and also for movement. The existence of these cells is exciting, as it sets the tone for more intensive studies to characterize their function and promote their differentiation.

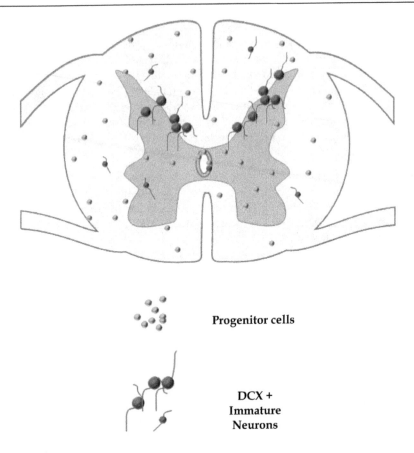

Progenitor cells

DCX +
Immature
Neurons

Fig. 6. Transverse section of an adult mouse spinal cord, depicting a model for progenitor cell and immature neuron location. Based on the work by Shechter et al, 2007, 2011, the majority of the GABAergic, BrdU(+)/ DCX(+) immature neurons reside in the gray matter of the dorsal horn. Under physiological conditions, the levels of these cells depend on the type of and exposure to sensory environmental enrichment. Image generated with motifolio.com©.

8. CB1R and adult spinal cord neurogenesis

Taking the adult brain as an example of endocannabinoid system involvement in progenitor cell proliferation and differentiation, there is a possibility that the spinal cord progenitors may also be modulated by this system. There is an overwhelming lack of published studies addressing the presence and roles of the endocannabinoid system in adult spinal cord progenitor cells. Of particular importance is that CB1R is widely distributed on cells throughout the spinal cord, but also in lamina X, which includes the putative progenitor cell niche. We have identified CB1R on adult spinal cord-derived Nestin(+) progenitor cells in primary cultures (**Figure 7**).

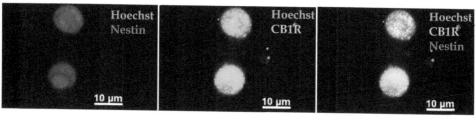

Fig. 7. Primary adult spinal cord cultures from rats contain Nestin(+) progenitor cells (red), which also express CB1R (green). The role of CB1R on these progenitors has not been examined, and further studies are needed to determine how the receptor is involved in progenitor cell quiescence, proliferation or differentiation. Image obtained after 6 days *in vitro* with 63X objective.

In response to injury, not only do progenitor cells proliferate in the spinal cord (Frisen, Johansson et al. 1995; Johansson, Momma et al. 1999; Namiki and Tator 1999; Shibuya, Miyamoto et al. 2002), but levels of endocannabinoids, receptors and enzymes are also altered as described earlier (in Section 4). Rigorous studies are needed to address if and how adult spinal cord progenitor cells respond to endogenous cannabinoid tone or to exogenously administered cannabinoids. Does endocannabinoid tone contribute to the non-neurogenic spinal cord environment? Are endo/exo-cannabinoids capable of promoting spinal cord neurogenesis or gliogenesis? These are just a few critical and novel avenues for potentially promoting neurogenesis in the adult spinal cord.

9. The effect of chronic cannabinergic drug use on the CNS- implications for the treatment of chronic pain

Cannabis is used both acutely and chronically for recreational or medicinal purposes. There is controversy regarding medical marijuana because of the documented cognitive side effects of chronic recreational use (Jager and Ramsey 2008; Hester, Nestor et al. 2009; Battisti, Roodenrys et al. 2010). However, all drugs come with a risk-benefit consideration, and a plethora of historical and emerging evidence indicates that the medicinal value of cannabis cannot be ignored. Many studies have demonstrated that endocannabinoids and application of exogenous cannabinoids (usually mixed CB1R/CB2R agonists) reduce pain sensation (Guindon and Hohmann 2009). Presently, such an approach is becoming more clinically accepted for treating chronic pain states (Aggarwal, Carter et al. 2009; Karst, Wippermann et al. 2010; Lynch and Campbell 2011). While CB2R activation attenuates nociception mostly by modulating the inflammatory response (Guindon and Hohmann 2008), the role of CB1R is more complex because its location on various cells along the pain pathways appears to contribute differently to nociception. Moreover, many cannabinergic drugs are not only mixed agonists, but may bind non-specifically to other receptors, including TRP-channels (Patwardhan, Jeske et al. 2006; Patil, Patwardhan et al. 2011).

The use of several CB1R knock-outs (global and conditional) has helped to clarify the role of these receptors in nociception. Recent worked demonstrated that cannabinoids mediate analgesia by activating CB1Rs located on peripheral nociceptors (dorsal root ganglia sensory neurons) (Agarwal, Pacher et al. 2007). Interestingly, by using *in vitro* spinal cord slices and *in vivo* recordings of dorsal horn neurons, activation of CB1Rs on spinal cord dorsal horn neurons actually enhances (not reduces) nociceptive responses (Pernia-Andrade, Kato et al. 2009; Zhang, Chen et al. 2010). Stimulation of spinal cord CB1Rs inhibits the release of GABA, glycine (Pernia-Andrade 2009), and opioids, while enhancing the release of substance P (Zhang, Chen et al. 2010). Therefore, CB1R activation may contribute to nociception by increasing excitability at the spinal cord level. Consequently, CB1R antagonists have shown anti-nociceptive efficacy in several experimental pain models (Costa, Trovato et al. 2005; Croci and Zarini 2007; Pernia-Andrade, Kato et al. 2009). On the contrary, another recent study also using *in vivo* recordings demonstrated that blocking spinal CB1Rs enhanced the evoked response of the spinal cord dorsal horn neurons in neuropathic rats, indicative of a pro-nociceptive role of the receptor (Sagar, Jhaveri et al. 2010). One explanation for these different results could be attributed to the anesthetic used. Pernia-Andrade et al 2009 used a mixture of pentobarbital with pancuronium (a muscle relaxant), while Sagar et al.'s study only used isoflurane. The use of a muscle relaxant would allow the use of lower levels of the anesthetic to achieve immobility (required for the *in vivo* recordings). It is possible that the level of anesthesia used in Sagar et al's 2010 recordings may have depressed the neuronal activity relevant to pain sensation. Consistent with this possibility is that there was no difference in the firing rate of dorsal horn neurons in anesthetized neuropathic and sham operated animals at various levels of stimulation.

The chronic use of mixed cannabinoid drugs should be further investigated in light of the fact that the majority readily cross the blood-brain barrier. These compounds may be capable of providing pain relief, but they may also be affecting other important cellular functions, such as neurogenesis in the brain and spinal cord. Neurogenesis from endogenous progenitor cells is associated with a wide range of functions, and perturbations of this process are correlated with disease symptoms. Interference of physiological neurogenesis may be a highly undesirable side-effect of chronic endocannabinoid system manipulation by the use of CB1R/CB2R agonists or antagonists. For example, following peripheral nerve injury or direct spinal cord injury, a specific loss of inhibitory GABAergic interneurons in the spinal cord dorsal horn is postulated to be a major contributor to chronic pain (Moore, Kohno et al. 2002; Scholz, Broom et al. 2005; Meisner, Marsh et al. 2010). Replacement of these neurons through neurogenesis is an attractive therapeutic strategy because it attempts to go beyond the management of symptoms; it targets an underlying biological phenomenon of neuronal death following injury. Given the controversy regarding how cannabinoids modulate neurogenesis, it is possible that while treatment with mixed cannabinoids can ameliorate pain, long term usage may prevent the replacement of damaged inhibitory neurons by blocking neurogenesis, and thus contribute to an underlying etiology of chronic pain. Hence understading the role of the individual CBRs in adult neurogenesis, but also during pain states, could help discern how to more susccesfully use these agents clinically.

10. Conclusions

CB1R expression on adult CNS-derived progenitor cells is not only indicative of endogenous cannabinoid modulation, but also points to potential consequences of cannabinoid pharmacotherapy on progenitor proliferation and differentiation- whether beneficial or deleterious. The complex results published about adult brain progenitors and the lack of data on adult spinal cord progenitors demonstrate that extensive basic research is still needed to understand how the endocannabinoid system affects these cells normally and in response to injury and disease.

11. References

Agarwal, N., P. Pacher, et al. (2007). "Cannabinoids mediate analgesia largely via peripheral type 1 cannabinoid receptors in nociceptors." Nat Neurosci 10(7): 870-879.
Aggarwal, S. K., G. T. Carter, et al. (2009). "Medicinal use of cannabis in the United States: historical perspectives, current trends, and future directions." J Opioid Manag 5(3): 153-168.
Aguado, T., K. Monory, et al. (2005). "The endocannabinoid system drives neural progenitor proliferation." Faseb J 19(12): 1704-1706.
Aguado, T., J. Palazuelos, et al. (2006). "The endocannabinoid system promotes astroglial differentiation by acting on neural progenitor cells." J Neurosci 26(5): 1551-1561.
Aldrich, M. R. (2006). "The Remarkable W.B. O'Shaughnessy" Retrieved January 29, 2011, from http://antiquecannabisbook.com/chap2B/Shaughnessy/Shaughnessy.htm.
Arevalo-Martin, A., D. Garcia-Ovejero, et al. (2008). "CB2 cannabinoid receptors as an emerging target for demyelinating diseases: from neuroimmune interactions to cell replacement strategies." Br J Pharmacol 153(2): 216-225.
Barnabe-Heider, F., C. Goritz, et al. (2010). "Origin of new glial cells in intact and injured adult spinal cord." Cell Stem Cell 7(4): 470-482.
Battisti, R. A., S. Roodenrys, et al. (2010). "Chronic use of cannabis and poor neural efficiency in verbal memory ability." Psychopharmacology (Berl) 209(4): 319-330.
Bisogno, T., F. Berrendero, et al. (1999). "Brain regional distribution of endocannabinoids: implications for their biosynthesis and biological function." Biochem Biophys Res Commun 256(2): 377-380.
Bisogno, T. and V. Di Marzo (2010). "Cannabinoid receptors and endocannabinoids: role in neuroinflammatory and neurodegenerative disorders." CNS Neurol Disord Drug Targets 9(5): 564-573.
Bouaboula, M., C. Poinot-Chazel, et al. (1995). "Activation of mitogen-activated protein kinases by stimulation of the central cannabinoid receptor CB1." Biochem J 312 (Pt 2): 637-641.
Brown, S. P., P. K. Safo, et al. (2004). "Endocannabinoids inhibit transmission at granule cell to Purkinje cell synapses by modulating three types of presynaptic calcium channels." J Neurosci 24(24): 5623-5631.
Carrier, E. J., C. S. Kearn, et al. (2004). "Cultured rat microglial cells synthesize the endocannabinoid 2-arachidonylglycerol, which increases proliferation via a CB2 receptor-dependent mechanism." Mol Pharmacol 65(4): 999-1007.
Caulfield, M. P. and D. A. Brown (1992). "Cannabinoid receptor agonists inhibit Ca current in NG108-15 neuroblastoma cells via a pertussis toxin-sensitive me   ism." Br J Pharmacol 106(2): 231-232.
Costa, B., A. E. Trovato, et al. (2005). "Effect of the cannabinoid CB1 receptor antagonist, SR141716, on nociceptive response and nerve demyelination in rodents with chronic constriction injury of the sciatic nerve." Pain 116(1-2): 52-61.

Croci, T. and E. Zarini (2007). "Effect of the cannabinoid CB1 receptor antagonist rimonabant on nociceptive responses and adjuvant-induced arthritis in obese and lean rats." Br J Pharmacol 150(5): 559-566.

Danilov, A. I., R. Covacu, et al. (2006). "Neurogenesis in the adult spinal cord in an experimental model of multiple sclerosis." Eur J Neurosci 23(2): 394-400.

Darmani, N. A. (2001). "Delta(9)-tetrahydrocannabinol and synthetic cannabinoids prevent emesis produced by the cannabinoid CB(1) receptor antagonist/inverse agonist SR 141716A." Neuropsychopharmacology 24(2): 198-203.

Devane, W. A., A. Breuer, et al. (1992). "A novel probe for the cannabinoid receptor." J Med Chem 35(11): 2065-2069.

Devane, W. A., F. A. Dysarz, 3rd, et al. (1988). "Determination and characterization of a cannabinoid receptor in rat brain." Mol Pharmacol 34(5): 605-613.

Devane, W. A., L. Hanus, et al. (1992). "Isolation and structure of a brain constituent that binds to the cannabinoid receptor." Science 258(5090): 1946-1949.

Di Marzo, V., M. Bifulco, et al. (2004). "The endocannabinoid system and its therapeutic exploitation." Nat Rev Drug Discov 3(9): 771-784.

El Manira, A. and A. Kyriakatos (2010). "The role of endocannabinoid signaling in motor control." Physiology (Bethesda) 25(4): 230-238.

El Manira, A., A. Kyriakatos, et al. (2008). "Endocannabinoid signaling in the spinal locomotor circuitry." Brain Res Rev 57(1): 29-36.

Farquhar-Smith, W. P., M. Egertova, et al. (2000). "Cannabinoid CB(1) receptor expression in rat spinal cord." Mol Cell Neurosci 15(6): 510-521.

Freund, T. F., I. Katona, et al. (2003). "Role of endogenous cannabinoids in synaptic signaling." Physiol Rev 83(3): 1017-1066.

Frisen, J., C. B. Johansson, et al. (1995). "Rapid, widespread, and longlasting induction of nestin contributes to the generation of glial scar tissue after CNS injury." J Cell Biol 131(2): 453-464.

Galve-Roperh, I., T. Aguado, et al. (2007). "The endocannabinoid system and neurogenesis in health and disease." Neuroscientist 13(2): 109-114.

Galve-Roperh, I., T. Aguado, et al. (2006). "Endocannabinoids: a new family of lipid mediators involved in the regulation of neural cell development." Curr Pharm Des 12(18): 2319-2325.

Gao, Y., D. V. Vasilyev, et al. (2010). "Loss of Retrograde Endocannabinoid Signaling and Reduced Adult Neurogenesis in Diacylglycerol Lipase Knock-out Mice." J Neurosci 30(6): 2017-2024.

Garcia-Ovejero, D., A. Arevalo-Martin, et al. (2009). "The endocannabinoid system is modulated in response to spinal cord injury in rats." Neurobiol Dis 33(1): 57-71.

Gerard, C. M., C. Mollereau, et al. (1991). "Molecular cloning of a human cannabinoid receptor which is also expressed in testis." Biochem J 279 (Pt 1): 129-134.

Gomez del Pulgar, T., G. Velasco, et al. (2000). "The CB1 cannabinoid receptor is coupled to the activation of protein kinase B/Akt." Biochem J 347(Pt 2): 369-373.

Grinspoon, L. (1993). Marihuana, the forbidden medicine. New Haven, Yale University Press.

Guindon, J. and A. G. Hohmann (2008). "Cannabinoid CB2 receptors: a therapeutic target for the treatment of inflammatory and neuropathic pain." Br J Pharmacol 153(2): 319-334.

Guindon, J. and A. G. Hohmann (2009). "The endocannabinoid system and pain." CNS Neurol Disord Drug Targets 8(6): 403-421.

Guzman, M., C. Sanchez, et al. (2001). "Control of the cell survival/death decision by cannabinoids." J Mol Med 78(11): 613-625.

Guzman, M., C. Sanchez, et al. (2002). "Cannabinoids and cell fate." Pharmacol Ther 95(2): 175-184.

Hamilton, L. K., M. K. Truong, et al. (2009). "Cellular organization of the central canal ependymal zone, a niche of latent neural stem cells in the adult mammalian spinal cord." Neuroscience 164(3): 1044-1056.

Hannila, S. S., M. M. Siddiq, et al. (2007). "Therapeutic approaches to promoting axonal regeneration in the adult mammalian spinal cord." Int Rev Neurobiol 77: 57-105.

Harkany, T., M. Guzman, et al. (2007). "The emerging functions of endocannabinoid signaling during CNS development." Trends Pharmacol Sci 28(2): 83-92.

Harkany, T., E. Keimpema, et al. (2008). "Endocannabinoid functions controlling neuronal specification during brain development." Mol Cell Endocrinol 286(1-2 Suppl 1): S84-90.

Hegyi, Z., G. Kis, et al. (2009). "Neuronal and glial localization of the cannabinoid-1 receptor in the superficial spinal dorsal horn of the rodent spinal cord." Eur J Neurosci 30(2): 251-262.

Herkenham, M., A. B. Lynn, et al. (1991). "Characterization and localization of cannabinoid receptors in rat brain: a quantitative in vitro autoradiographic study." J Neurosci 11(2): 563-583.

Herodotus (1824). The History of Herodotus. R. Larcher, Mitford, Schweighaeuser. Oxford, Talboys and Wheeler. Volume 2.

Hester, R., L. Nestor, et al. (2009). "Impaired error awareness and anterior cingulate cortex hypoactivity in chronic cannabis users." Neuropsychopharmacology 34(11): 2450-2458.

Hofstetter, C. P., N. A. Holmstrom, et al. (2005). "Allodynia limits the usefulness of intraspinal neural stem cell grafts; directed differentiation improves outcome." Nat Neurosci 8(3): 346-353.

Horky, L. L., F. Galimi, et al. (2006). "Fate of endogenous stem/progenitor cells following spinal cord injury." J Comp Neurol 498(4): 525-538.

Horner, P. J., A. E. Power, et al. (2000). "Proliferation and differentiation of progenitor cells throughout the intact adult rat spinal cord." J Neurosci 20(6): 2218-2228.

Huang, C. C., S. W. Lo, et al. (2001). "Presynaptic mechanisms underlying cannabinoid inhibition of excitatory synaptic transmission in rat striatal neurons." J Physiol 532(Pt 3): 731-748.

Hugnot, J. P. and R. Franzen (2011). "The spinal cord ependymal region: a stem cell niche in the caudal central nervous system." Front Biosci 16: 1044-1059.

Jager, G. and N. F. Ramsey (2008). "Long-term consequences of adolescent cannabis exposure on the development of cognition, brain structure and function: an overview of animal and human research." Curr Drug Abuse Rev 1(2): 114-123.

Jiang, W., Y. Zhang, et al. (2005). "Cannabinoids promote embryonic and adult hippocampus neurogenesis and produce anxiolytic- and antidepressant-like effects." J Clin Invest 115(11): 3104-3116.

Jin, K., L. Xie, et al. (2004). "Defective adult neurogenesis in CB1 cannabinoid receptor knockout mice." Mol Pharmacol 66(2): 204-208.

Johansson, C. B., S. Momma, et al. (1999). "Identification of a neural stem cell in the adult mammalian central nervous system." Cell 96(1): 25-34.

Karst, M., S. Wippermann, et al. (2010). "Role of cannabinoids in the treatment of pain and (painful) spasticity." Drugs 70(18): 2409-2438.

Katona, I., B. Sperlagh, et al. (1999). "Presynaptically located CB1 cannabinoid receptors regulate GABA release from axon terminals of specific hippocampal interneurons." J Neurosci 19(11): 4544-4558.

Kirby, M. T., R. E. Hampson, et al. (1995). "Cannabinoids selectively decrease paired-pulse facilitation of perforant path synaptic potentials in the dentate gyrus in vitro." Brain Res 688(1-2): 114-120.

Knerlich-Lukoschus, F., M. Noack, et al. (2011). "Spinal cord injuries induce changes in CB1 cannabinoid receptor and C-C chemokine expression in brain areas underlying circuitry of chronic pain conditions." J Neurotrauma 28(4): 619-634.

Lynch, M. E. and F. Campbell (2011). "Cannabinoids for Treatment of Chronic Non-Cancer Pain; a Systematic Review of Randomized Trials." Br J Clin Pharmacol.

Mackie, K. (2005). "Cannabinoid receptor homo- and heterodimerization." Life Sci 77(14): 1667-1673.

Mackie, K., W. A. Devane, et al. (1993). "Anandamide, an endogenous cannabinoid, inhibits calcium currents as a partial agonist in N18 neuroblastoma cells." Mol Pharmacol 44(3): 498-503.

Mackie, K. and B. Hille (1992). "Cannabinoids inhibit N-type calcium channels in neuroblastoma-glioma cells." Proc Natl Acad Sci U S A 89(9): 3825-3829.

Mailleux, P., M. Verslijpe, et al. (1992). "Initial observations on the distribution of cannabinoid receptor binding sites in the human adult basal ganglia using autoradiography." Neurosci Lett 139(1): 7-9.

Marichal, N., G. Garcia, et al. (2009). "Enigmatic central canal contacting cells: immature neurons in "standby mode"?" J Neurosci 29(32): 10010-10024.

Martin, B. R. and J. L. Wiley (2004). "Mechanism of action of cannabinoids: how it may lead to treatment of cachexia, emesis, and pain." J Support Oncol 2(4): 305-314; discussion 314-306.

Matsuda, L. A., S. J. Lolait, et al. (1990). "Structure of a cannabinoid receptor and functional expression of the cloned cDNA." Nature 346(6284): 561-564.

Mechoulam, R. (2000). "Looking back at Cannabis research." Curr Pharm Des 6(13): 1313-1322.

Mechoulam, R., S. Ben-Shabat, et al. (1995). "Identification of an endogenous 2-monoglyceride, present in canine gut, that binds to cannabinoid receptors." Biochem Pharmacol 50(1): 83-90.

Mechoulam, R. and Y. Gaoni (1965). "Hashish. IV. The isolation and structure of cannabinolic cannabidiolic and cannabigerolic acids." Tetrahedron 21(5): 1223-1229.

Mechoulam, R. and Y. Gaoni (1965). "A Total Synthesis of Dl-Delta-1-Tetrahydrocannabinol, the Active Constituent of Hashish." J Am Chem Soc 87: 3273-3275.

Mechoulam, R. and L. Hanus (2000). "A historical overview of chemical research on cannabinoids." Chem Phys Lipids 108(1-2): 1-13.

Meisner, J. G., A. D. Marsh, et al. (2010). "Loss of GABAergic interneurons in laminae I-III of the spinal cord dorsal horn contributes to reduced GABAergic tone and neuropathic pain after spinal cord injury." J Neurotrauma 27(4): 729-737.

Meletis, K., F. Barnabe-Heider, et al. (2008). "Spinal cord injury reveals multilineage differentiation of ependymal cells." PLoS Biol 6(7): e182.

Melis, M., M. Pistis, et al. (2004). "Endocannabinoids mediate presynaptic inhibition of glutamatergic transmission in rat ventral tegmental area dopamine neurons through activation of CB1 receptors." J Neurosci 24(1): 53-62.

Ming, G. L. and H. Song (2011). "Adult neurogenesis in the mammalian brain: significant answers and significant questions." Neuron 70(4): 687-702.

Molina-Holgado, E., J. M. Vela, et al. (2002). "Cannabinoids promote oligodendrocyte progenitor survival: involvement of cannabinoid receptors and phosphatidylinositol-3 kinase/Akt signaling." J Neurosci 22(22): 9742-9753.

Moore, K. A., T. Kohno, et al. (2002). "Partial peripheral nerve injury promotes a selective loss of GABAergic inhibition in the superficial dorsal horn of the spinal cord." J Neurosci 22(15): 6724-6731.

Munro, S., K. L. Thomas, et al. (1993). "Molecular characterization of a peripheral receptor for cannabinoids." Nature 365(6441): 61-65.

Namiki, J. and C. H. Tator (1999). "Cell proliferation and nestin expression in the ependyma of the adult rat spinal cord after injury." J Neuropathol Exp Neurol 58(5): 489-498.

Navarrete, M. and A. Araque (2008). "Endocannabinoids mediate neuron-astrocyte communication." Neuron 57(6): 883-893.

Nogueiras, R., A. Diaz-Arteaga, et al. (2009). "The endocannabinoid system: role in glucose and energy metabolism." Pharmacol Res 60(2): 93-98.

O'Shaughnessy, W. B. (1842). On the preparations of the Indian Hemp, or Gunjah. Transactions of the Medical and Physical Society of Calcutta. Calcutta, William Rushton and Co. VIII: 40.

Obermair, F. J., A. Schroter, et al. (2008). "Endogenous neural progenitor cells as therapeutic target after spinal cord injury." Physiology (Bethesda) 23: 296-304.

Ohori, Y., S. Yamamoto, et al. (2006). "Growth factor treatment and genetic manipulation stimulate neurogenesis and oligodendrogenesis by endogenous neural progenitors in the injured adult spinal cord." J Neurosci 26(46): 11948-11960.

Onaivi, E. S., C. M. Leonard, et al. (2002). "Endocannabinoids and cannabinoid receptor genetics." Prog Neurobiol 66(5): 307-344.

Ong, W. Y. and K. Mackie (1999). "A light and electron microscopic study of the CB1 cannabinoid receptor in the primate spinal cord." J Neurocytol 28(1): 39-45.

Palazuelos, J., T. Aguado, et al. (2006). "Non-psychoactive CB2 cannabinoid agonists stimulate neural progenitor proliferation." Faseb J 20(13): 2405-2407.

Patil, M., A. Patwardhan, et al. (2011). "Cannabinoid receptor antagonists AM251 and AM630 activate TRPA1 in sensory neurons." Neuropharmacology 61(4): 778-788.

Paton, W. D. (1975). "Pharmacology of marijuana." Annu Rev Pharmacol 15: 191-220.

Patwardhan, A. M., N. A. Jeske, et al. (2006). "The cannabinoid WIN 55,212-2 inhibits transient receptor potential vanilloid 1 (TRPV1) and evokes peripheral antihyperalgesia via calcineurin." Proc Natl Acad Sci U S A 103(30): 11393-11398.

Pazos, M. R., E. Nunez, et al. (2005). "Functional neuroanatomy of the endocannabinoid system." Pharmacol Biochem Behav 81(2): 239-247.

Pernia-Andrade, A. J., A. Kato, et al. (2009). "Spinal endocannabinoids and CB1 receptors mediate C-fiber-induced heterosynaptic pain sensitization." Science 325(5941): 760-764.

Pertwee, R. G. (1997). "Pharmacology of cannabinoid CB1 and CB2 receptors." Pharmacol Ther 74(2): 129-180.

Robbe, D., G. Alonso, et al. (2001). "Localization and mechanisms of action of cannabinoid receptors at the glutamatergic synapses of the mouse nucleus accumbens." J Neurosci 21(1): 109-116.

Rodriguez, J. J., K. Mackie, et al. (2001). "Ultrastructural localization of the CB1 cannabinoid receptor in mu-opioid receptor patches of the rat Caudate putamen nucleus." J Neurosci 21(3): 823-833.

Romero-Sandoval, A., N. Nutile-McMenemy, et al. (2008). "Spinal microglial and perivascular cell cannabinoid receptor type 2 activation reduces behavioral hypersensitivity without tolerance after peripheral nerve injury." Anesthesiology 108(4): 722-734.

Rueda, D., B. Navarro, et al. (2002). "The endocannabinoid anandamide inhibits neuronal progenitor cell differentiation through attenuation of the Rap1/B-Raf/ERK pathway." J Biol Chem 277(48): 46645-46650.

Sagar, D. R., M. D. Jhaveri, et al. (2010). "Endocannabinoid regulation of spinal nociceptive processing in a model of neuropathic pain." Eur J Neurosci.

Salio, C., S. Doly, et al. (2002). "Neuronal and astrocytic localization of the cannabinoid receptor-1 in the dorsal horn of the rat spinal cord." Neurosci Lett 329(1): 13-16.

Sanchez, C., I. Galve-Roperh, et al. (1998). "Involvement of sphingomyelin hydrolysis and the mitogen-activated protein kinase cascade in the Delta9-tetrahydrocannabinol-induced stimulation of glucose metabolism in primary astrocytes." Mol Pharmacol 54(5): 834-843.

Sanudo-Pena, M. C., K. Tsou, et al. (1997). "Endogenous cannabinoids as an aversive or counter-rewarding system in the rat." Neurosci Lett 223(2): 125-128.

Schlicker, E. and M. Kathmann (2001). "Modulation of transmitter release via presynaptic cannabinoid receptors." Trends Pharmacol Sci 22(11): 565-572.

Scholz, J., D. C. Broom, et al. (2005). "Blocking caspase activity prevents transsynaptic neuronal apoptosis and the loss of inhibition in lamina II of the dorsal horn after peripheral nerve injury." J Neurosci 25(32): 7317-7323.

Scotter, E. L., M. E. Abood, et al. (2010). "The endocannabinoid system as a target for the treatment of neurodegenerative disease." Br J Pharmacol 160(3): 480-498.

Shechter, R., K. Baruch, et al. (2011). "Touch gives new life: mechanosensation modulates spinal cord adult neurogenesis." Mol Psychiatry 16(3): 342-352.

Shechter, R., Y. Ziv, et al. (2007). "New GABAergic interneurons supported by myelin-specific T cells are formed in intact adult spinal cord." Stem Cells 25(9): 2277-2282.

Shibuya, S., O. Miyamoto, et al. (2002). "Embryonic intermediate filament, nestin, expression following traumatic spinal cord injury in adult rats." Neuroscience 114(4): 905-916.

Shihabuddin, L. S., P. J. Horner, et al. (2000). "Adult spinal cord stem cells generate neurons after transplantation in the adult dentate gyrus." J Neurosci 20(23): 8727-8735.

Song, H., C. F. Stevens, et al. (2002). "Astroglia induce neurogenesis from adult neural stem cells." Nature 417(6884): 39-44.

Sugiura, T., S. Kondo, et al. (1995). "2-Arachidonoylglycerol: a possible endogenous cannabinoid receptor ligand in brain." Biochem Biophys Res Commun 215(1): 89-97.

Suh, H., W. Deng, et al. (2009). "Signaling in adult neurogenesis." Annu Rev Cell Dev Biol 25: 253-275.

Sullivan, J. M. (1999). "Mechanisms of cannabinoid-receptor-mediated inhibition of synaptic transmission in cultured hippocampal pyramidal neurons." J Neurophysiol 82(3): 1286-1294.

Szabo, B. and E. Schlicker (2005). "Effects of cannabinoids on neurotransmission." Handb Exp Pharmacol(168): 327-365.

Tsou, K., S. Brown, et al. (1998). "Immunohistochemical distribution of cannabinoid CB1 receptors in the rat central nervous system." Neuroscience 83(2): 393-411.

Tsou, K., K. Mackie, et al. (1999). "Cannabinoid CB1 receptors are localized primarily on cholecystokinin-containing GABAergic interneurons in the rat hippocampal formation." Neuroscience 93(3): 969-975.

Van Sickle, M. D., L. D. Oland, et al. (2001). "Cannabinoids inhibit emesis through CB1 receptors in the brainstem of the ferret." Gastroenterology 121(4): 767-774.

Van Sickle, M. D., L. D. Oland, et al. (2003). "Delta9-tetrahydrocannabinol selectively acts on CB1 receptors in specific regions of dorsal vagal complex to inhibit emesis in ferrets." Am J Physiol Gastrointest Liver Physiol 285(3): G566-576.

Vessal, M., A. Aycock, et al. (2007). "Adult neurogenesis in primate and rodent spinal cord: comparing a cervical dorsal rhizotomy with a dorsal column transection." Eur J Neurosci 26(10): 2777-2794.

Waksman, Y., J. M. Olson, et al. (1999). "The central cannabinoid receptor (CB1) mediates inhibition of nitric oxide production by rat microglial cells." J Pharmacol Exp Ther 288(3): 1357-1366.

Wang, Y., X. Cheng, et al. (2011). "Astrocytes from the contused spinal cord inhibit oligodendrocyte differentiation of adult oligodendrocyte precursor cells by increasing the expression of bone morphogenetic proteins." J Neurosci 31(16): 6053-6058.

Wartmann, M., D. Campbell, et al. (1995). "The MAP kinase signal transduction pathway is activated by the endogenous cannabinoid anandamide." FEBS Lett 359(2-3): 133-136.

Weiss, S., C. Dunne, et al. (1996). "Multipotent CNS stem cells are present in the adult mammalian spinal cord and ventricular neuroaxis." J Neurosci 16(23): 7599-7609.

Wilson, R. I. and R. A. Nicoll (2002). "Endocannabinoid signaling in the brain." Science 296(5568): 678-682.

Wolf, S. A., A. Bick-Sander, et al. (2010). "Cannabinoid receptor CB1 mediates baseline and activity-induced survival of new neurons in adult hippocampal neurogenesis." Cell Commun Signal 8: 12.

Yamamoto, S., M. Nagao, et al. (2001). "Transcription factor expression and Notch-dependent regulation of neural progenitors in the adult rat spinal cord." J Neurosci 21(24): 9814-9823.

Yamamoto, S., N. Yamamoto, et al. (2001). "Proliferation of parenchymal neural progenitors in response to injury in the adult rat spinal cord." Exp Neurol 172(1): 115-127.

Zhang, G., W. Chen, et al. (2010). "Cannabinoid CB1 receptor facilitation of substance P release in the rat spinal cord, measured as neurokinin 1 receptor internalization." Eur J Neurosci 31(2): 225-237.

Zhang, J., C. Hoffert, et al. (2003). "Induction of CB2 receptor expression in the rat spinal cord of neuropathic but not inflammatory chronic pain models." Eur J Neurosci 17(12): 2750-2754.

4

Molecular Pharmacology of Nucleoside and Nucleotide HIV-1 Reverse Transcriptase Inhibitors

Brian D. Herman and Nicolas Sluis-Cremer
University of Pittsburgh, Department of Medicine,
Division of Infectious Diseases, Pittsburgh,
USA

1. Introduction

In 1985, 3'-azido-thymidine (AZT, zidovudine) was identified as the first nucleoside analog with activity against human immunodeficiency virus type 1 (HIV-1) (Mitsuya et al., 1985, 1987; Mitsuya & Broder, 1986), the etiologic agent of acquired immunodeficiency syndrome (Barre-Sinoussi et al., 1983; Gallo et al., 1984). This seminal discovery showed that HIV-1 replication could be suppressed by small molecule chemotherapeutic agents, and provided the basis for the field of antiviral drug discovery. Zidovudine was approved by the United States of America Food and Drug Administration for the treatment of HIV-1 infection in 1987. In the 26 years since, an additional seven nucleoside or nucleotide analogs have been approved, while several others are in clinical development. This chapter will provide a summary of the molecular pharmacology of these compounds.

2. Mechanism of action

Retroviruses such as HIV-1 carry their genomic information in the form of (+)strand RNA, but are distinguished from other RNA viruses by the fact that they replicate through a double-stranded DNA that is integrated into the host cell's genomic DNA (Temin & Mizutani, 1970; Baltimore, 1970; DeStefano et al., 1993). While the conversion of viral RNA into double-stranded DNA intermediate is a complex process, all chemical steps are catalyzed by the multi-functional viral enzyme reverse transcriptase (RT). HIV-1 RT exhibits two types of DNA polymerase activity, an RNA-dependent DNA polymerase activity that synthesizes a (-)strand DNA copy of the viral RNA, and a DNA-dependent DNA polymerase activity that generates the (+)strand DNA (Peliska & Benkovic, 1992; Cirno et al., 1995). RT also has ribonuclease H activity that degrades the RNA in the intermediate (+)RNA/(-)DNA duplex (Ghosh et al., 1997).

Once metabolized by host cell enzymes to their triphosphate forms (described in more detail below), nucleoside analogs inhibit HIV-1 reverse transcription. As such, they are typically referred to as nucleoside RT inhibitors (NRTI). NRTI-triphosphates (NRTI-TP) inhibit RT-catalyzed proviral DNA synthesis by two mechanisms (Goody et al., 1991). First, they are competitive inhibitors for binding and/or catalytic incorporation with respect to the analogous natural dNTP substrate. Second, they terminate further viral DNA synthesis due to the lack of a 3'-OH group. Chain termination is the principal mechanism of NRTI antiviral action (Goody et al., 1991). In theory, NRTI-TPs should be ideal antivirals. Each HIV virion carries only two copies of genomic RNA. There are about 20,000 nucleotide incorporation events catalyzed by RT during the synthesis of complete viral DNA, thus providing about 5000 chances for chain-termination by any given NRTI. Since HIV-1 RT lacks a formal proof-reading activity, a single NRTI incorporation event should effectively terminate reverse transcription. In reality, however, NRTIs are less potent than might be expected. The two primary reasons responsible for this are: (i) HIV-1 RT can effectively discriminate between the natural dNTP and NRTI-TP, and the extent of this discrimination is dramatically modulated by nucleic acid sequence (Isel et al., 2001); and (ii) HIV-1 RT can excise the chain-terminating NRTI-monophosphate (NRTI-MP) by using either pyrophosphate (pyrophophorolysis) or ATP as a substrate (Meyer et al., 1998; Goldschmidt & Marquet, 2004).

3. NRTI approved for clinical use

3.1 Zidovudine

Zidovudine was first synthesized in 1964 as a potential anticancer drug, but was not further developed for human use because of toxicity concerns. However, as described in the Introduction, it was found to have potent anti-HIV activity and, in 1987, was the first antiviral drug to be approved for clinical use. Zidovudine is a thymidine analog in which the 3'-OH group has been replaced with an azido (-N3) group (Figure 1). Zidovudine permeates the cell membrane by passive transport and not via a nucleoside carrier transporter (Zimmerman et al., 1987). It has good oral bioavailability and shows efficient penetration into the central nervous system. Zidovudine is efficiently metabolized to its 5'-MP form by cytosolic thymidine kinase (Ho & Hitchcock, 1989). The phosphorylation of zidovudine-MP to zidovudine-DP is catalyzed by thymidinylate monophosphate kinase (dTMP kinase; Furman et al., 1986). Interestingly, the apparent Michaelis constant (K_m) of zidovudine-MP for dTMP kinase is almost equivalent to that of dTMP, however its maximum kinetic rate (V_{max}) is only 0.3 % that of dTMP (Furman et al., 1986). Therefore, zidovudine-MP acts as a substrate inhibitor of dTMP kinase and limits its own conversion to the 5'-DP form. In this regard, there is a marked accumulation of zidovudine-MP and only low levels of the 5'-DP- and 5'-TP derivatives are detected in human T-lymphocytes (Balzarini et al., 1989). Cellular nucleoside diphosphate kinase (NDP kinase) is likely responsible for the further conversion of zidovudine-DP to zidovudine-TP. Zidovudine is metabolized to its 5'-O-glucuronide in the liver, kidney, and intestinal mucosa (Barbier et al., 2000). Because of the extensive glucuronidation of ZDV, other drugs that are also glucuronidated or that inhibit this process cause an increase in zidovudine plasma levels. Fourteen percent of the parent compound and 74% of the glucuronide have been recovered from the urine after oral administration in normal subjects (Ruane et al., 2004). Renal excretion of zidovudine is by both glomerular filtration and active tubular secretion. In some cells zidovudine can be metabolized to the highly toxic reduction product 3'-amino-thymidine (Weidner & Sommadossi, 1990).

3.2 Stavudine

Like zidovudine, stavudine (2′,3′-didehydro-3′-deoxythymidine, d4T) is a thymidine analog that undergoes metabolic activation by the sequential action of thymidine kinase and dTMP kinase (Figure 1). However, stavudine is inefficiently phosphorylated to its 5′-MP form by thymidine kinase (August et al., 1988; Zhu et al., 1990). As such, this first phosphorylation step is rate-limiting and most intracellular stavudine is not phophorylated (Balzarini et al., 1989). Maximal plasma concentrations of stavudine are achieved within 2 hours of oral administration and increase linearly as the dose increases, with an absolute bioavailability approaching 100 % (Rana & Dudley, 1997)). The drug distributes into total body water and appears to enter cells by non-facilitated diffusion (passive transport). Penetration into the central nervous system, however, is far less than zidovudine. Stavudine is cleared quickly with a terminal plasma half-life of 1-1.6 hours by both renal and nonrenal processes (Dudley et al., 1992).

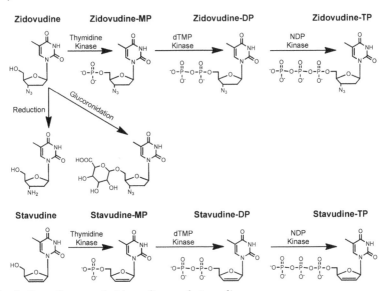

Fig. 1. Metabolic pathways of zidovudine and stavudine

3.3 Didanosine

Initially, 2′,3′-dideoxyadenosine (ddA) was evaluated as a clinical candidate but was ultimately discovered to cause nephrotoxicity. ddA is acid labile and oral administration leads to exposure to the acidic pH of the stomach and degradation to adenine (Masood et al., 1990). Adenine is further metabolized to 2,8-dihydroxyadenine which causes nephrotoxicity by crystallization in the kidney. Interestingly, ddA was shown to be metabolized to 2′,3′-dideoxyinosine (ddI, didanosine) by adenosine deaminase (Figure 2), and that much of the antiviral activity of ddA resides in didanosine (Cooney et al., 1987). Furthermore, the administration of didanosine avoids the production of adenine and the resulting nephrotoxicity. Didanosine is phosphorylated to didanosine-MP by cytosolic 5′-nucleotidase, which uses either inosine monophosphate (IMP) or guanosine monophosphate (GMP) as phosphate donors (Johnson & Fridland, 1989). Didanosine-MP is then converted to ddAMP by adenylosuccinate synthetase and 5' adenosine monophosphate-activated protein (AMP) kinase (Ahluwalia et al., 1987). The enzymes involved in phosphorylation of ddAMP to ddADP and ddATP have not been identified, although AMP kinase and NDP kinase have been proposed to play a role. ddATP is the active metabolite that is recognized by HIV-1 RT and incorporated into the nascent viral DNA chain causing chain-termination. No evidence has been provided for the formation of didanosine-DP or didanosine-TP. Didanosine is hydrolyzed to hypoxanthine by purine nucleoside phosphorylase (PNP) and further anabolized by hypoxanthine-guanine phosphoribosyl transferase to IMP (Ahluwalia et al., 1987). ATP and GTP are formed from IMP through the classical purine nucleotide biosynthetic pathways.

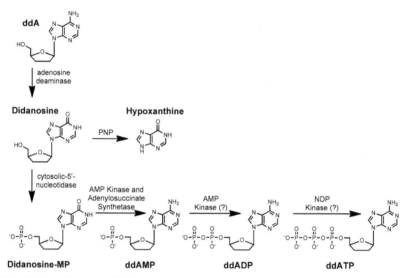

Fig. 2. Metabolic pathways of ddA and didanosine

3.4 Lamivudine and emtricitabine

The structurally related cytidine analogs lamivudine ((-)-3'-thia-2',3'-dideoxycytidine; 3TC) and ematricitabine ((-)-3'-thia-5-flouro-2',3'-dideoxycytidine; FTC) both contain the unnatural L-enantiomer ribose with a sulfur atom replacing the C3' position (Figure 3). Emtricitabine has an additional 5-flouro moiety on the cytosine ring. Lamivudine and emtricitabine are both metabolized to their respective 5'-mono- and di- and triphosphate derivatives by deoxycytidine kinase, deoxycytidine monophosphate kinase, and 5'-nucleoside diphosphate kinase, respectively (Chang et al., 1992; Cammack et al., 1992; Stein & Moore 2001; Darque et al., 1999; Bang & Scott, 2003). There is no evidence that lamivudine or emtricitabine are deaminated to their uridine analogs by cellular cytidine or deoxycytidine deaminases (Starnes & Cheng, 1987). Formation of the free base by cellular pyrimidine phosphorylases has also not been observed. Lamivudine-DP and emtricitabine-TP accumulate to higher levels in peripheral blood mononuclear cells than their monophosphate forms. It has been suggested that conversion of lamivudine-DP to lamivudine-TP is rate limiting. Lamivudine and emtricitabine are rapidly absorbed through the GI tract with peek plasma levels of 85-93% achieved within 2 hours post oral administration. Lamivudine has a plasma half-life of 5-7 hours and is eliminated unmetabolized by active organic cationic excretion (Johnson et al., 1999). Emtricitabine persists in plasma with a half-life of 10 hours and is eliminated primarily in urine by glomerular filtration and active tubular secretion but approximately 14% is eliminated in feces. Oxidation of the 3'-thiol by unidentified enzymes yields 3'-sulfoxide diasteriomers and 2'-O-glucuronidation also occurs.

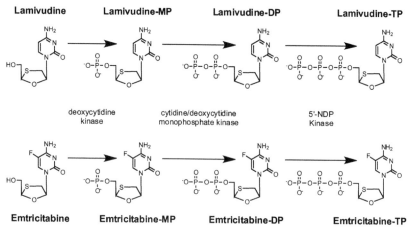

Fig. 3. Metabolic pathways of lamivudine and emtricitabine

3.5 Abacavir

Abacavir (1S,4R)-4-[2-amino-6-(cyclopropylamino)-9H-purin-9-yl]cyclopent-2-en-1-yl]methanol) is a prodrug of carbovir (2-Amino-1,9-dihydro-9-[(1R,4S)-4-(hydroxymethyl)-2-cyclopenten-1-yl]-6H-purin-6-one), a deoxyguanosine analog (Figure 4; Daluge et al., 1997). Abacavir permeates T lymophoblastoid cell lines by passive diffusion. Abacavir is phosphorylated to abacavir-MP by adenosine phosphotransferase (Faletto et al., 1997). A yet unidentified cytosolic deaminase then converts abacavir-MP to carbovir-MP. Phosphorylation to the diphosphate derivative occurs via guanidinylate monophosphate kinase. The final phosphorylation step can be catalyzed by a number of cellular enzymes including 5'-nucleotide diphosphate kinase, pyruvate kinase, and creatine kinase (Faletto et al., 1997). A linear dose relationship with carbovir-mono-, di-, and tri- phosphate derivatives over a 1000-fold dose range in vitro suggests there are no rate limiting steps in abacavir anabolism. The active metabolite carbovir-TP has been shown to persist with an elimination half-life of greater than 20 hours (McDowell et al., 2000). Abacavir bioavailability is ~83 % and is rapidly absorbed after oral dosing reaching peak plasma levels within 1 hour (Chittick et al., 1999). However, abacavir is extensively catabolized in the liver and only 1.2% is excreted as unchanged abacavir in urine. Abacavir oxidation by alcohol dehyrogenases to form the 5'-carboxylic acid derivative represents 36% of metabolites recovered from urine, while the 5'-O-glucuronide corresponds to 30% of metabolites from urine (Chittick et al., 1999). Fecal excretion also accounts for approximately 16 % of the given dose. Abacavir is not metabolized by cytochrome P450 enzymes and does not inhibit these enzymes.

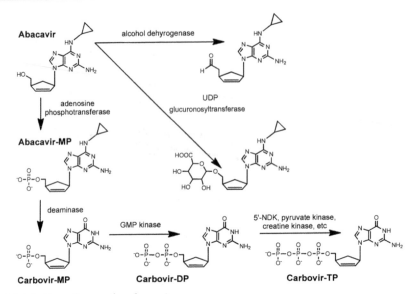

Fig. 4. Metabolic pathways for abacavir

3.6 Tenofovir and tenofovir disoproxil fumerate

The acyclic nucleoside phosphonate tenofovir (R-9-(2-phosphonylmethoxypropyl)-adenine) has no sugar ring structure but contains an acyclic methoxypropyl linker between the base N9 atom and a non-hydrolyzable C-P phosphonate bond. Thus tenofovir represents the only currently approved *nucleotide* HIV inhibitor. Tenofovir is poorly absorbed by the oral route and is therefore administered as a lipophilic orally bioavailable prodrug tenofovir disoproxil fumerate (TDF), a fumaric acid salt of the bis-isopropoxycarbonyloxymethyl ester of tenofovir (Figure 5). TDF is readily absorbed by the gastrointestinal epithelial cells with an oral bioavailability of 25% (Barditch-Crovo et al., 2001). Administration with a high fat meal increases absorption to 40%. Degradation of TDF to its monoester and subsequently to tenofovir occurs readily in the intestinal mucosa by the action of carboxylesterases and phosphodiesterases, respectively. The mono- or bis-ester forms of tenofovir are not observed in plasma suggesting efficient release of tenofovir following oral administration of TDF (Naesens et al., 1998). Following oral administration tenofovir has a long terminal half-life of 17 hours. The phosphonic acid linkage is chemically and metabolically stable and phosphorolysis back to the nucleoside does not occur (Naesens et al., 1998). Tenofovir is rapidly converted intracellularly to tenofovir-monophosphate and the active tenofovir-diphosphate forms by adenylate monophosphate kinase and 5′-nucleoside diphosphate kinase, respectively (Robbins et al., 1998). Tenofovir is not subject to intracellular deamination or deglycosylation. This stability results in a very long intracellular half-life for tenofovir-diphosphate of 15 hours in activated lymphocytes and 50 hours in resting lymphocytes (Robbins et al., 1998). Tenofovir is eliminated by glomerular filtration and active tubular secretion by organic anion transporter mediated uptake and MRP4 mediated efflux (Ray et al., 2006). At 72 hours post oral administration 70 - 80 % is recovered from urine as unchanged tenofovir. Tenofovir does not inhibit cytochrome P450 enzymes.

However, the mono- and di-phosphate forms both inhibit purine nucleoside phosphorylase which is responsible for base removal of didanosine to form hypoxanthine.

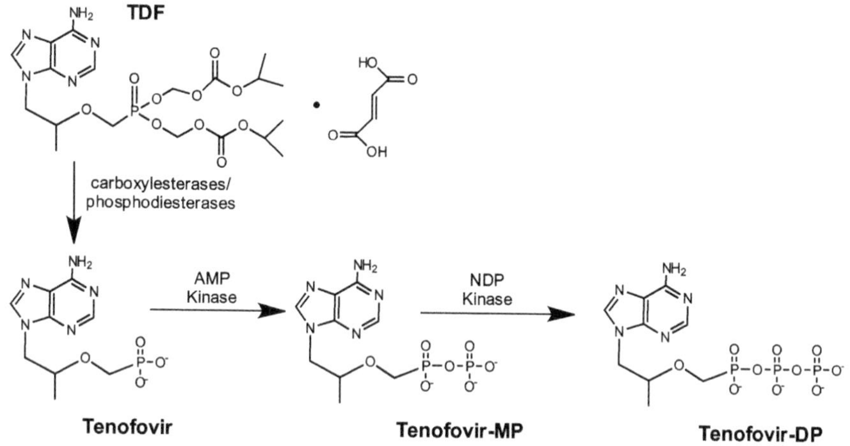

Fig. 5. Metabolic pathways of tenofovir and TDF

4. NRTI in the pipeline

Despite the widespread clinical success of NRTI-containing therapy, the currently FDA approved NRTIs display important limitations including the selection of drug resistance mutations that display cross-resistance to other NRTI, toxicity-related adverse events, and drug-drug interactions (for review see Cihlar & Ray, 2010). Thus, there is a need for novel NRTI that overcome these limitations. Here we will discuss the pharmacology of several novel drug candidates.

4.1 Apricitabine

Apricitabine (ATC) is the (-)-enantiomer of 2'-deoxy-3'-oxa-4'-thiocytidine, a deoxycytidine analog that is currently in phase II/III clinical trials (Figure 6). Both the (+) and (-)-enantiomers of apricitabine demonstrate potent inhibition of HIV-1 replication, however the (+)-enantiomer demonstrated significant mitochondrial and cellular toxicity in pre-clinical studies that was not observed with the (-) enantiomer (de Muys et al., 1999; Taylor et al., 2000). Racemic conversion of (-)-apricitabine to (+)-apricitabine is not observed in vivo (Holdich et al., 2006). Orally administered ATC is absorbed quickly, reaching maximal plasma levels within 2 hours with a plasma half-life of 3 hours. Maximal peripheral blood mononuclear cell (PBMC) intracellular concentrations of apricitabine -TP are achieved 3.5 – 4 hours after oral administration in healthy and HIV-infected patients. The intracellular half-life is 6 – 7 hours (Sawyer & Struthers-Semple, 2006; Cahn et al., 2008; Holdich et al., 2007). Apricitabine is not metabolized by hepatocytes in vitro, however a deaminated metabolite was observed likely due to gastrointestinal metabolism (Nakatani-Freshwater et al., 2006). This metabolite is excreted renally and does not demonstrate antiviral or pharmacologic effects. Apricitabine had no effect on cytochrome P450 or glucouronidase but was a weak inhibitor of P-glycoprotein (Sawyer & Cox, 2006). The first phosphorylation of apricitabine is mediated by deoxycytidine kinase, the enzyme also responsible for the initial phosphorylation of lamivudine and emtricitabine (de Muys et al., 1999). The possibility of competition for deoxycytidine kinase was examined in PBMC. Co-administration of apricitabine with lamivudine or emtricitabine leads to a dose-dependent decrease in apricitabine phosphorylation, whereas lamivudine and emtricitabine phosphorylation was not affected by apricitabine (Bethell et al., 2007). In healthy volunteers given apricitabine and lamivudine, the intracellular PBMC levels of apricitabine-TP were decreased 75% compared to apricitabine alone (Holdich et al., 2006). Consequently, administration of apricitabine in combination with lamivudine or emtricitabine is not recommended. Similarly, lamivudine and emtricitabine co-administration is also contraindicated. Apricitabine-MP is sequentially phosphorylated to the di- and tri-phosphate forms by cytidine or deoxycytidine monophosphate kinase and 5'-nucleotide diphosphate kinase, respectively.

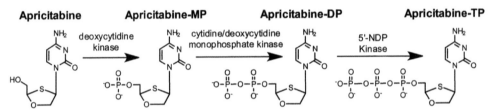

Fig. 6. Metabolic pathway of apricitabine

4.2 Festinavir

Festinavir (2',3'-didehydro-3'-deoxy-4'-ethynylthymidine; 4'-Ed4T) is a 4'-ethynyl analog of stavudine that is 5-10 fold more potent (Figure 7) (Haraguchi et al., 2003; Nitanda et al., 2005). Festinavir shows decreased cellular toxicity compared to stavudine, with little or no inhibition of host polymerases (Yang et al., 2007; Dutschman et al., 2004). Stepwise phosphorylation of festinavir occurs via the same enzymes as stavudine. Thymidine kinase 1 phosphorylates festinavir to festinavir-MP with 4-fold greater efficiency than stavudine (Hsu et al., 2007). The efficiency of festinavir-MP phosphorylation by thymidinylate monophosphate kinase is approximately 10 % of that seen for stavudine-MP or zidovudine-MP. Conversion from festinavir-DP to festinavir-TP appears to be catalyzed by multiple enzymes including nucleoside diphosphate kinase, pyruvate kinase, creatine kinase, and 3-phosphoglycerate kinase (Hsu et al., 2007). In contrast to other thymidine analogs which are readily catabolized by thymidine phosphorylase, festinavir catabolism cannot be detected. Furthermore, festinavir efflux from the cell is much less efficient than that of zidovudine. The festinavir nucleoside form alone is effluxed by a yet to be identified cellular transporter, while zidovudine and zidovudine-MP are effluxed from the cell. A Phase 1a study investigated the pharmacokinetic profile of a single oral dose between 10 and 900 mg and found a linear dose response in plasma with no apparent effects from food (Paintsil et al., 2009). A Phase 1b/2a study of festinavir oral monotherapy in 32 patients was recently completed. The results indicated that festinavir was safe (few festinavir related adverse events), well tolerated, and demonstrated dose dependent decreases in viral load between 0.87 and 1.36 logs (Cotte et al., 2010).

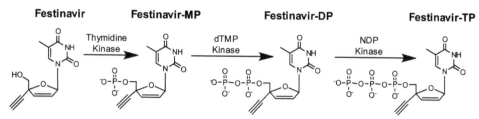

Fig. 7. Metabolic pathway of festinavir

4.3 Amdoxovir

The purine nucleoside analog 1-β-D-dioxolane guanosine (DXG) has potent activity against HIV and hepatitis B virus (Kim et al., 1993). However, it demonstrates poor solubility and limited oral bioavailability in monkeys (Chen et al., 1996). The analog 1-β-D-2,6-diaminopurine dioxolane (amdoxovir; Figure 8) also exhibits antiviral activity and is more water soluble and orally bioavailable (Chen et al., 1999; Kim et al., 1993)). Amdoxovir serves as a prodrug for DXG by deamination at the 6-position by adenosine deaminase (Gu et al., 1999). *In vitro*, amdoxovir bound adenosine deaminase as efficiently as adenosine, however amdoxovir was deaminated 540-fold slower than adenosine (Furman et al., 2001). Only DXG-triphosphate was detected in PBMC and CEM cells following exposure to DXG or amdoxovir (Rajagopalan et al., 1994; Rajagopalan et al., 1996). DXG is phosphorylated to DXG-MP by 5'-nucleotidase using IMP as a phosphate donor (Feng et al., 2004). DXG-diphosphate is then generated by guanosine monophosphate kinase (GMP kinase). DXG-DP acts as substrate for phosphorylation to the active DXG-TP for several enzymes including nucleotide diphosphate kinase (NDP kinase), 3-phosphoglycerate kinase (3-PG kinase, creatine kinase, and pyruvate kinase. Amdoxovir is rapidly converted to DXG in monkeys,

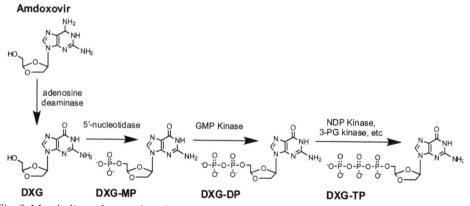

Fig. 8. Metabolic pathway of amdoxovir

woodchucks, and rats with approximately 61 % of the dose converted to DXG (Chen et al., 1996; Chen et al., 1999; Rajagopalan et al., 1996). The oral bioavailability of amdoxovir is estimated to be 30% (Chen et al., 1999). Following oral administration of amdoxovir to HIV-infected patients, peak plasma levels of amdoxivir and DXG were reached within 2 hours

(Thompson et al., 2005). Amdoxovir was eliminated from plasma with half-life of 1 - 2 hours by conversion to DXG, whereas DXG demonstrated a longer half-life of 4 - 7 hours. In animal studies amdoxovir toxicities included obstructive nephropathy, uremia, islet cell atrophy, hyperglycemia, and lens opacities (Rajagopalan et al., 1996). In a phase I/II clinical study 4 of 18 patients developed nongradeable lens opacities (Thompson et al., 2005). In other studies most adverse events were minor and included nausea, headache, and diarrhea (Gripshover et al., 2006; Murphy et al., 2008).

4.4 GS-7340

GS-7340   (9-[(R)-2-[[(S)-[[(S)-1-(isopropoxycarbonyl)ethyl]amino]phenoxyphosphinyl]-methoxy]propyl]adenine) is a novel isopropylalaninyl phenyl ester prodrug of tenofovir designed to increase intracellular delivery of the active tenofovir-DP metabolite by masking the charged phosphonate (Figure 9; Eisenberg et al 2001). Preclinical studies demonstrated 200-fold improved plasma stability and 400-fold increased accumulation of tenofovir and active tenofovir-DP in lymphatic tissues and peripheral blood mononuclear cells (PBMC) compared to tenofovir (Lee et al., 2005; Eisenberg et al., 2001). GS-7340 has 1000-fold improved potency *in vitro* over tenofovir. Following rapid target cell uptake, GS-7340 is hydrolyzed at the carboxy ester bond in lysozomes by the serine protease cathepsin A and other serine and cysteine proteases (Birkus et al., 2007; 2008). The resulting partially stable product spontaneously releases phenol by intramolecular cyclization and hydrolysis to a negatively charged, cell impermeable tenofovir-alanine intermediate (Balzarini et al., 1996). Formation of tenofovir-alanine is faster in resting PBMC compared to activated PBMC, while metabolism to parent tenofovir by a phosphoamidase and downstream phosphorylation to tenofovir-MP and tenofovir-DP is much faster in activated PBMC. A recent clinical study comparing 50 mg and 150 mg doses of GS-7340 with 300 mg TDF was conducted to determine the efficacy, safety and pharmacokinetics over 14 days (Markowitz et al., 2011). Viral loads were reduced -1.71-log and -1.57-log for 150 mg and 50 mg doses, respectively, compared to 0.94-log for TDF. PBMC levels of tenofovir were 4 – 33- times greater with GS-7340 than those for TDF at day 14 while plasma levels of tenofovir were decreased up to 88% at 24 hours with administration of GS-7340 compared to TDF. No serious adverse events were reported while the most frequent complaint was mild to moderate headache and nausea.

4.5 CMX-157

Like GS-7340, CMX-157 is an alternative prodrug of tenofovir designed to increase cell penetration by the natural lipid uptake pathways (Figure 9; Hostetler et al., 1997; Painter et al., 2004). CMX-157 contains a hexadecyloxypropyl (HDP) lipid conjugation which mimics lysophosphatidylcholine. CMX-157, unlike TDF is not cleaved to free tenofovir in the intestinal mucosa and thus circulates in plasma as the tenofovir-HDP lipid conjugate (Painter et al., 2007). Tenofovir-HDP is not a substrate for human organic anion transporters and therefore is subject to decreased renal excretion and increased intracellular drug exposure compared to TDF (Tippin et al., 2010). Free tenofovir is liberated intracellularly by hydrolytic removal of the HDP lipid by phospholipases. Intracellular activation to the active tenofovir-DP form is achieved in the same manner as TDF. CMX-157 delivers > 30-fold increased active metabolite tenofovir-DP in PBMC than tenofovir. Higher intracellular concentrations of CMX-157 provide >300-fold greater activity against clinical isolates than tenofovir with EC_{50} values < 1 nM (Lanier et al., 2010). It has additionally been proposed that CMX-157 may bind cell free virions by direct lipid insertion into the viral envelope resulting in facilitated delivery to target cells (Painter et al., 2007). CMX-157 recently completed a Phase I clinical trial to evaluate safety, tolerability and pharmacokinetics. CMX-157 was well tolerated with no drug-related adverse events. Plasma levels increased linearly with dose and active TFV-DP was detected up to six days post administration of a 400 mg dose suggesting the possibility of a once weekly dosing regimen.

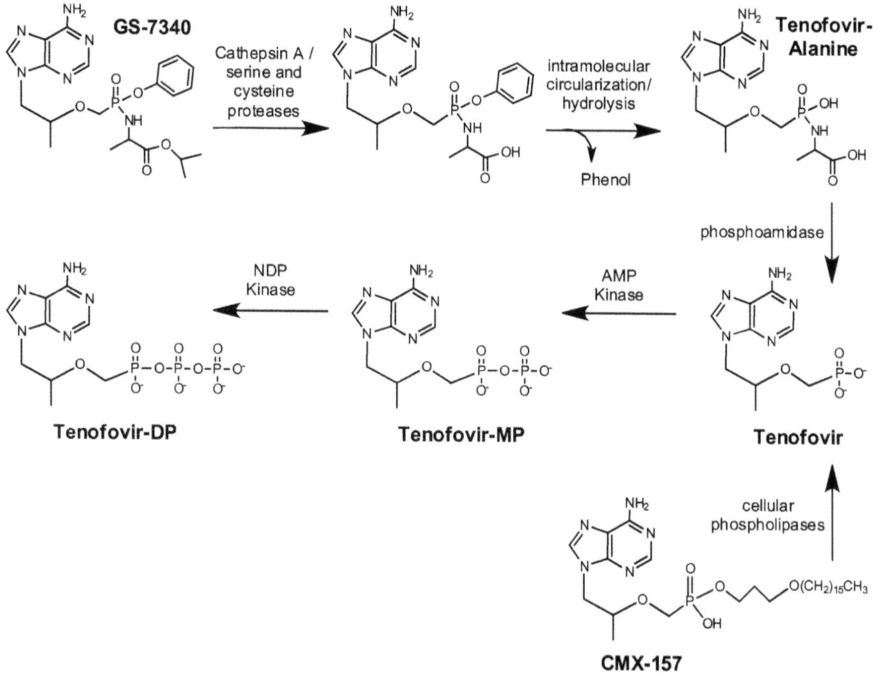

Fig. 9. Intracellular metabolism of GS-7340 and CMX-157

5. Conclusions

Nucleoside and nucleotide reverse transcriptase inhibitors have remained the backbone of antiretroviral therapy. The absolute dependence of NRTI on host cellular enzymes for activation is a unique property of this drug class. The eight approved NRTI and numerous experimental NRTI display great diversity for all of these factors, thus presenting pharmacological advantages and challenges that are unique to the NRTI class. The complex relationships between NRTIs and host cell enzymes have necessitated detailed studies of the *in vitro* and *in vivo* pharmacologic properties of novel NRTIs in pre-clinical development. Current drug discovery efforts increasingly utilize NRTI prodrugs in order to accelerate NRTI phosphorylation or otherwise improve pharmacologic properties. Further understanding of the cellular pharmacology of NRTI is crucial for the development of novel drugs for increased potency, improved safety and tolerability, and decreased resistance.

6. Acknowledgements

Research in the Sluis-Cremer laboratory was supported by grants AI081571, GM068406 and AI071846 from the National Institutes of Health (NIH), United States of America. Brian Herman was supported by an NIH training grant (T32 AAI 49820).

7. References

Ahluwalia, G., Cooney, D.A., Mitsuya, H., Fridland, A., Flora, K.P., Hao, Z., Dalal, M., Broder, S. & Johns, D.G. (1987). Initial studies on the cellular pharmacology of 2',3'-dideoxyinosine, an inhibitor of HIV infectivity. *Biochem. Pharmacol.* 36(22): 3797-800.

August, E.M., Marongiu, M.E., Lin, T.,S. & Prusoff, W.H. (1988). Initial studies on the cellular pharmacology of 3'-deoxythymidin-2'-ene (d4T): a potent and selective inhibitor of human immunodeficiency virus. *Biochem. Pharmacol.*, 37(23): 4419-22.

Baltimore, D. (1970) Viral RNA-dependent DNA polymerase. *Nature* 226: 1209-1211.

Balzarini, J., Herdewijn, P. & De Clercq, E. (1989). Differential patterns of intracellular metabolism of 2',3'-didehydro-2',3'-dideoxy-thymidine (D4T) and 3'-azido-2',3'-dideoxythymidine (AZT), two potent anti-HIV compounds. *J. Biol. Chem.* 264: 6127-33.

Balzarini, J., Karlsson, A., Aquaro, S., Perno, C.F., Cahard, D., Naesens, L., De Clercq, E. & McGuigan, C. (1996). Mechanism of anti-HIV action of masked alaninyl d4T-MP derivatives. *Proc. Natl. Acad. Sci. U.S.A.* 93: 7295–7299.

Bang, L. & Scott, L.J. (2003). Emtricitabine: an antiretroviral agent for HIV infection. *Drugs.* 63: 2413–2424.

Barbier, O., Turgeon, D., Girard, C., Green, M.D., Tephly, T.R., Hum, D.W. & Bélanger, A. (2000). 3'-azido-3'-deoxythimidine (AZT) is glucuronidated by human UDP-glucuronosyltransferase 2B7 (UGT2B7). *Drug Metab. Dispos.* 28(5): 497-502.

Barditch-Crovo, P., Deeks, S.G., Collier, A., Safrin, S., Coakley, D.F., Miller, M., Kearney, B.P., Coleman, R.L., Lamy, P.D., Kahn, J.O., McGowan, I. & Lietman, P.S. (2001). Phase I/II trial of the pharmacokinetics, safety and antiretroviral activity of tenofovir disoproxil fumarate in human immunodeficiency virus-infected adults. *Antimicrob Agents Chemother.* 2001; 45: 2733-9.

Barre-Sinoussi, F., Chermann, J.C., Rey, F., Nugeyre, M.T., Chamaret, S., Gruest, J., Dauguet, C., Axler-Blin, C., Vezinet-Brun, F., Rouzioux, C., Rozenbaum,W., & Montagnier, L., (1983) Isolation of a T-lymphotropic retrovirus from a patient at risk for acquired immune deficiency syndrome (AIDS). *Science* 220: 868–871.

Bethell, R., de Muys, J., Lippens, J., Richard, A., Hamelin, B., Ren, C. & Collins, P. (2007). In vitro interactions between apricitabine and other deoxycytidine analogues. *Antimicrob. Agents Chemother.* 51: 2948 -53.

Birkus, G., Kutty, N., He, G.X., Mulato, A., Lee, W., McDermott, M. & Cihlar, T. (2008). Activation of 9-[(R)-2-[[(S)-[[(S)-1-(Isopropoxycarbonyl)ethyl]amino] phenoxyphosphinyl]-ethoxy]propyl]adenine (GS-7340) and other tenofovir phosphonoamidate prodrugs by human proteases. *Mol. Pharmacol.* 74(1): 92-100.

Birkus, G., Wang, R., Liu, X., Kutty, N., MacArthur, H., Cihlar, T., Gibbs, C., Swaminathan, S., Lee, W. & McDermott, M. (2007). Cathepsin A is the major hydrolase catalyzing the intracellular hydrolysis of the antiretroviral nucleotide phosphonoamidate prodrugs GS-7340 and GS-9131. *Antimicrob. Agents Chemother.* 51(2): 543-50.

Cahn, P., Rolon, M., Cassetti, I., Shiveley, L., Holdich, T. & Sawyer, J. (2008). Multiple-dose pharmacokinetics of apricitabine, a novel nucleoside reverse transcriptase inhibitor, in patients with HIV-1 infection. *Clin. Drug. Invest.* 28: 129 -38.

Cammack, N., Rouse, P., Marr, C.L., Reid, P.J., Boehme, R.E., Coates, J.A., Penn, C.R. & Cameron, J.M. (1992). Cellular metabolism of (-) enantiomeric 2,-deoxy-3,-thiacytidine. *Biochem. Pharmacol.* 43: 2059-2064.

Chang, C.N., Skalski, V., Zhou, J.H. & Cheng, Y.C. (1992). Biochemical pharmacology of (+)- and (-)-2',3'-dideoxy-3'-thiacytidine as anti-hepatitis B virus agents. *J. Biol. Chem.* 267(31): 22414-20.

Chen, H., Boudinot, F.D., Chu, C.K., Mcclure, H.M. & Schinazi, R.F. (1996). Pharmacokinetics of (-)-beta-D-2-aminopurine dioxolane and (-)-beta-D-2-amino-6-chloropurine dioxolane and their antiviral metabolite (-)-beta-D-dioxolane guanine in rhesus monkeys. *Antimicrob. Agents Chemother.* 40(10): 2332-6.

Chen, H., Schinazi, R.F., Rajagopalan, P., Gao, Z., Chu, C.K., McClure, H.M. & Boudinot, F.D. (1999). Pharmacokinetics of (-)-beta-D-dioxolane guanine and prodrug (-)-beta-D-2,6-diaminopurine dioxolane in rats and monkeys. *AIDS Res. Hum. Retroviruses.* 15(18): 1625-30.

Chittick, G.E., Gillotin, C., McDowell, J.A., Lou, Y., Edwards, K.D., Prince, W.T. & Stein, D.S. (1999). Abacavir: absolute bioavailability, bioequivalence of three oral formulations, and effect of food. *Pharmacotherapy.* 19(8): 932-42.

Cihlar, T. & Ray, A.S. (2010). Nucleoside and nucleotide HIV reverse transcriptase inhibitors: 25 years after zidovudine. *Antiviral Res.* 85(1):39-58.

Cirno, N.M., Cameron, C.E., Smith, J.S., Rausch, J.W., Roth, M.J., Benkovic, S.J. & Le Grice, S.F.J. (1995) Divalent cation modulation of the Ribonuclease h functions of human immunodeficiency virus reverse transcriptase. *Biochemistry* 34: 9936-9943.

Cooney, D.A., Ahiuwalia, G., Mitsuya, H., Fridland, A., Johnson, M., Hao, Z., Dalal, M., Balzarini, J., Broder, S. & Johns, D.G. (1987). Initial studies on the cellular pharmacology of 2',3'-dideoxyadenosine, an inhibitor of HTLV-III infectivity. *Biochem. Pharmacol.* 36: 1765-1768.

Cotte, L., Dellamonica, P., Raffi, F., Yazdanpanah, L.Y., Molina, J. M., Boue, F., & Urata, Y. (2010). A Phase-Ib/IIa Dose-Escalation Study of OBP-601 (4'-ethynyl-d4T, Festinavir) in Treatment-Experienced, HIV-1-Infected Patients. *50th Interscience Conference on Antimicrobial Agents and Chemotherapy* (ICAAC 2010). Boston, MA. U.S.A. September 12-15, 2010.

Daluge, S.M., Good, S.S., Faletto, M.B., Miller, W.H., St Clair, M.H., Boone, L.R., Tisdale, M., Parry, N.R., Reardon, J.E., Dornsife, R.E., Averett, D.R. & Krenitsky, T.A. (1997). 1592U89, a novel carbocyclic nucleoside analog with potent, selective anti-human immunodeficiency virus activity. *Antimicrob. Agents Chemother.* 41(5): 1082-93.

Darque, A., Valette, G., Rousseau, F., Wang, L.H., Sommadossi, J.P. & Zhou, X.J. (1999). Quantitation of intracellular triphosphate of emtricitabine in peripheral blood mononuclear cells from human immunodeficiency virus-infected patients. *Antimicrob. Agents Chemother.* 43: 2245-2250.

de Muys, J.M., Gourdeau, H., Nguyen-Ba, N., Taylor, D.L., Ahmed, P.S., Mansour, T., Locas, C., Richard, N., Wainberg, M.A. & Rando, R.F. (1999). Anti-human immunodeficiency virus type 1 activity, intracellular metabolism, and pharmacokinetic evaluation of 2'-deoxy-3'-oxa-4'-thiocytidine. *Antimicrob. Agents. Chemother.* 43(8): 1835-44.

DeStefano, J.J., Bambara, R.A., & Fay, P.J. (1993) Parameters that influence the binding of human immunodeficiency virus reverse transcriptase to nucleic acid structures. *Biochemistry* 32: 6908-6915.

Dudley, M.N., Graham, K.K., Kaul, S., Geletko, S., Dunkle, L., Browne, M. & Mayer, K. (1992). Pharmacokinetics of stavudine in patients with AIDS or AIDS-related complex. *J. Infect. Dis.* 166: 480–485.

Dutschman, G.E., Grill, S.P., Gullen, E.A., Haraguchi, K., Takeda, S., Tanaka, H., Baba, M. & Cheng, Y.C. (2004). Novel 4'-substituted stavudine analog with improved antihumanimmunodeficiency virus activity and decreased cytotoxicity. *Antimicrob. Agents Chemother.* 48: 1640–1646.

Eisenberg, E.J., He, G.X. & Lee, W.A. (2001). Metabolism of GS-7340, a novel phenyl monophosphoramidate intracellular prodrug of PMPA, in blood. *Nucleosides Nucleotides Nucleic Acids.* 20: 1091-8.

Faletto, M.B., Miller, W.H., Garvey, E.P., St Clair, M.H., Daluge, S.M. & Good, S.S. (1997). Unique intracellular activation of the potent anti-human immunodeficiency virus agent 1592U89. *Antimicrob. Agents Chemother.* 41(5): 1099-107.

Feng, J.Y., Parker, W.B., Krajewski, M.L., Deville-Bonne, D., Veron, M., Krishnan, P., Cheng, Y.C. & Borroto-Esoda, K. (2004). Anabolism of amdoxovir: phosphorylation of dioxolane guanosine and its 5'-phosphates by mammalian phosphotransferases. *Biochem. Pharmacol.* 68(9): 1879-88.

Furman, P.A., Fyfe, J.A., St Clair, M.H., Weinhold, K., Rideout, J.L., Freeman, G.A., Lehrman, S.N., Bolognesi, D.P., Broder, S., Mitsuya H, et al. (1986). Phosphorylation of 3'-azido-3'-deoxythymidine and selective interaction of the 5'-triphosphate with human immunodeficiency virus reverse transcriptase. *Proc. Natl. Acad. Sci. U. S. A.* 83(21): 8333-7.

Furman, P.A., Jeffrey, J., Kiefer, L.L., Feng, J.Y., Anderson, K.S., Borroto-Esoda, K., Hill, E., Copeland, W.C., Chu, C.K., Sommadossi, J.P., Liberman, I., Schinazi, R.F. & Painter, G.R. (2001). Mechanism of action of 1-beta-D-2,6-diaminopurine dioxolane, a prodrug of the human immunodeficiency virus type 1 inhibitor 1-beta-D-dioxolane guanosine. *Antimicrob. Agents Chemother.* 45(1): 158-65.

Gallo, R.C., Salahuddin, S.Z., Popovic, M., Shearer, G.M., Kaplan, M., Haynes, B.F., Palker, T.J., Redfield, R., Oleske, J., Safai, B., et al., (1984) Frequent detection and isolation of cytopathic retroviruses (HTLV-III) from patients with AIDS and at risk for AIDS. *Science* 224, 500–503.

Ghosh M., Williams, J., Powell, M.G., Levin, J.G., & Le Grice, S.F.J. (1997) Mutating a conserved motif of the HIV-1 reverse transcriptase palm subdomain alters primer utilization. *Biochemistry* 36: 5758-5768.

Goldschmidt, V. & Marquet, R. (2004). Primer unblocking by HIV-1 reverse transcriptase and resistance to nucleoside RT inhibitors (NRTIs). *Int. J. Biochem. Cell Biol.* (9): 1687-705.

Goody, R.S., Müller, B. & Restle, T. (1991). Factors contributing to the inhibition of HIV reverse transcriptase by chain-terminating nucleotides in vitro and in vivo. *FEBS Lett.* 291(1):1-5.

Gripshover, B.M., Ribaudo, H., Santana, J., Gerber, J.G., Campbell, T.B., Hogg, E., Jarocki, B., Hammer, S.M. & Kuritzkes, D.R.; A5118 Team. (2006). Amdoxovir versus placebo with enfuvirtide plus optimized background therapy for HIV-1-infected

Gu, Z., Wainberg, M.A., Nguyen-Ba, N., L'Heureux, L., de Muys, J.M., Bowlin, T.L. & Rando, R.F. (1999) Mechanism of action and in vitro activity of 1',3'-dioxolanylpurine nucleoside analogues against sensitive and drug-resistant human immunodeficiency virus type 1 variants. *Antimicrob. Agents Chemother.* 43(10): 2376-82.

Haraguchi, K., Takeda, S., Tanaka, H., Nitanda, T., Baba, M., Dutschman, G.,E. & Cheng, Y.C. (2003). Synthesis of a highly active new anti-HIV agent 2',3'-didehydro-3'-deoxy-4'-ethynylthymidine. *Bioorg. Med. Chem. Lett.* 13(21): 3775-7.

Ho, H.,T. & Hitchcock, M.,J. (1989). Cellular pharmacology of 2',3'-dideoxy-2',3'-didehydrothymidine, a nucleoside analog active against human immunodeficiency virus. *Antimicrob. Agents Chemother.* 33(6): 844-9.

Holdich, T., Shiveley, L. & Sawyer, J. (2006). Pharmacokinetics of single oral doses of apricitabine, a novel deoxycytidine analogue reverse transcriptase inhibitor, in healthy volunteers. *Clin. Drug. Invest.* 26: 279 -86.

Holdich, T., Shiveley, L.A. & Sawyer, J. (2007). Effect of lamivudine on the plasma and intracellular pharmacokinetics of apricitabine, a novel nucleoside reverse transcriptase inhibitor, in healthy volunteers. *Antimicrob Agents Chemother.* 51: 2943 -2947.

Hostetler, K.Y., Beadle, J.R., Kini, G.D., Gardner, M.F., Wright, K.N., Wu, T.H. & Korba, B.A. (1997). Enhanced oral absorption and antiviral activity of 1-O-octadecyl-sn-glycero-3-phospho-acyclovir and related compounds in hepatitis B virus infection, in vitro. *Biochem. Pharmacol.* 53: 1815–1822.

Hsu, C.H., Hu, R., Dutschman, G.E., Yang, G., Krishnan, P., Tanaka, H., Baba, M. & Cheng, Y.C. (2007). Comparison of the phosphorylation of 4'-ethynyl 2',3'-dihydro-3'-deoxythymidine with that of other anti-human immunodeficiency virus thymidine analogs. *Antimicrob. Agents Chemother.* 51(5): 1687-93.

Johnson, M.A. & Fridland, A. (1989). Phosphorylation of 2',3'-dideoxyinosine by cytosolic 5'-nucleotidase of human lymphoid cells. *Mol. Pharmacol.* 36: 291-5.

Johnson, M.A., Moore, K.H., Yuen, G.J., Bye, A. & Pakes, G.E. (1999). Clinical pharmacokinetics of lamivudine. *Clin. Pharmacokinet.* 36(1):41-66.

Kim, H.O., Schinazi, R.F., Nampalli, S., Shanmuganathan, K., Cannon, D.L., Alves, A.J., Jeong, L.S., Beach, J.W. & Chu, C.K. (1993). 1,3-dioxolanylpurine nucleosides (2R,4R) and (2R,4S) with selective anti-HIV-1 activity in human lymphocytes. *J. Med. Chem.* 36(1): 30-37.

Lanier, E.R., Ptak, R.G., Lampert, B.M., Keilholz, L., Hartman, T., Buckheit, Jr., R.W., Mankowski, M.K., Osterling, M.C., Almond, M.R. & Painter, G.R. (2010). Development of hexadecyloxypropyl tenofovir (CMX157) for treatment of infection caused by wild-type and nucleoside/nucleotide-resistant HIV. *Antimicrob Agents Chemother.* 54(7): 2901-9.

Lee, W.A., He, G.X., Eisenberg, E., Cihlar, T., Swaminathan, S., Mulato, A. & Cundy, K.C. (2005). Selective intracellular activation of a novel prodrug of the human immunodeficiency virus reverse transcriptase inhibitor tenofovir leads to preferential distribution and accumulation in lymphatic tissue. *Antimicrob. Agents Chemother.* 49(5): 1898-906.

Markowitz, M., Zolopa, A., Ruane, P., Squires, K., Zhong, L., Kearney, B.P. & Lee, W. (2011). GS-7340 Demonstrates Greater Declines in HIV-1 RNA than Tenofovir Disoproxil Fumarate During 14 Days of Monotherapy in HIV-1 Infected Subjects. *18th Conference on Retroviruses and Opportunistic Infections* March 2, 2011 Boston, MA., Abstract # 152LB.

Masood, R.W., Ahluwalia, G.S., Cooney, D.A., Fridland, A., Marquez, V.E., Driscoll, J.S., Hao, Z., Mitsuya, H., Perno, C.F., Broder, S., et al. (1990). 2'-Fluoro-2',3'-dideoxyarabinosyladenine: a metabolically stable analogue of the antiretroviral agent 2',3'-dideoxyadenosine. *Mol. Pharmacol.* 37: 590-6.

McDowell, J.A., Lou, Y., Symonds, W.S. & Stein, D.S. (2000). Multiple-dose pharmacokinetics and pharmacodynamics of abacavir alone and in combination with zidovudine in human immunodeficiency virus-infected adults. *Antimicrob. Agents Chemother.* 44(8): 2061-7.

Meyer, P.R., Matsuura, S.E., So, A.G. & Scott, W.A. (1998). Unblocking of chain-terminated primer by HIV-1 reverse transcriptase through a nucleotide-dependent mechanism. *Proc. Natl. Acad. Sci. U.S.A.* 95(23): 13471-6.

Mitsuya, H., & Broder, S. (1986) Inhibition of the in vitro infectivity and cytopathic effect of human T-lymphotrophic virus type III/lymphadenopathy-associated virus (HTLV-III/LAV) by 2',3'-dideoxynucleosides. *Proc. Natl. Acad. Sci. U. S. A.* 83: 1911–1915.

Mitsuya, H., Jarrett, R.F., Matsukura, M., Veronese, F.D., DeVico, A.L., Sarngadharan, M.G., Johns, D.G., Reitz, M.S., & Broder, S. (1987) Long-term inhibition of human T-lymphotropic virus type III/lymphadenopathy-associated virus (human immunodeficiency virus) DNA synthesis and RNA expression in T cells protected by 2',3'-dideoxynucleosides in vitro. *Proc. Natl. Acad. Sci. U. S. A.* 84: 2033–2037.

Mitsuya, H., Weinhold, K.J., Furman, P.A., St Clair, M.H., Nusinoff-Lehrman, S., Gallo, R.C., Bolognesi, D., Barry, D.W., & Broder, S. (1985) 3'-azido-3'-deoxythymidine (BW A509U): an antiviral agent that inhibits the infectivity and cytopathic effect of human T-lymphotropic virus type III/lymphadenopathy-associated virus in vitro. *Proc. Natl. Acad. Sci. U. S. A.* 82: 7096–7100.

Murphy, R., Zala, C., Ochoa, C., Tharnish, P., Mathew, J., Fromentin, E., Asif, G., Hurwitz, S.J., Kivel, N.M., & Schinazi, R.F. (2008). Pharmacokinetics and potent anti-HIV-1 activity of amdoxovir plus zidovudine in a randomized double-blind placebo-controlled study. *15th Conference on Retroviruses and Opportunistic Infections.* February 3-6, 2008. Boston, MA. Abstract 794.

Naesens, L., Bischofberger, N., Augustijns, P., Annaert, P., Van den Mooter, G., Arimilli, M.N., Kim, C.U., De Clercq, E., (1998). Antiretroviral efficacy and pharmacokinetics of oral bis-(isopropyloxycarbonyloxymethyl)-9-(2-phosphonylmethoxypropyl)adenine in mice. *Antimicrob. Agents Chemother.* 42: 1568–1573.

Nakatani-Freshwater, T., Babayeva, M., Dontabhaktuni, A. & Taft, D.R. (2006). Effects of trimethoprim on the clearance of apricitabine, a deoxycytidine analog reverse transcriptase inhibitor, and lamivudine in the isolated rat perfused kidney. *J. Pharmacol. Exper. Ther.* 319: 941 -947.

Nitanda, T., Wang, X., Kumamoto, H., Haraguchi, K., Tanaka, H., Cheng, Y.C. & Baba, M. (2005). Anti-human immunodeficiency virus type 1 activity and resistance profile of 2',3'-didehydro-3'-deoxy-4'-ethynylthymidine in vitro. *Antimicrob. Agents Chemother.* 49: 3355–3360.

Painter, G.R., Almond, M.R., Trost, L.C., Lampert, B.M., Neyts, J., De Clercq, E., Korba, B.E., Aldern, K.A., Beadle, J.R. & Hostetler, K.Y. (2007). Evaluation of hexadecyloxypropyl-9-R-[2-(phosphonomethoxy)propyl]-adenine, CMX157, as a potential treatment for human immunodeficiency virus type 1 and hepatitis B virus infections. *Antimicrob. Agents Chemother.* 51: 3505–3509.

Painter, G.R. & Hostetler, K.Y. (2004). Design and development of oral drugs for the prophylaxis and treatment of smallpox infection. *Trends Biotechnol.* 22: 423–427.

Paintsil, E., Mastuda, T., Ross, J., Schofield, J., Cheng, Y.C., Urata, Y., (2009). A Singledose escalation study to evaluate the safety, tolerability, and pharmacokinetics of OBP-601, a novel NRTI, in healthy subjects. In: *16th Conference on Retroviruses and Opportunistic Infections*, February 2009, Montreal, Canada. Abstract 568.

Peliska, J.A. & Benkovic, S.J. (1992) Mechanism of DNA strand transfer reactions catalyzed by HIV-1 reverse transcriptase. *Science* 258: 1112-1118.

Rajagopalan, P., Boudinot, F. D., Chu, C.K., McClure, H.M., & Schinazi, R.F. (1994). Pharmacokinetics of (2)-β-D-2,6-diaminopurine dioxolaneand its metabolite guanosine in rhesus monkeys. *Pharm. Res.* 11(Suppl.): 381–386.

Rajagopalan, P., Boudinot, F.D., Chu, C.K., Tennant, B.C., Baldwin, B.H. & Schinazi, R.F. (1996). Pharmacokinetics of (2)-β-D-2,6-diaminopurinedioxolane and its metabolite, dioxolane guanosine, in woodchucks (Marmotamonax). *Antivir. Chem. Chemother.* 7: 65–70.

Rana, K.Z. & Dudley, M.N. (1997). Clinical pharmacokinetics of stavudine. *Clin. Pharmacokinet.* 33:276–284.

Ray, A. S., Cihlar, T., Robinson, K. L., Tong, L., Vela, J. E., Fuller, M. D., Wieman, L. M., Eisenberg, E. J. & Rhodes, G. R. (2006). Mechanism of active renal tubular efflux of tenofovir. *Antimicrob. Agents Chemother.* 50: 3297–3304.

Robbins, B.L., Srinivas, R.V., Kim, C., Bischofberger, N., Fridland, A. (1998). Anti-human immunodeficiency virus activity and cellular metabolism of a potential prodrug of the acyclic nucleoside phosphonate 9-R-(2-phosphonomethoxypropyl)adenine (PMPA), bis(isopropyloxymethylcarbonyl)PMPA. *Antimicrob. Agents Chemother.* 42: 612–617.

Ruane, .P.J, Richmond, G.J., DeJesus, E., Hill-Zabala, C.E., Danehower, S.C., Liao, Q., Johnson, J. & Shaefer, M.S. (2004). Pharmacodynamic effects of zidovudine 600 mg once/day versus 300 mg twice/day in therapy-naïve patients infected with human immunodeficiency virus. *Pharmacotherapy.* 24(3): 307-12.

Sawyer, J. & Cox, S. (2006). In vitro pharmacology of Apricitabine, a new NRTI for HIV. *XVI International AIDS Conference,* August 2006, Toronto, Canada, abstract CDB0046.

Sawyer, J. & Struthers-Semple, C. (2006). Pharmacokinetics of apricitabine in healthy volunteers and HIV-infected individuals. *XVI International AIDS Conference,* August 2006, Toronto, Canada, Abstract TUPE0077.

Starnes, M.C. & Cheng, Y.C. (1987). Cellular metabolism of 2',3'-dideoxycytidine, a compound active against human immunodeficiency virus in vitro. *J Biol. Chem.* 262(3): 988-91.

Stein, D.S. & Moore, K.H. (2001). Phosphorylation of nucleoside analog antiretrovirals: a review for clinicians. *Pharmacotherapy.* (1):11-34.

Taylor, D.L., Ahmed, P.S., Tyms, A.S., Wood, L.J., Kelly, L.A., Chambers, P., Clarke, J., Bedard, J., Bowlin, T.L., Rando, R.F. (2000). Drug resistance and drug combination features of the human immunodeficiency virus inhibitor, BCH-10652 [(+/-)-2'-deoxy-3'-oxa-4'-thiocytidine, dOTC]. *Antivir. Chem. Chemother.* 11(4): 291-301.

Temin, H. & Mizutani, S. (1970) RNA-dependent DNA polymerase in virions of Rous sarcoma virus. *Nature* 226: 1211-1232.

Thompson, M.A., Kessler, H.A., Eron, J.J. Jr., Jacobson, J.M., Adda, N., Shen, G., Zong, J., Harris, J., Moxham, C. & Rousseau, F.S.; DAPD-101 Study Group. (2005). Short-term safety and pharmacodynamics of amdoxovir in HIV-infected patients. *AIDS* 19: 1607–1615.

Tippin, T.K., Lampert, B.M., Painter, G.R. & Lanier, E.R. (2010). CMX001 & CMX157 Are Not Substrates of Human Organic Anion Transporters hOAT1 and hOAT3. *FIP Pharmaceutical Sciences World Congress and AAPS Meeting* November 16, 2010 New Orleans, LA.

Weidner, D.,A. & Sommadossi, J.P. (1990). 3'-Azido-3'-deoxythymidine inhibits globin gene transcription in butyric acid-induced K-562 human leukemia cells. *Mol. Pharmacol.* 38(6): 797-804.

Yang, G., Dutschman, G.E., Wang, C.J., Tanaka, H., Baba, M., Anderson, K.S. & Cheng, Y.C. (2007). Highly selective action of triphosphate metabolite of 4'-ethynyl D4T: a novel anti-HIV compound against HIV-1 RT. *Antiviral Res.* 73: 185–191.

Zhu, Z., Ho, H.T., Hitchcock, M.J. & Sommadossi, J.P. (1990). Cellular pharmacology of 2',3'-didehydro-2',3'-dideoxythymidine (D4T) in human peripheral blood mononuclear cells. *Biochem. Pharmacol.* 39(9): R15-9.

Zimmerman, T.P., Mahony, W.B. & Prus, K.L. (1987). 3'-Azido-3'-deoxythymidine. An unusual nucleoside analogue that permeates the membrane of human erythrocytes and lymphocytes by nonfacilitated diffusion. *J. Biol. Chem.* 262: 5748-54.

5

Interactions Between Glutamate Receptors and TRPV1 Involved in Nociceptive Processing at Peripheral Endings of Primary Afferent Fibers

You-Hong Jin[1], Motohide Takemura[2],
Akira Furuyama[3] and Norifumi Yonehara[4]
[1]Department of Anatomy the Affiliated Stomatological,
Hospital of Nanchang University, Nanchang, Jiangxi Province,
[2]Department of Oral Anatomy and Neurobiology,
Osaka University Graduate School of Dentistry,
[3]Departments of Oral Physiology
[4]Oral Medical Science (Division of Dental Pharmacology),
Ohu University School of Dentistry, Koriyama, Fukushima,
[1]China
[2,3,4]Japan

1. Introduction

Glutamate (Glu) is a main excitatory neurotransmitter in the central nervous system. Concerning the existence of Glu in the small-diameter afferent fibers, their central (Westlund et al., 1989; Keast and Stephensen, 2000) and peripheral (Westlund et al., 1992; Keast and Stephensen, 2000) processes as well as dorsal root ganglion (DRG) cells (Battaglia and Rustioni, 1988; Keast and Stephensen, 2000) contain Glu. Recently, Glu has been shown to have a role in transduction of sensory input at the periphery (Carlton, 2001).

Electron microscope studies demonstrate that Glu receptors are transported from the DRG cell bodies into central and/or peripheral primary afferent terminals (Liu et al., 1994). The N-methyl-D-aspartic acid (NMDA), α-amino-3-hydroxy-5methyl-4-isoxazole propionic acid (AMPA) and kainate receptors (NMDA/AMPA-kainate receptors) are localized on unmyelinated axons at the dermal-epidermal junction in the glabrous and hairy skin of the rat (Carlton et al., 1995; Coggeshall and Carlton, 1998), and in human hairly skin (Kinkelin et al., 2000). Approximately 20% of the fibers were immunostained in one of the receptor subtypes. As Sato et al. (1993) reported that virtually all DRG cells as well as their central (Laurie et al., 1995; Zou et al., 2002) and peripheral (Carlton et al., 1995) processes are positively labeled for the NMDA receptor, it is highly likely that two or more of the ionotropic Glu receptors are colocalized.

Behavioral evidence supports a role for peripheral Glu receptors in normal nociceptive transmission. Intraplantar injection of L-Glu into the hindpaw evokes hyperalgesia in rats (Follenfant and Nakamura-Craig, 1992; Carlton et al., 1995). Futhermore, intraplantar injection of the specific Glu receptors agonists NMDA, AMPA or kainate results in mechanical hyperalgesia and allodynia that can be blocked by appropriate antagonists (Zhou et al., 1996). Hyperalgesia is induced by binding the released glutamate to NMDA receptor (Leem et al., 2001; Du et al., 2003), group I mGluR (Bhave et al., 2001; Zhou et al., 2001; Hu et al., 2002; Walker et al., 2001; Lee et al., 2007), but not group II mGluR (Yang and Gereau IV, 2003).

In addition to these behavioral and anatomical data, Omote et al. (1998) showed that subcutaneous administration of inflammatory substances such as formalin induced the release of peripheral EAAs (Glu and aspartate) on the ipsilateral side. We have already reported that local application of capsaicin cream evoked a marked increase in Glu level in the s.c. perfusate. In addition, electrical stimulation of the sciatic nerve or noxious heat stimulation (50°C) also caused increase of Glu level in the s.c. space, and this capsaicin-evoked Glu release was significantly decreased by daily high-dose pretreatment with capsaicin for three consecutive days (Jin et al., 2006).

The capsaicin receptor, transient receptor potential vanilloid 1 (TRPV1), is located in a neurochemically heterogeneous population of small diameter primary afferent neurons (Tominaga et al., 1998). This receptor is sensitive to high temperature in the noxious range of 43°C to 50°C (Hardy, 1953; Beitel and Dubner, 1976; Caterina et al., 1997). Furthermore, repeated exposure to high-dose capsaicin selectively produces a prolonged influx of cations leading to desensitization of small-diameter sensory neurons to subsequent noxious stimulation (Yonehara et al., 1987; Lynn, 1990; Zhou et al., 1998; Caterina and Julius, 2001), while myelinated Aβ fibers are insensitive to capsaicin (Jancso et al., 1977; Nagy et al., 1983; Michael and Priestly, 1999).

There is an evidence suggesting possibility that capsaicin-evoked pain responses might be regulated by peripheral GluRs. In this connection, Lam et al. (2005) demonstrated that peripheral NMDA receptor modulate jaw muscle electromyographic activity induced by capsaicin injection into the temporomandibular joint of rats.

This study, therefore, has been done to elucidate at large in what manner Glu receptors and Glu existing in the peripheral endings of small-diameter afferent fibers and their extracellular space, respectively, are involved in development and/or maintenance of nociception evoked by capsaicin. Additionally, in order to demonstrate a link between the increase of Glu levels in the extracellular space following noxious stimulation and pain behavior, the changes in thermal withdrawal latency and the expression of c-Fos protein in the dorsal horn were determined following subcutaneous (s.c.) injection of drugs associated with Glu receptors with/without capsaicin.

2. Materials and methods

All surgical and experimental procedures for animals were reviewed and approved by the Ohu University Intramural Animal Care and Use Committee and conformed to the guidelines of the International Association for the Study of Pain (Zimmermann, 1983).

Interactions Between Glutamate Receptors and TRPV1 Involved in Nociceptive Processing at Peripheral
Endings of Primary Afferent Fibers

105

2.1 Experimental procedures

Adult male Sprague-Dawley rats weighing between 200-300 g (CLEA Japan, INC. Tokyo, Japan) were used in all experiments. Rats were on a 12 hrs light/dark cycle and received food and water ad libitum.

2.2 Release of Glu into the subcutaneous space

Animals were anesthetized with urethane (1 g/kg i.p.). A single loop catheter whose tip was covered with a 5000 molecular weight dialysis membrane (MS 0045, PSS® SELECT, Florida) was introduced into the s.c. space of the instep using a 2.2 mm outer diameter polyethylene tube as a guide. Ringer's solution was perfused at 15 µl/min through this catheter with a micro syringe pump (EP-60, Eicom, Kyoto, Japan) and perfusate was collected into the tubes placed in an ice bath at intervals of 20 min. The samples were kept at -80°C until analysis.

2.3 Amino acid analysis

Amino acids in the dialysate were analyzed by a high-performance liquid chromatography (HPLC) system for automated analysis of amino acids using o-phthalaldehyde derivatization and fluorescence detection. Amino acids were quantified by reverse-phase chromatography using a C_{18} octadecylsilyl (ODS) silica-gel column (EICOMPAK SC-50DS 2.1 mm x 150 mm) with pre-column (EICOM PREPAKSET-AC 3 mm x 4 mm). An HPLC system (HTEC500, EICOM) attaching this column consists of a pump connected with a degasser, a sampling injector with a sample processor and a cool pump, a fluorescence HPLC monitor and a personal computer with the data processor (Power Chrom; EPC-500, EICOM). The mobile phase used for separation of amino acids was 100 mM, pH 6 phosphate buffer containing 30% methanol and 10 µM EDTA. The flow rate was 0.23 ml/min. Peak areas of unknown substances were compared to those of control compounds for quantitation.

To determine the effect of drugs on the level of Glu, the average amounts of Glu concentration in two 20-min fractions collected over periods of 40 min before and after local application of capsaicin cream were obtained and expressed as percentages of the control value before stimulation.

2.4 Drug administration

While the animals were inside the small cage, drugs were administered into the s.c. left hindpaw in a volume of 50 µl using a 100 µl Hamilton syringe (Reno, NV, USA) with a 30-gauge needle without any anesthesia. The needle was inserted into the plantar skin proximal to the midpoint of the hindpaw. Capsazepine (30mg/kg) was injected in the volume of 50 µl into the s.c. of the neck.

2.5 Behavioral assessments

The Plantar Test (model 7370; Ugo Basile, Verese, Italy) was used in accordance with previously described methods (Yonehara et al., 1997) to determine whether the rats were hyperalgesic. In brief, prior to testing, the animals were placed in a small cage on a glass plate. They were not restrained and could move about and explore freely. Radiant heat was beamed onto the plantar surface of the hindpaw. The intensity of the beam was controlled and adjusted prior to the experiments, and the cutoff latency was set at 24 sec. The beam was applied to the test and control foot in turns and the latency of the withdrawal reflexes was recorded. The mean of the four responses was determined (Figs 4-8), and the ratio of the test foot latency divided by control foot latency, multiplied by 100, was calculated and termed the "percentage withdrawal latency" (Fig.3), at hourly intervals, from 1 hr before injection of the drugs to 6 h after the injection, except for 15 min after the injection

2.6 c-Fos immunohistochemistry

Two hours after the drug injection, animals were deeply anesthetized with sodium-pentobarbital and perfused transcardially with 100ml of 0.9% saline followed by 500 ml of 4% paraformaldehyde in 0.1 M phosphate buffer (PB; pH 7.4) and the spinal cord was taken out, postfixed in the same fixative overnight at 4°C, and then immersed into 20% sucrose in 0.1M PB at 4°C until it sank. Serial transverse 60 μm thick sections at L4-6 were cut using a freezing microtome and collected in 0.02 M phosphate buffered saline (PBS). Sections were washed in PBS for 30 min and blocked with 1% normal goat serum for 30 min and then incubated in a rabbit antibody against c-Fos (1:7000 dilution; Santa Cruz Biotech, Santa Cruz, CA, USA) for 60 min in room temperature and then for 12 hrs at 4°C. After washing in PBS for 30 min, sections were incubated in biotinylated goat anti-rabbit antiserum, and washed in PBS for 30 min and then immunohistochemically stained for 60 min using avidin-biotin-peroxidase complex (Vectastain, Vector Laboratories, Burlingame, CA, USA). To visualize peroxidase activity, sections were immersed in 0.05% diaminobenzidine tetrahydrochloride, 0.1% ammonium nickel sulfate and 0.01% hydrogen peroxide in 0.05 M Tris-HCl buffer (pH 7.2). Sections were washed in PBS for 30 min and then mounted on gelatin-coated slides, air-dried and coverslipped. The c-Fos-immunoreactive cells of 10 best-labeled sections were counted in the L5 spinal dorsal horn. In all these tests a double blind procedure was used to prevent the observers from knowing the experimental groups.

2.7 Drugs

The list of drugs and chemicals were as follows: as Glu receptors agonist, L-glutamic acid; selective NMDA receptor agonist, NMDA; AMPA receptor agonist, α-amino-3-hydroxy-4-isoxazoleproprionic acid (AMPA); selective group 1 mGlu receptor agonist, (S)-3,5-dihydroxyphenylglycine ((S)-3,5-DHPG); group II mGlu receptor agonist, (2S,1'S,2'S)-2-(carboxycyclopropyl) glycine (L-CCG-I); selective group III mGlu receptor agonist, L-(+)-2-amino-4-phosphonobutyric acid (L-AP4). The following drugs were used for Glu receptors antagonists, selective non-competitive NMDA receptor antagonist, (5S,10R)-(+)-5-Methyl-10,11-dihydro-5H-dibenzo[a,d] cyclo-hepten-5, 10-imine hydrogen maleate ((+)-MK-801 hydrogen maleate); competitive kainite/AMPA receptor antagonist, 6-Cyano-7-nitroquinoxaline-2,3-dione disodium (CNQX) and 2,3-Dioxo-6-nitro-1,2,3,4-tetrahydrobenzo[f]quinoxaline-7-sulfonamide disodium salt (NBQX); group 1 mGlu receptor selective non-competitive mGlu$_1$ receptor antagonist, 7-(hydroxyimino) cyclopropa[b]chromen-1a-carboxylate ethyl ester (CPCCOEt); group 1 mGlu receptor mGlu5 subtype-selective antagonist, 2-Methyl-6-(phenylethynyl)pyridine hydrochloride (MPEP); group II mGlu receptor antagonist, ((2S,3S,4S)-2-methyl-2-(carboxycyclopropyl)glycine

Interactions Between Glutamate Receptors and TRPV1 Involved in Nociceptive Processing at Peripheral
Endings of Primary Afferent Fibers

107

(MCCG); selective group III mGlu receptor antagonist, (RS)-α-methylserine-O-phoephate (MSOP). These compounds of Glu receptors were obtained from Tocris (Ballwin, MO, USA). 8-Methyl-N-vanillyl-6-noneamide (capsaicin) was obtained from Sigma Chemical Co. (USA). All other chemicals were obtained from Wako Pure Chemical Industries, Ltd. (Osaka, Japan).

In accordance with the product material safety data sheets, L-glutamate acid, L-CCG-I and L-AP4 were diluted in NaOH; and MK801, NMDA, (S)-3, 5,-DHPG, MCCG and MSOP were diluted in water. CNQX, CPCCOEt and MPEP were diluted in dimethyl sulphoxide. The other drugs except for these were dissolved in saline. Capsaicin was prepared as a 10 mg/ml solution in saline containing 10% ethanol and 10% Tween 80. The pH of all solutions was adjusted to 7.4. Capsazepine was dissolved in dimethyl formamide and then diluted with saline. O-phthalaldehyde was dissolved in methanol and adjusted to 4 mM with 0.1 M, pH 9.5 carbonate buffer.

2.8 Statistical analysis

All data are shown as mean ± S.E.M. In the study of Glu release, statistical analyses were performed using posthoc test of Fisher's protected least significant difference and $P<0.05$ was considered to be statistically significant. In the behavioral study, statistical analyses were performed with Dunnett's test for multiple comparison subsequent to analyses of variance. In the c-Fos immunohistochemichal study, a Student's test was used to test significant differences of the c-Fos expression between the treatments.

2.9 Abbreviations

AMPA; α-amino-3-hydroxy-4-isoxazole proprionic acid, Cap+MK801; Capsaicin combined with MK801, Cap+CNQX; Capsaicin combined with CNQX, Cap+NBQX; Capsaicin combined with NBQX, Cap+CPCCOEt; Capsaicin combined with CPCCOEt, Cap+MCCG; Capsaicin combined with MCCG, Cap+MSOP; Capsaicin combined with MSOP, CNQX; 6-Cyano-7-nitroquinoxaline-2,3-dione disodium, CPCCOEt; 7-(hydroxyimino) cyclopropa[b]chromen-1a-carboxylate ethyl ester, (S)-3,5-DHPG; (S)-3,5- dihydroxyphenylglycine, DRG; dorsal root ganglion, Glu, glutamate; L-CCG-I; (2S,1'S,2'S)-2-(carboxycyclopropyl) glycine, L-AP4; L-(+)-2-amino-4-phosphonobutyric acid, MCCG; (2S,3S,4S)-2-methyl-2-(carboxycyclopropyl) glycine, mGluRs; metabotropic glutamate receptors, (+)-MK-801; (5S,10R)-(+)-5-Methyl-10,11-dihydro-5H-dibenzo[a,d] cyclo-hepten-5, 10-imine hydrogen maleate, MPEP; 2-Methyl-6-(phenylethynyl) pyridine hydrochloride, MSOP; (RS)-α-methylserine-O-phoephate, NBQX; 2,3-Dioxo-6-nitro-1,2,3,4-tetrahydrobenzo[f]quinoxaline-7-sulfonamide disodium salt, NMDA; N-methyl-D-aspartic acid.

3. Results

3.1 Basal Glu release

The concentration of Glu in the perfusate was initially high, but gradually decreased with time reaching a stable level after 2 hrs of perfusion, which was then maintained for at least 4.5 h. Glu was present at 1.95 ± 0.25 μM (n=10, S.E.M.) in the resting state which is defined here as the mean of the two 20-min fraction collected from 80 min after starting perfusion to 120 min (fraction 5~6 in control group in Fig.1).

3.2 Effects of capsazepine on capsaicin-evoked Glu release

The s.c. injection of capsaicin (3 mM) in the vicinity of the perfusion side evoked a significant increase in Glu release (Fig.1). The average concentration of the released Glu was 4.86 ± 0.48 µM/20 min in 2 fractions collected after the injection of capsaicin. This augmentation of Glu release was last over 2 h. This effect was remarkably suppressed by preadministration of capsazepine (30 mg/kg, s.c.) 30 min before capsaicin injection (Fig.1). In the group of pretreatment with capsazepine, the average concentrations of the released Glu were 2.25 ± 0.4 µM/20 min and 2.36 ± 0.31 µM/20 min in 2 fractions collected after the injection of vehicle or capsaicin, respectively. S.c. injections of vehicle or capsazepine alone did not produce any significant changes in the levels of Glu in the perfusates.

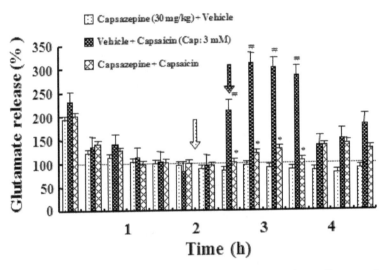

Fig. 1. Effect of capsazepine on the capsaicin-induced glutamate release. Capsazepine (s.c.) was injected subcutaneously into the neck 30 min before capsaicin treatment. Capsazepine (30 mg/kg) or vehicle for capsazepine, and capsaicin (3 mM) or vehicle for capsaicin were subcutaneously injected at the time indicated by the arrows, (⊡) and (⊠), respectively. All data are presented as the mean ± S.E.M. obtained from 10 animals. #P<0.05 compare with the value prior to s.c. administration of capsaicin+vehicle. *P<0.05 compared with capsaicin+vehicle (for capsazepine) group at each time measured.

3.3 Effects of iGluRs antagonists injection on capsaicin-evoked Glu release

The combined injection of capsaicin with MK801(1 mM) (Cap + MK-801) or NBQX (5 mM) (Cap + NBQX) into the perfusion region showed far less Glu release than injection of capsaicin alone (Fig 2-A). The average concentration of the released Glu was 1.20 ± 0.1 µM/ 20 min or 1.70 ± 0.1 µM/ 20min in 2 fractions collected after the co-injection of MK-801 or NBQX with capsaicin, respectively. These inhibitory effects of iGluRs antagonists sustained over 2.5 h.

Interactions Between Glutamate Receptors and TRPV1 Involved in Nociceptive Processing at Peripheral
Endings of Primary Afferent Fibers

109

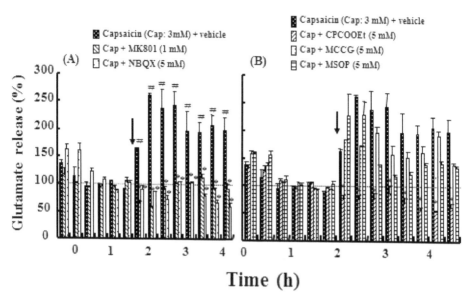

Fig. 2. Effect of the ionotropic (A) and metabotropic (B) glutamate receptor antagonists on
the capsaicin-induced glutamate release. The glutamate receptor antagonists were
subcutaneously injected together with capsaicin at the time indicated by the arrow. All data
are presented as the mean ± S.E.M. obtained from 10 animals. #$P<0.05$ compare with the
value prior to s.c. administration of capsaicin+vehicle. *$P<0.05$ compared with
capsaicin+vehicle group at each time measured. MK801, selective non-competitive NMDA
receptor antagonist; NBQX, competitive kainate/AMPA receptor antagonist; CPCOOEt,
group 1 mGlu receptor selective non-competitive mGlu$_1$ receptor antagonist; MCCG, group
II mGlu receptor antagonist; MSOP, selective group III mGlu receptor antagonist.

3.4 Effects of mGluRs antagonists injection on capsaicin-induced Glu release

At the doses employed, CPCCOEt (5 mM) (Cap + CPCCOEt) showed remarkable inhibition
in capsaicin-evoked Glu release. The average concentration of the released Glu was 1.46 ±
0.1 μM/ 20 min after the co-injection of CPCCOEt with capsaicin. S.c. combined injection of
MCCG (5 mM) (Cap + MCCG) or MSOP (5 mM) (Cap + MSOP) with capsaicin did not show
significant decrease in Glu release compared to capsaicin injection alone. The average
concentration of the released Glu was 3.68 ± 0.38 μM / 20 min or 4.31 ± 0.60 μM/ 20min in 2
fractions collected after the co-injection of MCCG or MSOP with capsaicin, respectively.
(Fig. 2-B)

3.5 Effects of capsazepine on capsaicin-induced thermal hypersensitivity

The mean withdrawal latencies to stimulation with radiant heat at pre-injection were 11.2 ±
0.3 s and 11.2 ± 0.3 s (n=40) on the left and right side, respectively (Fig.3-A). The withdrawal

latency did not significantly change after injection of vehicle or low dose of capsaicin (0.6 mM). A quarter and one h after injection of capsaicin (3 mM and 6 mM), withdrawal latency to irradiation decreased to much shorter than that of vehicle injection, which was recorded at the same interval (P<0.05), and then recovered gradually to the level of vehicle injection by 4 h after injection of capsaicin. Pretreatment of capsazepine (30 mg/kg, s.c.) produced a marked inhibition against capsaicin-induced thermal hyperalgesia (Fig.3-B). We did not observed any signs of motor deficiency or other side effects for any of the doses of any drugs in all paradigms described here and below.

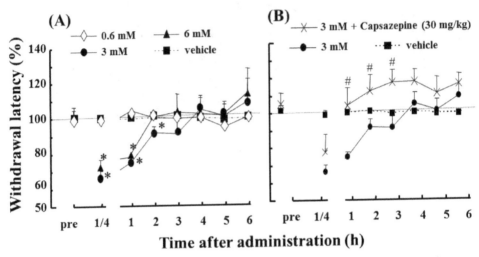

Time after administration (h)

Fig. 3. Time course of withdrawal latencies in response to noxious heat stimulation after s.c. injection of capsaicin, and co-injection of capsazepine with capsaicin. The data for each group (10 animals) are presented as the means ± S.E.M. The withdrawal latency per animal at respective time points was calculated as the average of the latencies obtained from 3 consecutive stimuli applied at intervals of 5 min. The value at time zero (pre) was obtained 1 h prior to s.c. injection of capsaicin. * and # P<0.05 significantly different from vehicle-treated group and capsaicin-treated group (3 mM), respectively.

3.6 Thermal sensitivity after injection of iGluRs agonists

S.c. injections of Glu, NMDA or AMPA produced dose-dependent decreases in withdrawal latency on the ipsilateral side 15 min after s.c. injection, and lasted for a few hours (Fig. 4). S.c. injection of vehicle did not produced any changes in thermal-withdrawal latency.

3.7 Thermal sensitivity after injection of mGluRs agonists

S.c. injection of (s)-DHPG caused a dose-dependent decrease in withdrawal latencies on the ipsilateral side from 15 min to 6 h, but L-CCG-I and L-AP4 did not show any significant changes (Fig. 5).

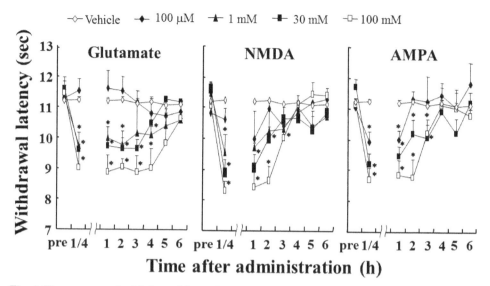

Fig. 4. Time course of withdrawal latencies in response to noxious heat stimulation after s.c.
injection of various concentration of the ionotropic glutamate receptor agonists; glutamate,
NMDA and AMPA. The data for each group (at least 10 animals) are presented as the means
± S.E.M. *P <0.05 significantly different from vehicle-treated group.

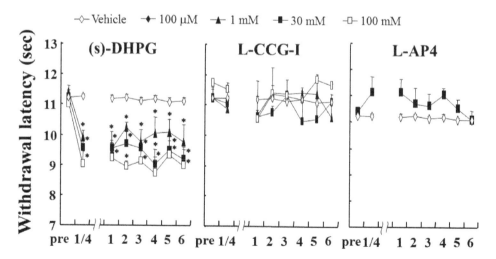

Fig. 5. Time course of withdrawal latencies in response to noxious heat stimulation after s.c.
injection of various concentration of the metabotropic glutamate receptor agonists; (s)-
DHPG, L-CCG-I and L-AP4. The data for each group (at least 10 animals) are presented as
the means ± S.E.M. *P <0.05 significantly different from vehicle-treated group.

3.8 Effect of iGluRs antagonists injection on capsaicin-induced thermal hypersensitivity

When MK801 or CNQX were injected together with capsaicin (Cap+MK801 or Cap+CNQX), a dose-dependent increase in withdrawal latency was observed. These analgesic effects of MK801 or CNQX on capsaicin-induced thermal hyperalgesia lasted for more than 6 h (Fig. 6). The single injection of MK801 or CNQX into the hindpaw did not show changes in withdrawal latencies compared to vehicle injection.

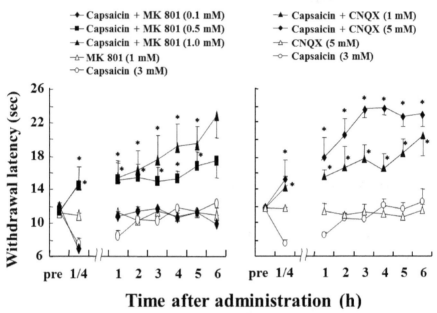

Fig. 6. Time course of withdrawal latencies in response to noxious heat stimulation after s.c. injection of capsaicin in combination with the ionotropic glutamate receptor antagonists; MK801 and CNQX. The data for each group (at least 10 animals) are presented as the means ± S.E.M. *P <0.05 significantly different from capsaicin (3 mM)-treated group.

3.9 Effect of mGluRs antagonists injection on capsaicin-induced thermal hypersensitivity

Following s.c. injection of CPCCOEt (5 mM), MPEP (30 mM), MCCG (5 mM), and MSOP (5 mM) into hindpaw, there was no changes in withdrawal latencies compared to vehicle injection (Figs. 7 and 8). When CPCCOEt or MPEP were injected together with capsaicin (Cap+CPCCOEt or Cap+MPEP), withdrawal latencies showed a dose-dependent increase from 15 min to 2~3 h after the injection compared with when capsaicin was injected alone (P<0.05) (Fig. 7). The heat insensitivity evoked in ipsilateral side following Cap+CPCCOEt and Cap+MPEP injection continued for 5 h or more. S.c. injection of MCCG or MSOP combined with capsaicin did not show any significant changes in withdrawal latencies compared to capsaicin injection alone (Fig. 8).

Interactions Between Glutamate Receptors and TRPV1 Involved in Nociceptive Processing at Peripheral Endings of Primary Afferent Fibers

113

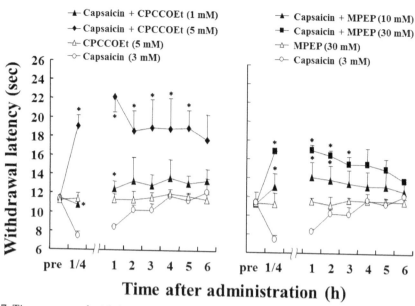

Fig. 7. Time course of withdrawal latencies in response to noxious heat stimulation after s.c. injection of capsaicin in combination with the metabotropic glutamate receptor antagonists; CPCCOEt and MPEP. The data for each group (at least 10 animals) are presented as the means ± S.E.M. *P <0.05 significantly different from capsaicin (3 mM)-treated group.

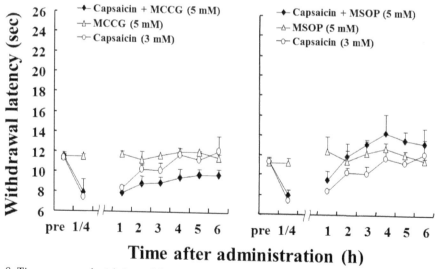

Fig. 8. Time course of withdrawal latencies in response to noxious heat stimulation after s.c. injection of capsaicin in combination with the metabotropic glutamate receptor antagonists; MCCG and MSOP. The data for each group (at least 10 animals) are presented as the means ± S.E.M

3.10 Basal c-Fos expression in dorsal horn after injection of vehicle, capsaicin and Glu into hindpaw

Immunoreactivity for c-Fos appeared gray-to-black and homogeneously labeled the oval or roundish nucleus of cells in spinal dorsal horn at L5 (Figs. 9-11). In all the experimental tests with injection of Glu, the maximum number of labeled cells occurred consistently in laminae I and II (I/II) of the spinal dorsal horn on the ipsilateral side (mean number ± S.E.M.=268 ± 21) (Figs. 9-11 and Table 1). Much smaller number of c-Fos immunopositive cells occurred in lamine III and IV (III/IV, 30 ± 7). The capsaicin-induced c-Fos expression in laminae I/II (489 ± 34) and laminae III/IV (63 ± 18) on the ipsilateral side was greater than that with Glu (Figs. 9, 10 and Table 1). The numbers of c-Fos-immunopositive cells on the contralateral side was modest either with glutamate (I/II, 16 ± 7; III/IV, 12 ± 6) or capsaicin (I/II, 44 ± 13; III/IV, 20 ± 9). In animals administered with vehicle, c-Fos-immunopositive cells were rarely distributed either in laminae I/II (60 ± 5) or in laminae III/IV (22 ± 8) on the ipsilateral side or on the contralateral side (I/II, 12 ± 4; III/IV, 7 ± 2) (Table 1).

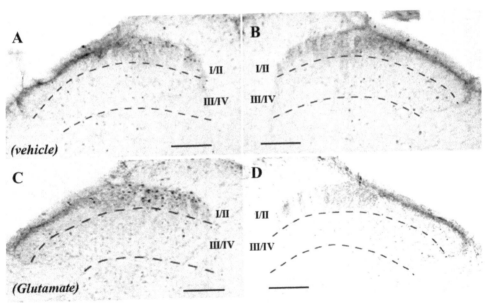

Fig. 9. Photomicrographs showing c-Fos-positive neurons in the dorsal horn of L5 2 h after hindpaw injection of vehicle and glutamate. A and C: ipisilateral side. B and D: contralateral side. Solid line indicates 100 μ m.

3.11 Effects of ionotropic Glu receptors antagonists injection on the capsaicin-induced c-Fos expression

Few c-Fos-immunopositive cells were found in laminae I/II and laminae III/IV of the ipsilateral dorsal horn after each single injection of ionotropic Glu receptors antagonists MK-801 (I/II, 79 ± 3; III/IV, 11 ± 7) and CNQX (I/II, 70 ± 8; III/IV, 7 ± 3) similar to vehicle

Interactions Between Glutamate Receptors and TRPV1 Involved in Nociceptive Processing at Peripheral
Endings of Primary Afferent Fibers

115

injection (I/II, 60 ± 5; III/IV, 22 ± 8). The numbers of capsaicin-induced c-Fos-immunopositive cells in laminae I/II (489 ± 34), but not in laminae III/IV (63 ± 18), were significantly decreased (P<0,005), when MK801 and CNQX were injected with capsaicin (Cap+MK801, I/II, 227 ± 32, III/IV, 14 ± 4; Cap+CNQX, I/II, 205 ± 40, III/IV, 11 ± 7) (Fig. 10 and Table 1). The numbers of capsaicin-induced c-Fos-immunopositive cells on the contralateral sides did not significantly change by any of drugs with/without capsaicin.

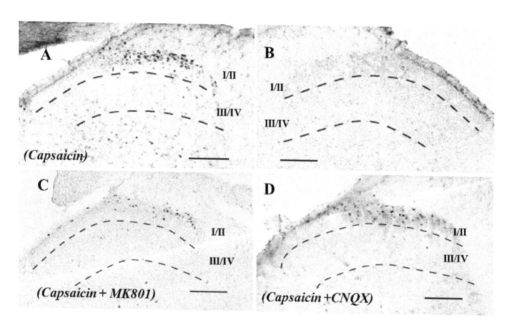

Fig. 10. Photomicrographs showing c-Fos-positive neurons in the dorsal horn of L5 2 h after hindpaw injection of capsaicin alone (A, B), combined with MK801 (C), and combined with MK801 CNQX (D). A, C and D: ipisilateral side. B: contralateral side. Solid line indicates 100 μ m.

3.12 Effects of metabotropic glu antagonists injeection on the capsaicin-induced c-Fos expression

Few c-Fos-immunopositive cells in the ipsilateral laminae I/II and III/IV, and fewer cells in the contralateral sides, were observed with single injection of CPCCOEt (I/II, 59 ± 8, III/IV, 1 ± 1), MCCG (I/II, 63 ± 10, III/IV, 3 ± 2) and MSOP (I/II, 66 ± 16, III/IV, 5 ± 3). Co-injection of CPCCOEt with capsaicin (Cap+CPCCOEt) significantly decreased the number of capsaicin-induced c-Fos-immunopositive cells in the ipsilateral laminae I/II (236 ± 58), but not in laminae III/IV (6 ± 4) and contralateral laminae I/II and III/IV. There was no significant change in the number of c-Fos-immunopositive cells in the ipsilateral laminae I/II, and III/IV by administration of MCCG combined with capsaicin (Cap+MCCG) or by administration of MSOP combined with capsaicin (Cap+MSOP; I/II, 383 ± 21, III/IV, 22 ± 3) compared to single injection of capsaicin, respectively (Fig. 11 and Table 1).

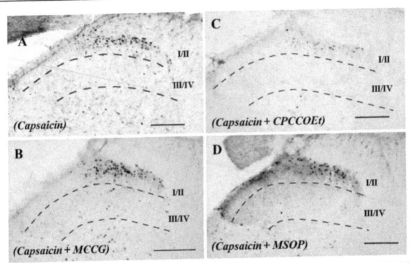

Fig. 11. Photomicrographs showing c-Fos-positive neurons in the dorsal horn of L5 2 h after hindpaw injection of capsaicin alone (A), combined with CPCCOEt (B), with MCCG (C), with MSOP (D). A, B, C and D: ipsilateral side. Solid line indicates 100 μ m.

Group	Ipsilateral		Contralateral	
	I/II-layer	III/IV-layer	I/II-layer	III/IV-layer
Vehicle	60 ± 5	22 ± 8	12 ± 4	7 ± 2
Capsaicin(Cap)	489 ± 34[*]	63 ± 18	44 ± 13	20 ± 9
Glutamate	283 ± 18[*]	36 ± 5	19 ± 8	12 ± 6
MK801	79 ± 3	11 ± 7	33 ± 12	9 ± 5
CNQX	70 ± 8	7 ± 3	14 ± 7	3 ± 2
CPCCOEt	59 ± 8	6 ± 3	10 ± 4	6 ± 2
MCCG	63 ± 10	5 ± 2	28 ± 11	5 ± 2
MSOP	66 ± 16	5 ± 3	9 ± 4	5 ± 3
Cap + MK801	227 ± 32[#]	14 ± 4	8 ± 6	3 ± 2
Cap + CNQX	205 ± 40[#]	11 ± 7	22 ± 12	3 ± 2
Cap + CPCCOEt	236 ± 58[#]	17 ± 11	12 ± 7	4 ± 3
Cap + MCCG	560 ± 85	27 ± 10	24 ± 9	3 ± 1
Cap + MSOP	383 ± 21	22 ± 3	18 ± 13	4 ± 1

Table 1. Mean value of c-Fos-positive neurons in the dorsal horn of L5 2 h after s.c. injection of Glu receptors agonists and antagonists. The value in each group was represented mean ± S.E.M. obtained from at least 10 animals, and the difference of the means was analyzed with the Student's t-test. * Significant difference at P< 0.05 between vehicle and capsaicin, or glutamate-treated group. #Significant difference at P< 0.05 between capsaicin and capsaicin+MK801, or capsaicin+CNQX, or capsaicin+CPCCOEt-treated group

Interactions Between Glutamate Receptors and TRPV1 Involved in Nociceptive Processing at Peripheral Endings of Primary Afferent Fibers

117

4. Discussion

We confirmed a large release of Glu immediately after the introduction of the catheter, followed by a rapid decrease, like in our previous study (Yonehara et al., 1987; Yonehara et al., 1992; Yonehara et al., 1995). Insertion of the polyethylene tube into the s.c. space of the rat instep did not evoke any inflammatory responses such as extravasation (Yonehara et al., 1995). All these data suggest that the basal levels of Glu in the s.c. perfusate were caused by neither acute noxious stimulation nor inflammation.

Topical application of capsaicin cream to the instep evoked a marked increase in Glu level in the s.c. perfusate, similar to the results in our previous study (Jin et al., 2006). In addition, electrical stimulation of the sciatic nerve or noxious heat stimulation (50°C) also caused an increase of Glu level in the s.c. space, and this capsaicin-evoked Glu release was significantly decreased by daily high-dose pretreatment with capsaicin for three consecutive days (Jin et al., 2006).

The TRPV1 is located in a neurochemically heterogeneous population of small diameter primary afferent neurons (Tominaga et al., 1998). Furthermore, repeated exposure to high-dose capsaicin selectively produces a prolonged influx of cations leading to desensitization of small-diameter sensory neurons to subsequent noxious stimulation (Yonehara et al., 1987; Lynn, 1990; Zhou et al., 1998; Caterina and Julius, 2001), while myelinated Aβ fibers are insensitive to capsaicin (Jancso et al., 1977; Nagy et al., 1983; Michael and Priestly, 1999). These findings and the present results suggest that the activation of capsaicin-sensitive afferent fibers by capsaicin causes release of Glu from the peripheral endings via activation of peripheral TRPV1, particularly from those of small-diameter fibers possibly through a mechanism such as the axon-reflex pathway, or autocrine and/or paracrine. It is reasonable to speculate that axon-reflex mechanism is involved in capsaicin-induced Glu release observed in Figs. 1 and 2, as only nociceptive afferent fibers have the axon-reflex mechanism which is localized on superficial tissues exposed to noxious influences (Celander and Folkow, 1953).

Amount of capsaicin-induced Glu release was remarkably decreased by concomitant administration of ionotropic Glu receptors antagonists; MK801 and NBQX, and mGluR I antagonist; CPCCOEt in the hindpaw, but not by administration of group II and III mGluR antagonist; MCCG and MSOP. These results suggest that peripheral ionotropic Glu receptors and group I mGluR appear to play a role in mediating capsaicin-evoked increases in Glu release. The Glu release through the activation of TRPV1 could then further activate ionotoropic Glu receptors and group I mGluR on the same neuronal terminal or adjacent neighboring peripheral terminals. In this connection, there were evidences supporting the co-localization of peripheral NMDA and TRPV1 receptors on the same primary afferent terminal (Lam et al., 2003; Lam et al., 2004).

Activation of peripheral Glu receptors could lead to enhance the Glu release in the peripheral tissues and might alter TRPV1 receptor responsiveness to reinforce nociceptive responses. As it is necessary to investigate the interaction between TRPV1 and glutamate receptors by using specific receptor antagonists of TRPV1 in detail, the mechanism to account for the antagonism of peripheral Glu receptors contributes to inhibit capsaicin-induced Glu release remains unanswered. However, it may be possible that glutamate receptors play a pivotal role for the activation of TRPV1 in the peripheral terminals. This idea is supported by the results that the intraplantar injection of ionotoropic Glu receptors and group I mGluR agonists evoked dose-dependent thermal hyperalgesia. Moreover, it is very interesting to note that injection of Glu receptors antagonists alone did not produce any changes on withdrawal latency, and intraplantar co-injection of ionotropic Glu receptors and group I mGluR antagonists with capsaicin not only antagonized capsaicin-induced hyperalgesia, but also resulted in remarkable longer withdrawal latency to heat irradiation.

Concerning the mechanism that ionotoropic Glu receptors and mGluR antagonists produced remarkable analgesic action in the presence of capsaicin, there is evidence that capsaicin injected into the rat temporomandibular joint evoked a dose-dependent increase in jaw muscle electromyographic activity. This capsaicin-evoked increase in electromyographic activity was attenuated by ipsilateral injection of NMDA receptor antagonists into the temporomandibular joint (Lam et al. 2005). This finding and our present results indicate that the activation of peripheral Glu receptors, especially ionotropic Glu receptors and group I mGluR could be indispensable in the mechanisms whereby capsaicin evokes nociceptive responses.

The ionotropic, and metabotropic subunits of Glu receptors are present in DRG cell bodies and on unmyelinated fibers in the glabrous skin of the mammalian foot (Carlton et al., 1995; Bhave et al., 2001; Carlton et al., 2001; Sato et al., 1993; Carlton et al., 2007). It is well established that the excitatory amino acids in the peripheral endings of small-diameter afferent fibers contribute to development and/or maintenance of pain in humans (Nordlind et al., 1993; Warncke et al., 1997) and in laboratory animals (Davidson et al., 1997; Cairns et al., 1998; Davidson et al., 1998). For example, peripherally applied NMDA and non-NMDA receptor antagonists attenuate or block nociceptive behaviors in several animal models of inflammation (Jackson et al., 1995; Lawand et al., 1997; Carlton et al., 1998).

In the present study, we examined the c-Fos expression in spinal cord dorsal horn following injection of drugs associated with glutamate receptors with/without capsaicin into the hindpaw. c-Fos is rapidly and transiently induced in cells of the spinal dorsal horn after noxious stimulation (Hunt et al., 1987, Strassman and Vos, 1993, Takemura et al., 2000), c-Fos has been widely used as a marker for analyzing nociceptive processing.

Our present data support the view that Glu receptors, in particular, ionotropic Glu receptors and group I mGluR existing in peripheral ending of capsaicin-sensitive afferent fibers play an important role on development and/or maintenance of pain following excitation of TRPV1. In addition, the formulation of the peripheral ionotoropic Glu receptors and group I mGluR antagonists that do not cross the blood brain barrier may be of potential benefit by reducing peripheral nociceptive excitability, and therefore they could provide a new therapeutic target to pain control in the periphery.

5. References

Battaglia, G., and Rustioni, A., 1988. Coexistence of glutamate and substance P in dorsal root ganglion neurons of the rat and monkey. J. Comp. Neurol. 277, 302-312.

Beitel, R.E., and Dubner, R., 1976. Response of unmyelinated (C) polymodal nociceptors to thermal stimuli applied to monkey's face. J. Neurophysiol. 39, 1160-1175.

Interactions Between Glutamate Receptors and TRPV1 Involved in Nociceptive Processing at Peripheral
Endings of Primary Afferent Fibers

119

Bhave, G., Karim, F., Carlton, S.M., and Gereau IV, R.W., 2001. Peripheral group I metabotropic glutamate receptors modulate nociception in mice. Nature 4, 417-423.

Cairns, B.E., Sessle, B.J., and Hu, J.W., 1998. Evidence that excitatory amino acid receptors within the temporomandibular joint region are involved in the reflex activation of the jaw muscles. J. Neurosci. 18, 8056-8064.

Carlton, S.M., Hargett, G.L., and Coggeshall, R.E., 1995. Localization and activation of glutamate receptors in unmyelinated axons of rat glabrous skin. Neurosci. Lett. 197, 25-28.

Carlton, S.M., Zhou, S., and Coggeshall, R.E., 1998. Evidence for the interaction of glutamate and NK1 receptors in the periphery. Brain Res. 790, 160-169.

Carlton, S.M., 2001. Peripheral excitatory amino acids. Current Opinion in Pharmacology, 1, 52-56.

Carlton, S.M., and Hargett, G.L., 2007. Colocalization of metabotropic glutamate receptors in rat dorsal root ganglion cells. J. Comp. Neurol. 501, 780-789.

Caterina, M.J., Schumacher, M.A., Tominaga, M., Rosen, T.A., Levine, J.D., and Julius, D., 1997. The capsaicin receptor: a heat-activated ion channel in the pain pathway. Nature. 389, 816-24.

Caterina, M.J., and Julius, D., 2001. The vanilloid receptor: a molecular gateway to the pain pathway. Annu. Rev. Neurosci. 24, 487-517.

Celander, O., and Folkow, B., 1953. The nature and the distribution of afferent fibers provided with the axon reflex arrangement. Acta Physiol. Scand. 29, 369-370.

Coggeshall, R.E., and Carlton, S.M., 1998. Ultrastructural analysis of NMDA, AMPA and kainate receptors on unmyelinated and myelinated axons in the periphery. J. Comp. Neurol. 391, 78-86.

Davidson, E.M., Coggeshall, R.E., and Carlton, S.M., 1997. Peripheral NMDA and non-NMDA glutamate receptors contribute to nociceptive behaviors in the rat formalin test. Neuroreport 8, 941-946.

Davidson, E.M., and Carlton, S.M., 1998. Intraplantar injection of dextrorphan, ketamine or memantine attenuates formalin-induced behaviors. Brain Res. 785, 136-142.

Du, J., Zhou, S., Coggeshall, R.E. and Carlton, S.M., 2003. N-methyl-d-aspartate-induced excitation and sensitization of normal and inflamed nociceptors. Neuroscience 118, 547–562.

Follenfant, R.L., and Nakamura-Craig, M., 1992. Glutamate induces hyperalgesia in the rat paw. Br. J. Pharmacol. 106, 49P

Hardy, J.D., 1953. Thresholds of pain and reflex ontraction as releated to noxious stimuli. J. Appl. Physiol. 5, 725-739.

Hu, H.-J., Bhave, G., and Gereau IV R.W., 2002. Prostaglandin and protein kinase A-dependent modulation of vanilloid receptor function by metabotropic glutamate receptor 5: Potential mechanism for thermal hyperalgesia. J Neurosci. 22, 7444–7452.

Hunt, S.P., Pini, A., and Evan, G., 1987. Induction of c-fos-like protein in spinal cord neurons following sensory stimulation. Nature 328, 632-634.

Jackson, D.L., Graff, C.B., Richardson, J.D., and Hargreaves, K.M., 1995. Glutamate participates in the peripheral modulation of thermal hyperalgesia in rats. Eur. J. Pharmacol. 284, 321-325.

Jancso, G., Kiraly, E., and Jancso-Gabor, A., 1977. Pharmacologically induced selective degeneration of chemosensitive primary sensory neurons. Nature 270, 741-743.

Jin, Y.H., Nishioka, H., Wakabayashi, K., Fujita, T., and Yonehara, N., 2006. Effect of morphine on the release of excitatory amino acids in the rat hind instep: pain is modulated by the interaction between the peripheral opioid and glutamate systems. Neuroscience 138, 1329-1339.

Keast, J.R., and Stephensen, T.M., 2000. Glutamate and aspartate immunoreactivity in dorsal root ganglion cells supplying visceral and somatic targets and evidence for peripheral axonal transport. J. Comp. Neurol. 424, 577-587.

Kinkelin, I., Brocker, E.-B., Koltzenburg, M., and Carlton, S.M., 2000. Localization of ionotropic glutamate receptors in peripheral axons of human skin. Neurosci. Lett. 283, 149-152.

Lam, D.K., Sessle, B.J. and Hu, J.W., 2003. Glutamate and capsaicin-induced activation primary afferents. (Abst) Program No. 294.6, Abstract Viewer/Itinerary Planner, Society for Neuroscience, Washington, DC (Online) .

Lam, D.K., Sessle, B.J. and Hu, J.W., 2004. Glutamate and capsaicin-evoked activity in deep craniofacial trigeminal nociceptive afferents. (Abst) Program No. 3817., Abstract Viewer/Itinerary Planner, International Association for Dental Research.

Lam, D.K., Sessle, B.J., Cairns, B.E. and Hu, J.W., 2005. Peripheral NMDA receptor modulation of jaw muscle elecromyographic activity induced by capsaicin injection into the temporomandibular joint of rats. Brain Res. 1046, 68-76.

Laurie, D.J., Putzke, J, Zieglgansberger, W, Seeburg, P.H. and Tolle, T.R., 1995. The distribution of splice variants of the NMDAR1 subunit mRNA in adult rat brain. Mol. Brain Res. 32, 94-108.

Lawand, N.B., Willis, W.D., and Westlund, K.N., 1997. Excitatory amino acid receptor involvement in peripheral nociceptive transmission in rats. Eur. J. Pharmacol. 324, 169-177.

Lee, K.S., Kim, J., Yoon, Y.W., Lee, M.G., Hong, S.K., Han, H.C., 2007. The peripheral role of group I metabotropic glutamate receptors on nociceptive behaviors in rats with knee joint inflammation. Neurosci. Lett. 416, 123–127.

Leem, J.W., Hwang, J.H., Hwang, S.J., Park, H., Kim, M.K., and Choi, Y., 2001. The role of peripheral N-methyl-d-aspartate receptors in Freund's complete adjuvant induced mechanical hyperalgesia in rats. Neurosci. Lett. 297, 155-158.

Liu, H., Wang, H., Sheng, M., Jan, L.Y., and Basbaum, A.I., 1994. Evidence for presynaptic N-methyl-D-aspartate autoreceptors in the spinal cord dorsal horn. Proc. Natl. Acad. Sci. USA 91, 8383-8387.

Lynn B., 1990. Capsaicin: Actions on nociceptive C-fibers and therapeutic potential. Pain 41, 61-69.

Michael, G.J., and Priestly, J.V., 1999. Differential expression of the mRNA for the vanilloid receptor subtype 1 in cells of the adult rat dorsal root and nodose ganglia and its downregulation by axotomy. J. Neurosci. 19, 1844-1854.

Nagy, J.I., Iversen, L.I., Goedert, M., Chapman, D., and Hunt, S.P., 1983. Dose-dependent effects of capsaicin on primary sensory neurons in the neonatal rat. J. Neurosci. 3, 399-406.

Interactions Between Glutamate Receptors and TRPV1 Involved in Nociceptive Processing at Peripheral
Endings of Primary Afferent Fibers

121

Nordlind, K., Johansson, O., Liden, S., and Hökfelt, T., 1993. Glutamate- and aspartate-like immunoreactivities in human normal and inflamed skin. Cell Path. Mol. Path. 64, 75-82.

Omote, K., Kawamata, T., Kawamata, M., and Namiki, A., 1998. Formalin-induced release of excitatory amino acids in the skin of the rat hindpaw. Brain Res. 787, 161-164.

Sato, K., Kiyama, H., Park, H.T., and Tohyama, M., 1993. AMPA, KA and NMDA receptors are expressed in the rat DRG neurones. Neuroreport 4, 1263-1265.

Strassman, A.M., and Vos, B.P., 1993. Somatotopic and laminar organization of Fos-like immunoreactivity in the medullary and upper dorsal horn induced by noxious facial stimulation in the rat. J. Comp. Neuro. 331, 495-516.

Takemura, M., Shimada, T., Sugiyo, S., Nokubi, T., and Shigenaga, Y., 2000. Mapping of c-Fos in the trigeminal sensory nucleus following high- and low-intensity afferent stimulation in the rat. Exp. Brain Res. 130, 113-123.

Tominaga, M., Caterina, M.J., Malmberg, A.B., Rosen, T.A., Gilbert, H., Skinner, K., Raumann, B.E., Basbaum, A.I., and Julius, D., 1998. The Cloned Capsaicin Receptor Integrates Multiple Pain-Producing Stimuli. Neuron 21, 531-543.

Walker, K., Reeve, A., Bowes, M., Winter J., Wotherspoon G., Davis A., Schmid, P., Gasparini, F., Kuhn R., and Urban, L., 2001. mGlu5 receptors and nociceptive function II. mGlu5 receptors functionally expressed on peripheral sensory neurones mediate inflammatory hyperalgesia. Neuropharmacol. 40, 10–19

Warncke, T., Jorum, E. and Stubhaug, A., 1997. Local treatment with the N-methyl-D-aspartate receptor antagonist ketamine, inhibits development of secondary hyperalgesia in man by a peripheral action. Neurosci. Lett. 227, 1-4.

Westlund, K.N., McNeill, D.L., and Coggeshall, R.E., 1989. Glutamate immnoreactivity in rat dorsal roots. Neurosci. Lett. 96, 13-17.

Westlund, K.N., Sun, Y.C., Sluka, K.A., Dougherty, P.M., Sorkin, L.S., and Willis, W.D., 1992. Neural changes in acute arthritis in monkeys. II. Increased glutamate immunoreactivity in the medial articular nerve. Brain Res. Rev. 17, 15-27.

Yanga, D., and Gereau IV, R.W., 2003. Peripheral group II metabotropic glutamate receptors mediate endogenous anti-allodynia in inflammation. Pain 106, 411–417.

Yonehara, N., Shibutani, T., and Inoki, R., 1987. Contribution of substance P to heat-induced edema in rat paw. J. Pharmacol. Exp. Ther. 242, 1071-1076.

Yonehara, N., Imai, Y., Chen, J.-Q., Takiuchi, S., and Inoki, R., 1992. Influence of opioids on substance P release evoked by antidromic stimulation of primary afferent fibers in the hind instep of rats. Regulatory Peptides 38, 13-22.

Yonehara, N., Saito, K., Oh-ishi, S., Katori, M., and Inoki, R., 1995. Contribution of bradykinin to heat-induced substance P release in the hind instep of rats. Life Science 56, 1679-1688.

Yonehara, N., Takemura, M., Yoshimura, M., Iwase, K., Seo, H.G., Taniguchi, N. and Shigenaga, Y., 1997. Nitric oxide in the rat spinal cord in Freund's adjuvant-induced hyperalgesia. Jpn. J. Pharmacol. 75, 327-335.

Zhou, L., Zhang, Q., Stein, C., and Schafer, M., 1998. Contribution of opioid receptors on primary afferent versus sympathetic neurons to peripheral opioid analgesia. J. Pharmacol. Exp. Ther. 286, 1000-1006.

Zhou, S., Bonasera, L., and Carlton, S.M., 1996. Peripheral administration of NMDA, AMPA or KA results in pain behaviors in rats. Neuroreport 7, 895-900.

Zhou, S., Komak, S., Du, J., and Carlton, S.M., 2001. Metabotropic glutamate 1a receptors on peripheral primary afferent fibers: their role in nociception. Brain Res. 913, 18-26.

Zou, X, Lin, Q, Willis, W.D., 2002. Role of protein kinase A in phosphorylation of NMDA receptor 1 subunits in dorsal horn and spinothalamic tract neurons after intradermal injection of capsaicin in rats. Neuroscience 115, 775-786.

Zimmermann, M., 1983. Ethical guidelines for investigations of experimental pain in conscious animals. Pain 16, 109-110.

6

Peroxisome Proliferator Activated Receptor Alpha (PPARα) Agonists: A Potential Tool for a Healthy Aging Brain

Jennifer Tremblay-Mercier

Université de Sherbrooke, Research Center on Aging
Canada

1. Introduction

1.1 Definitions and considerations

Cognitive decline related to advancing age includes many sub-categories of diseases, some more or less well defined and understood. First, there is "normal" cognitive decline, which is gradual and progressive during aging and seems inevitable. When cognitive decline is large enough to disrupt the activities of daily life, a state of dementia is diagnosed. There are several types of dementia according to the etiology of cognitive decline: vascular dementia, which results from a circulatory disorder causing an obstruction of cerebral blood vessels which leads to the progressive degeneration of brain cells due to a lack of oxygen. Vascular dementia represents 20% of all cases of dementia. Lewis body dementia is an accumulation of α-synuclein protein within the cell and it represents 5 to 15% of neurodegenerative diseases. Frontotemporal dementia as the name suggests, is a degeneration of the region of the frontal and temporal anterior cortex. The reasons for this degeneration are not fully understood. Alzheimer's disease (AD) represents the majority of cases of dementia (65%) although its etiology is not known exactly, or rather multi-factorial.

The most accepted theory in the medical community to explain the origin of AD is currently the accumulation of β-amyloid protein in the form of plaques accompanied by neurofibrillary tangles of tau protein that cause neuronal death and loss of brain matter. However, this theory is challenged for many reasons. The high profile failures of anti-amyloid interventions and lack of agreement on which form the β-amyloid is toxic and the mechanism by which this occurs force the scientific community to consider amyloid only as one part of a multi-factorial disease process including a variety of aggravating factors. A recent paper entitled "Changing perspectives on Alzheimer's Disease: Thinking outside the amyloid Box" resume this thinking (D'Alton & George, 2011).

1.2 Alzheimer's disease diagnosis

The clinical diagnosis of AD is based on clinical examination and confirmed by neuropsychological tests and is diagnosed through exclusion. That means if the person presents a certain profile of cognitive decline and does not match certain criteria (Table 1) the patient is put into the broad category of "probable" AD (Whitehouse, 2008). Within this category there are "typical" Alzheimer and those who are called "atypical" which means that their profile may include some features of vascular dementia or components of Lewis Body dementia. In 2011, the use of brain imaging (Positrons Emission Tomography (PET) and Magnetic Resonance Imaging (MRI)) can optimize the basic clinical diagnosis (clinical and neuropsychological data) of atypical profile, if this kind of technological platform is available. However, it is only at death that the diagnosis can be confirmed by neuropathological brain examination of the abundance of β-amyloid plaques and neurofibrillary tangle, even if the amyloid theory is increasingly questioned. Not surprisingly, neuropathological diagnosis of post-mortem brain does not always correlate with the clinical diagnosis. One classic example is the "Nun Study" from Chicago (Snowdon et al., 1997), in this study, several participants showed abundant neurofibrillary tangles and β-amyloid plaques at the post-mortem analysis, but had not received a clinical diagnosis of AD and were mentally intact during their life. The opposite was also seen i.e. that a person with a clinical AD diagnostic presented an intact brain (no neuropathology) at death.

Diagnosis of probable AD will be posed only :
IF THE PATIENT DOES NOT PRESENT:
Hypothyroidism; other metabolic problem
Vascular problem
Vitamine deficit (Vitamin B12)
Hypercalcemia
Hydrocephalus
Head injury
Psychiatric disorders (depression, schizophrenia)
Structural brain lesion (tumor, injury, blood clot)
Other degenerative disease (Parkinson disease)
Simulation or factitious disorder
Dehydration or other sources of confusion / delirium
Brain infection (HIV, encephalitis, meningitis, syphilis)
Chronic effects of various substances (alchool, drugs)

Table 1. Alzheimer's Disease: diagnosis of exclusion (Adapted from Whitehouse, 2008)

The mismatch between clinical diagnosis and aβ and tau neuropathology at death shakes the causation link and suggests the importance of other aspects in the etiology of the cognitive decline associated with aging.

1.3 Physiopathology: Focus on brain metabolism

In addition to the abnormal protein (aβ, tau, α-synuclein) present in the demented brains, there is also a decrease in brain glucose metabolism in the majority of dementia. The brain is one of the most metabolically active organs. Despite representing about 2% of adult body weight, the brain uses about 23 % of the body's total energy needs. The brain gets its energy from glucose to 97% making it the main energy substrate. Every day, an average human brain consumes approximately 16% of the total oxygen consumption and metabolizes approximately 110 to 145 g of glucose. Over 90% of used glucose is oxidized to ensure the supply of ATP which is vital for the cells and maintenance of synaptic transmission (Henderson, 2008). The determination of the brain glucose metabolism pattern is used in the differential diagnosis of dementia using Position Emission Tomography (PET) imaging with an analog of glucose; [18]fluorodeoxyglucose ([18]FDG). The cerebral glucose hypometabolism in cases of AD has been known since the 1980s with the beginning of PET imaging and represents about 20% reduction but varies between 8 and 49% (reviewed in Cunnane et al., 2011).

In the case of AD, several evidences shows that brain glucose hypometabolism is present in certain regions well before the first clinical signs of cognitive decline, so it is not simply the result of neuronal loss but rather would be responsible for this loss. For example, in a clinical study containing 20 AD patients and 20 young adults (20-39 years old) at risk of developing AD (carrier of the Apolipoprotein E4 allele; ApoE4), small areas of cortical glucose hypometabolism were present in the young participants, especially in the posterior cingulate, parietal, temporal and prefrontal cortex. These hypometabolic regions were the same in the AD patients but in a more extensive way. This reduction in brain glucose metabolism may be the earliest brain abnormalities yet found in living persons at risk for AD (Reiman et al., 2004).

It is still unclear as to whether or not healthy aging (no cognitive impairment) is associated with reduction in brain glucose metabolism. Cunnane and colleages reviewed the literature on this specific question and they found out that eight studies showed that cerebral glucose metabolism does not decline with healthy aging and nine studies have demonstrated that it does in a proportion of about 18% (Cunnane et al., 2011.)

The reason for this alteration in brain glucose metabolism is not clearly elucidated. It could be a problem in the glucose transport, glucose availability, or a dysfunction in the production of energy derived from glucose. Mitochondria play a central role in producing ATP as the central source of cellular energy, so a dysfunction at the mitochondria level is conceivable.

The brain uses glucose as main energy source but can also use ketones as an alternative energy source in situations of glucose deprivation (fasting, intense physical activity). Ketones refer to 3 molecules: acetoacetate, β-hydroxybutyrate (β-OHB) and acetone. In starvation conditions, up to 60% of the human brain energy requirements can be met by ketones (Owen, 1967). Whether ketone brain metabolism is also decreasing in healthy aging or in AD is not yet known, but Cunnane's team developed a ketone radiotracer (^{11}C-acetoacetate) especially to be able to study brain ketone metabolism in the elderly; studies are ongoing. Based on the fact that ketones are energetic molecules and used by the brain as an alternative to glucose, some studies have demonstrated the ability of ketones to improve some cognitive dysfunction in diabetic hypoglycemia (Page et al., 2009) and even in case

AD (Henderson et al., 2009). Although brain ketone metabolism is less known in the elderly population, fundamental and clinical studies suggests that they could represents an interesting therapeutic potential for cognitive decline (reviewed in Veech et al., 2001)

1.4 Risk factors: Importance of the metabolic condition

In addition to understanding the physiopathology underlying the cognitive decline it is important to know the factors that increase the risk of being affected by a decline in cognitive function to help prevent them. Aging is the main factor and it often say that it is inevitable. It is true that the passage of time cannot be slowing down, but individuals can play a role in modifying their "biological" age or their metabolic condition. Effectively, aging naturally tends to reduce the cognitive functioning but also worsen the metabolic condition. At advanced age, the prevalence of hypertension, dyslipidemia, inflammation, atherosclerosis and diabetes increase. To prevent these metabolic problems, it is highly documented that the adoption of a healthy lifestyle (physical activities and equilibrate diet) through the lifespan is an efficient way (Colcombe et al., 2003, Peters, 2009.) It turns out that having a bad metabolic condition raises up the risk to develop a cognitive disorder (Frisardi et al., 2010) Peripheral problems and brain disorders are often dissociated but a close relationship exist between these two entities.

Having type II diabetes is associated with the increased risk of developing a cognitive disorder. More than 80% of AD patients have type II diabetes or present an abnormal glucose level. Insulin resistance and hyperinsulinemia, two characteristics of type II diabetes, have been shown to have a high correlation with memory impairment and risk for AD. The rising insulin level that occurs with aging is also a strong predicator of cognitive impairments, in non-diabetics. (Landreth et al., 2008). The Italian Longitudinal study on aging shows that patients with mild cognitive impairment who were also afflict by metabolic syndrome had a higher risk of progression to dementia compared with those without metabolic syndrome. Hypertriglyceridemia was the major component of metabolic syndrome related to dementia (Solfrizzi et al., 2009). Genetic studies and epidemiological observations strongly suggest a relationship between dyslipidemia and AD. Elevated serum cholesterol levels have been reported to correlate with an increased incidence of AD (Landreth et al., 2008). Longitudinal studies have reported that obesity and chronic hypertension are also associated with higher risk of cognitive decline (reviewed in Frisardi et al., 2010).

Then, improvement in those metabolic parameters could modify the individual risk for dementia. Preventive activities during the lifespan are primordial but changing individual behaviour is a long term challenge for the public health. The use of metabolic regulator as a secondary prevention may become essential in individuals at middle age who presents a poor metabolic condition (high blood glucose, deteriorated lipids profile, hypertension, etc.) not only to prevent heart diseases but precisely to delay the first signs of cognitive decline. Given that tertiary prevention of AD dementia which refers to anticholinesterase drugs is known to modestly delay progression of dementia because its probaby too late to correct the existing damage, primary and secondary prevention are essentials (Haan & Wallace 2004) (figure 1).

It is well known that if you want to avoid a pulmonary cancer you should not smoke cigarettes, but the population feels armed less in front of neurodegenerative disorders and should not: progression to dementia can be prevented or modified (Haan et Wallace 2004).

2. PPARα

2.1 Mecanisms, pathways, activators

Peroxisome Proliferator Activated Receptor alpha (PPARα) is a nuclear receptor present in tissues where fatty acids catabolism is at elevated rate, especially in liver but also in heart, kidney, skeletal muscles, enterocytes and astrocytes. This receptor is activated by fatty acids and their derivates and among the synthetic ligands; by compounds of the fibrate family. PPARα regulates gene expression by associating with his ligand in the cytoplasm of cells; the complex then migrates into the nucleus and binds with the 9-cis retinoic acid receptor (RXR). The heterodimer (PPARα/RXR) recognizes specific response elements (peroxisome proliferator response element; PPRE) presents in the promoter regions of genes and binds to activate or repress (figure 2).

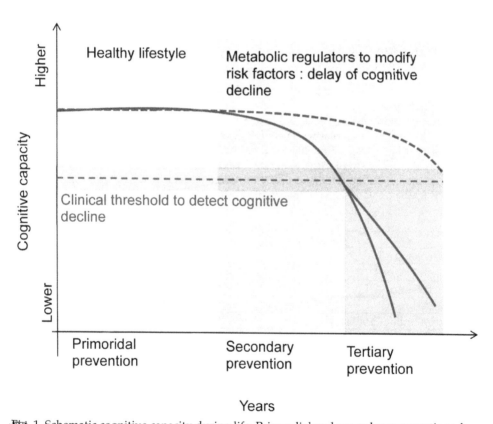

Years

Fig. 1. Schematic cognitive capacity during life. Primordial and secondary preventions, by regulating metabolic condition, may maintain cognitive capacity above the clinical threshold of cognitive decline. Tertiary prevention can modestly help to delays progression of dementia once it is installed. Progression of cognitive capacity in Alzheimer's disease (___) and in cognitively healthy elderly (_ _).

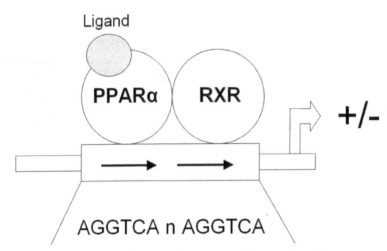

Fig. 2. Following activation with the ligand, PPARα binds a specific DNA sequence (PPRE) in the promoter region of target genes.

PPARα regulates gene associated with lipids, glucose and energy metabolism and exert an anti-inflammatory activity (table 2). Fibrates are first-line drugs used for over 40 years to treat hypertriglyceridemia and their mode of action is entirely via the activation of PPARα. Effectively, fibrates reduces plasma level of triglycerides by 30-50%, slightly increase HDL-cholesterol by up to 5-15 % and usually reduces LDL-cholesterol by 15 to 20% (Chapman et al., 2006). By the activation of PPARα, fibrates are effective to stimulate lipolysis, to increase cellular and mitochondrial fatty acid uptake, to promote fatty acid oxidation, to reduce TG production by the liver, to increase the VLDL clearance and to increase the HDL-cholesterol synthesis.

Genes	Expression	Functions
Apolipoprotein CIII	↓	VLDL clearance inhibition
Lipoprotein Lipase	↑	Lipolysis
Apolipoprotein AI AII	↑	HDL cholesterol synthesis
SR-BI/CLA-1 receptor	↑	Cholesterol efflux
Fatty Acid Binding Protein	↑	Fatty acids entry into the cell
AcylCoA Synthase	↑	Fatty acids entry into the mitochondria
AcetylCoA carboxylase	↓	Fatty acids synthesis
Fibrinogen	↓	Blood clotting
C reactive protein	↓	Inflammation
Interleukin 6	↓	Inflammation
Cyclooxygenase-2	↓	Arachidonic acid metabolism
VCAM-1	↓	Adhesion molecules

Table 2. Target genes regulated by PPARα (Goldenberg et al., 2008). Abbreviations: VLDL: very low density lipoprotein. SR-BI/CLA1: class B scavenger receptor. VCAM-1: vascular cell adhesion molecule 1.

Clofibrate is a first generation fibrate and was used for numerous years before the arrival of the second generation comprising bezafibrate and fenofibrate which are more selective and causes fewer side effects (figure 3). Clofibric acid and fenobibric acid (active metabolites of clofibrate and fenofibrate) activate PPARα and PPARγ but they are 10 times more selective to PPARα. Bezafibrate activates PPARα but can also be linked to PPARγ and PPARδ.

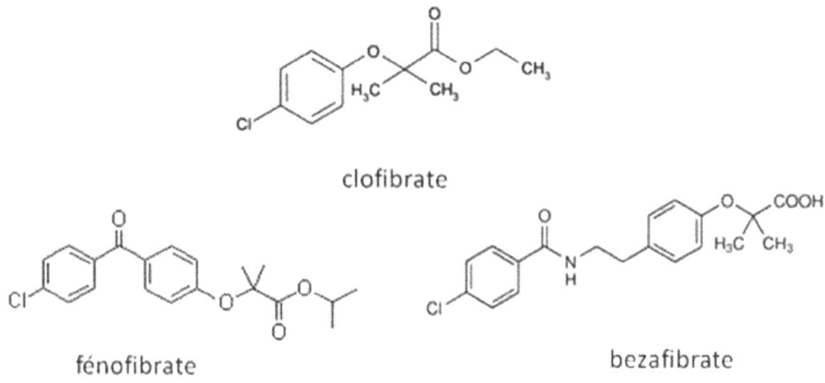

clofibrate

fénofibrate

bezafibrate

Fig. 3. Structures of clofibrate, fenofibrate and bezafibrate.

2.2 How can PPARα stimulation help cognitive functioning?

The impact of PPARα agonists on cognition was not deeply investigated at a large scale level but some observational studies are interesting. In a large Europeean study (8582 subjects) fibrate use tended (p=0.07) to be associated with a reduction in the prevalence of dementia. Dementia included AD (65%), vascular dementia (12%), mixed dementia (11%) and other form of dementia (11.7%). Prevalence of dementia was 1.5% among fibrates user and 2.3% among non-user (Dufouil et al., 2005). In another observational study Rodriguez et al, showed that in a population of 845 individuals, 20.1% of the cohort were demented (based on Clinical dementia Rating) and the proportion of lipid lowering drugs user within the demented population was lower compared to the non-demented (3.5% versus 10.8%) which suggest that lipid lowering drugs may be protective (Rodriguez et al., 2002). In an older study, reducing triglycerides with gemfibrozil (a fibrate) appeared to improve cerebral perfusion and cognitive performance compared to untreated group (Rogers RL et al., 1989). Next sections will focused on how fibrates intake can be protective for the aging brain.

2.3 Insulin resistance

Insulin is produce by the pancreas and control blood glucose level by allowing the transport of glucose molecules from the circulation into cells. Insulin resistance occur when the cells (insulin receptors) are progressively unable to have a proper insulin response resulting in an inadequate entry of glucose in the cells. By a compensatory mechanism, pancreas will secretes more insulin. If the higher amount of insulin is still inefficient to control blood glucose, the person with high insulin and high glucose level will present a situation of pre-diabetes and insulin resistance. Eventually, pancreas will decrease the insulin secretion, consequence of a pancreatic cell stress and damage, and insulin level will gradually drop and glucose will stay high: type II diabetes is then diagnose. If not treated well, diabetic patient will present high circulating glucose level that can causes deleterious effects including cardiovascular disease, kidney disease, nerve damage, retinopathy, etc. This condition will also lead to deficits in cellular energy production, increased oxidative stress and reduced neuronal survival.

For a long period of time, brain glucose metabolism was known to be independent of insulin action since brain glucose transporters (GLUT-1 and GLUT-3) are insensitive to insulin. Recent literature shows that GLUT-4 responds to insulin and that insulin is produce within the brain in various regions especially in the hippocampus which is associated with learning and memory. Insulin receptors are also presents in the brain (de la Monte et al., 2006). Given that brain cells are dependent on a high glucose supply, brain and peripheral insulin may then play an essential role in brain glucose homeostasis.

Evidences showed a physiological link between insulin and cognition. Reports have documented that brain insulin receptor signaling is reduced in AD brain (reviewed in Rupinder K et al., 2011). Production as well as neuronal insulin receptors was also greatly lower in AD brain compared to age-matched controls (Zhu et al., 2005). Interestingly, in AD patients, peripheral administration of insulin improved memory and cognition, reduced brain atrophy and dementia severity (Burns et al., 2007). In an experimental animal model, intracerebral streptozotocine injection was used to deplete brain insulin, but not pancreatic insulin. This brain specific depletion was associated with progressive neurodegeneration with similar features of AD. This same experiment demonstrates that early treatment with PPARα agonist can effectively prevent this experimentally induced neurodegeneration and the related deficits in learning and memory. This same research team also showed that AD is associated with major impairments in insulin gene expression and that abnormality increase with the severity of dementia. They suggest that AD brain may represent a brain specific form of diabetes; type 3 diabetes (de la Monte et al, 2006).

Hyperlipidemia and fatty acids overload (lipotoxicity) contribute to insulin resistance phenomenon (Reviewed in Carpentier, 2008). By their reducing action on triglycerides and their role in enhancement of fatty acids β-oxidation, PPARα activators should improve insulin sensibility. At human level, findings from a study deriving from Bezafibrate Infarction Prevention trial (BIP) suggest that treatment with fibrate reduce the incidence by 30% and delay the onset of type II diabetes. However, there is not a clear consensus regarding the direct impact of fibrate on insulin sensibility, but from studies reviewed, 10 showed an improvement (Tenenbaum et al., 2007, Cree et al., 2007, Kim et al., 2003, Damci et al., 2003, Jonkers et al., 2001, Idzio-Wallus, 2001, Yong et al., 1999, Kobayashi et al., 1988, Murakami et al. 1984, Ferrari et al., 1977) and 6 a reduction in sensibility or no change (Anderlova et al., 2007, Rizos et al., 2002, Whitelaw et al., 2002, Asplund-Carlson, 1996, Sane et al., 1995, Skrha et al., 1994) . In a recent study (2010) bezafibrate treatment for 12 weeks in a mild hypertriglyceridemic population showed a postprandial insulin response 26% lower after bezafibrate, suggesting the beneficial impact of fibrate on insulin sensitivity (figure 4; Tremblay-Mercier et al., 2010). Further clinical studies measuring insulin sensibility are warranted to confirm the real insulin-sensitizing potential of fibrates and the subsequent impact on brain glucose metabolism and further impact on cognition.

2.4 Ketone production

Ketones are the alternative fuel for the brain when glucose availability is low to insure an optimal brain functioning. They are the product of triglycerides lipolysis, β-oxidation of fatty acids and ketogenesis (figure 5). The majoritary of ketones are synthesised in the liver. Studies have shown that astocytes have the capacity to produce ketones from fatty acids and the ketogenic system (Auestad et al. 1991; Guzman & Blazquez, 2001). Acetyl CoA resulting from the β-oxidation of fatty acids, undergo the Krebs cycle but if the metabolic context is favorable for the ketone body formation, acetyl CoA will be redirected in the ketogenesis pathway.

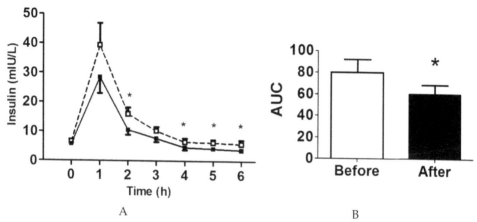

A   B

Fig. 4. A) Insulin concentration (mIU/L) during 6 hours. Breakfast was taken between time 0 and time 1 with no further meal. Before (-□-) and after (-■-), 12 weeks on bezafibrate. B) Area under the curve of the insulin curves were lower after bezafibrate treatment. Data are expressed by mean ± SEM. n=12, * p≤0.05. (Adapted from Tremblay-Mercier, 2010)

Under normal conditions (regular meals) ketogenesis is at a low rate (ketone bodies concentration <0.1 mmol/L), because a slight rise in blood glucose and the following increase in insulin concentration inhibits lipolysis and ketogenesis. After their production, β-OHB and acetoacetate will reach skeletal muscles, brain and heart by the systemic circulation to provide energy. Ketones will then be retransformed into acetyl CoA by the reaction called ketolysis (figure 6). Liver cannot use ketones as energetic molecules because the enzyme β-ketoacyl-CoA transferase is not present in the liver, so ketolysis can not occur (figure 6). Ketones pass through the blood brain barrier (BBB) by facilitated transport following the concentration gradient by the monocarboxylate transporter 1 (MCT-1), as well as pyruvate and lactate. The rate of cerebral ketone metabolism depends primarily on the concentration in blood. Cerebral ketone metabolism is also regulated by the permeability of the BBB, which depends on the abundance of MCT-1. An increase in ketone body concentration up regulates the expression of MCT-1 transporter (Leino et al. 2001; Pifferi et al., 2011).

In vitro experiments show that β-OHB protects hippocampal neurons in culture against the toxicity of the protein β-amyloid 1-42, found in the senile plaques in AD patients. This protective effect may be partly due to the fact that the ketone metabolism does not require the action of the enzyme pyruvate dehydrogenase (PDH) which is affected by the toxic effect of β-amyloid protein and essential for the conversion of glucose into energy (Kashiwaya et al., 2000). Rats and human studies also showed that ketones decreased damages associated with free radical (Sullivan et al., 2004)

Ketone production can be stimulated by fasting but also by the administration of a ketogenic diet. This classic ketogenic diet contains a 4:1 ratio by weight of lipids to combined glucose and protein; this high fat intake forces the body to burn fatty acids rather than glucose. The therapeutic ketogenic diet was developed for treatment of pediatric epilepsy refractory to anticonvulsant in the 1920s. This diet is very effective to treat epilepsy in 30-50% of cases but is very hard to apply in a daily basis and causes significant side effects (Cross et al., 2007). Another dietary way to stimulate ketogenesis is by the ingestion of medium chain triglycerides (MCTs), which provokes an acute elevation in ketone body concentration. Those triglycerides are composed of saturated fatty acids from 6 to 12 carbons and are absorbed across the intestinal barrier and directly enter the portal vein. This allows for much quicker absorption and utilization of MCTs compared to long chain triglycerides. MCTs are transported into the mitochondria independent of the carnitine palmitoyltransferase (CPT), which is necessary for the mitochondrial absorption of long chain fatty acids. After a single dose of MCTs, a significant raise (176%) in ketone bodies concentration occur within one hour but rapidly drops to baseline values (within 2 hours) so the effect is transient (Courchesne-Loyer et al., in preparation).

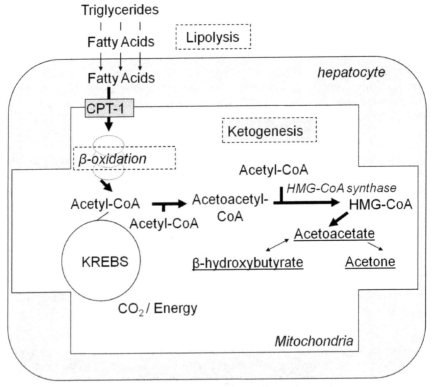

Fig. 5. Ketogenesis pathway. CPT-1: Carnitine palmitoyltransferase 1.

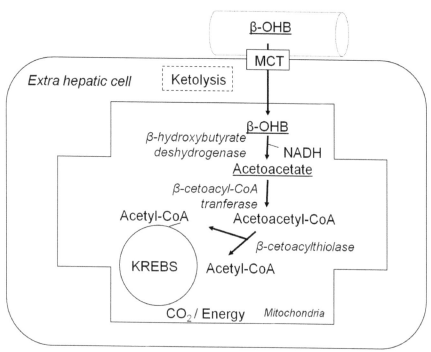

Fig. 6. Ketolysis pathway. β-OHB: β-hydroxybutyrate

Several human studies show that a slight raise in ketones concentration can maintain normal brain function even when plasma glucose would normally be low enough to result in acute cognitive and functional deficits. For example, Page and colleagues in 2009, administered MCTs to type 1 diabetics patient in hypoglycemic crisis and they observed an acute improvement in cognitive functions. Levels of ketones after the ingestion of MCTs were about 0.3-0.4 mM and were sufficient to have an impact on cognitive functioning (Page et al. 2009). Another team showed that a daily supplementation with MCTs for 90 days increased the ketogenic response to 400% and showed a score improvement at different cognitive tests in AD patients (Henderson et al, 2009). In 2004, Reger and colleagues conducted a study with 20 AD patients and showed that high β-OHB concentrations obtained after MCTs administration are positively correlated with ameliorations in the paragraph recall test which is involving memory cognitive function (figure 7).

Ketogenic diet and MCT ingestion, provides low glucose, low insulin environment and/or susbtrates for ketogenesis and are effective in raising ketones concentrations but need a change in eating habits. Another way to increase ketone bodies production without modifying eating habits is to up regulate the enzymes implicated in the pathway. As mentioned earlier fibrate drugs, via PPARα, stimulates the transcription of genes encoding for triglyceride lipolysis and fatty acid β-oxidation. As well, fibrate increase the transcription for the key enzyme in the ketogenesis which is the HMG CoA synthase. This enzyme catalyses the reaction between acetoacetyl CoA and acetyl CoA to form HMG-CoA (figure 4). Few studies on rats have demonstrated an increase in the production of ketone

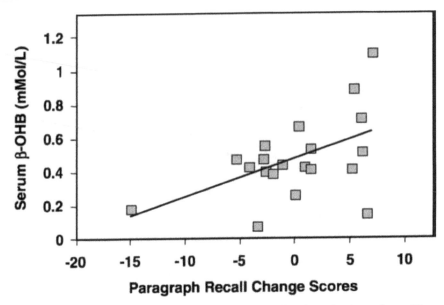

Fig. 7. Relationship between β-hydroxybutyrate (β-OHB) levels at the time of cognitive testing and the change in paragraph recall; $r = 0.50$, $P = 0.02$ (Reger et al., 2004).

bodies by the liver following a fibrate treatment which concord with studies on hepatocytes. In rats treated with clofibrate, PPARα stimulation leads to an upregulation of MCT-1 (König et al., 2008). At the human level the first study to investigate ketone metabolism following a fibrate therapy was done at the Research Center on Aging in Sherbrooke, Quebec, Canada. This study suggests that treatment with bezafibrate has a mild ketogenic potential; postprandial β-OHB response was 58% higher after bezafibrate treatment for 12 weeks. With bezafibrate treatment, the level of ketones (β-OHB) was low during fasting (early in the morning) but was rising during the experimental day to reach 0.3-0.4 mM β-OHB at the end of the day (Tremblay-Mercier et al., 2010). Perhaps in conjunction with a fibrate, joint administration of a dose of MCT, would maintain a moderate level of circulating ketones to insure the delivery to the brain to maintain the energetic homeostasis (Tremblay-Mercier et al., 2010). Preliminary results concerning cerebral ketone metabolism with the tracer ^{11}C-acetoacetate shows that brain ketones uptake is proportional to physiologic plasma ketones concentration as expected by anterior studies (Cunnane et al,. 2011). Further studies with this tracer will help to better understand the impact of fibrate on ketogenesis and the repercussion on brain metabolism in elderly and in cognitively impaired patients.

2.5 Mitochondrial function

Mitochondria are the central organelle in the generation of cellular energy via the Krebs cycle and the electron transport chain. They may be a key players in the cerebral low glucose metabolism observed in AD. Effectively, in the diseased brain, the numbers of neuronal mitochondria are greatly reduced. Several studies have demonstrated aberrations in the electron transport complexes and Krebs cycle in AD (Atamna & Frey, 2007). Mitochondrial perturbations are also seen in normal aging. Those perturbations decrease activities of complex I and IV of the electron transport chain which lead to an elevated reactive oxygen species production. Increased free radicals and peroxidative damage is also seen in AD (Cunnane et al., 2011). Mitchondria dysfunction seems to contribute to the early stage and to the development of various neurodegenerative diseases (Gibson et al., 2010). Numerous studies have suggested that the activation of PPAR may improve mitochondrial functions. PPARγ stimulation is likely to be more effective than PPARα in inducing mitochondrial biogenesis and seems to be effective to potentiate glucose utilization leading to improved cellular and cognitive function (Rupinder et al., 2011). Fibrates are more selective to PPARα but they also have an action on PPARγ. PPARα play a role in the oxidative stress observed in aging. Effectively, level of PPARα correlated negatively with lipid peroxide levels which are actually reduced following a bezafibrate administration (Pineda Torra et al., 1999). Therapeutic strategies targeted at preventing, delaying or treating mitochondrial dysfunction should contribute to the prevention or treatment of age related neurodegeneratives diseases (Atamna & Frey, 2007), and fibrates may be an interesting target to consider.

2.6 Cardiovascular condition /inflammation

There is a close link between cardiovascular condition and cognitive status. High blood pressure, obesity, hyperlipidemia and diabetes are among the principal risk factors for cardiovascular disease. Having those conditions also increase the risk of developing cognitive decline. Vascular risk factors may impair cognitive functions and are related to the occurrence of AD, hypertension and type II diabetes present the strongest association, especially when these factors are assessed in middle age. Atherosclerosis is also believed to be involved in development of dementia, particularly, vascular dementia. Some investigations have shown the importance of inflammation in the pathogenesis of AD, (Akiyama et al., 2000). Hypercholesterolemia, oxidative stress and inflammation have emerged as the dominant mechanism in the development of both atherosclerosis and AD (Steinberg, 2002).Genetic studies and epidemiological observations strongly suggest a relationship between dyslipidemia and AD. Elevated serum cholesterol levels have been reported to correlate with an increased incidence of AD.

Based on its efficiency to reduce plasma triglycerides and to increase HDL cholesterol and it lowering action on LDL-cholesterol, major randomized intervention trials involving fibrate therapy were done to evaluate the drug efficiency to prevent cardiac events. These studies showed that a treatment with a fibrate has beneficial effects by reducing myocardial infarction and coronary event (Goldenberg et al., 2008). The Bezafibrate Infarction Prevention (BIP) trial in 2000 showed that bezafibrate also prevent atherosclerosis and significantly attenuates the risk of long term major cadiovascular events (Tennenbaum et al., 2005). PPARα is also involved in the anti-inflammatory response by his inhibition of NFκB transcription and by decreasing the production of pro-inflammatory IL-6, prostaglandins and C- reactive protein. Fibrates are known to be efficient molecules to prevent cardiovascular disease, knowing that cardiovascular disease and cognitive decline share the same risk factors, preventing cardiovascular disease with fibrate therapy should help preserving cognitive functioning during aging.

3. Conclusions

Fibrates act as synthetic ligands for PPARα and are commonly used to treat hypertriglyceridemia and to prevent coronary heart disease. PPARα is also involved in the anti-inflammatory response and in improvement of mitochondrial function. Fibrate therapy reduces the incidence and delays the onset of type II diabetes and seems to improve insulin sensibility in humans (Goldenberg et al., 2008). A recent clinical study suggests that in hypertriglyceridemic individuals, bezafibrate increase the production of ketone bodies, the alternative energy source for the brain (Tremblay-Mercier et al., 2010). Thus, by reducing triglycerides, enhancing glucose availability, providing alternative brain fuel and improving cardiovascular profile, PPARα agonist could have relevant impact on the maintenance of a good cognitive health later in life (figure 8). Fibrate therapy may have potential as pharmacological agents aiming to reduce the risk of AD and future research are needed to determine if secondary prevention with fibrate therapy is able to delay the apparition of cognitive decline.

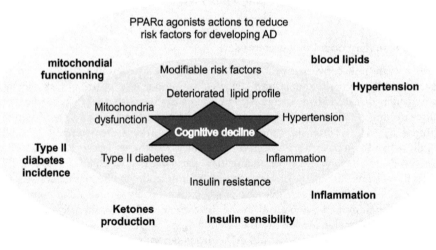

Fig. 8. Summary diagram on the PPARα agonist's action on modifiable risk factors for cognitive decline.

4. Acknowledgment

This chapter was possible because of the collaboration of Stephen Cunnane's laboratory, and was based on this following work:

Tremblay-Mercier, J. (2009) Étude des fibrates en tant qu'agent stimulateurs de la synthèse des cétones, des substrats énergétiques pour le cerveau vieillissant. Master's thesis, the Medecine and Health Science Faculty of Université de Sherbrooke , Sherbrooke, Qc, Canada, 19 January 2009.

Tremblay-Mercier, J., Tessier, D. Plourde, M. Fortier, M. Lorrain, D. Cunnane, S.C. (2010). Bezafibrate mildly stimulates ketogenesis and fatty acid metabolism in hypertriglyceridemic subjects. *J Pharmacol Exp Ther*, Vol. 334 No.1 pp. 341-346.

5. References

Akiyama, H. Barger, S. Barnum, S. (2000) Inflammation and Alzheimer's disease. *Neurobiol Aging*, Vol. 2, No. 3, pp. 383-421.

Anderlova, K. Dolezalova, R. Housova, J. Bosanska, L. Haluzikova, D. Kremen, J. Skrha, J. Haluzik, M. (2007) Influence of PPAR-alpha agonist fenofibrate on insulin sensitivity and selected adipose tissue-derived hormones in obese women with type 2 diabetes. *Physiol Res* Vol. 56 pp. 579-86.

Asplund-Carlson, A. (1996) Effects of gemfibrozil therapy on glucose tolerance, insulin sensitivity and plasma plasminogen activator inhibitor activity in hypertriglyceridaemia. *J Cardiovasc Risk*, Vol.3, pp.385-390.

Atamna, H. Frey, WH. (2007) Mechanism of mitochondrial dysfunction and energy deficiency in Alzheimer's disease. *Mitochondrion*, Vol. 7, pp. 297-310, ISSN 1567-7249

Auestad, N. Korsak, R. A. Morrow, J.W. Edmond J. (1991). Fatty acid oxidation and ketogenesis by astrocytes in primary culture. *J Neurochem,*Vol. 56, No. 4, (April 1991) pp. 1376-1386.

Blennow, K., M. J. de Leon, et al. (2006). Alzheimer's disease, *Lancet*, Vol. 368 No. 9533 (July 2006) pp. 387-403.

Burns, J.M. Donnelly, J.E. Anderson, H.S. Mayo, M.S. Spencer-Gardner, L. Thomas, G. Cronk, B.B. Haddad, Z. Klima, D. Hansen, D. Brooks, W.M. (2007) Peripheral insulin and brain structure in early Alzheimer disease. Neurology, Vol. 969, pp. 1094-1101

Carpentier, A. (2008) Postprandial fatty acid metabolism in the development of lipotoxicity and type 2 diabetes, *Diabetes & Metabolism,* Vol. 34. Pp. 697-107 ISSN 1262-3636

Colcombe, S. Erikson, K. Raz, N. Webb, A.G. Cohen, N.J. McAuley, E. Kramer, A.F. (2003) Aerobic fitness reduces brain tissue loss in ageing humans. *Journal of Gerontology*, Vol. 58, pp. 176-180. Courchesne-Loyer et al., in preparation

Cree, M.G. Newcomer, B.R. Read, L.K. Sheffield-Moore, M. Paddon-Jones, D. Chinkes, D. Aarsland, A. Wolfe, R.R. (2007) Plasma triglycerides are not related to tissue lipids and insulin sensitivity in elderly following PPAR-alpha agonist treatment. *Mech Ageing Dev* Vol.128, pp.558-565.

Cross, H. Ferrie, C. Lascelles, K. Livingstone, J. Mewasingh, L. (2007) Old versus new antiepileptic drug; the SANAD study. *Lancet,* Vol. 370, pp. 314-16.

Cunnane, S. Nugent, S. Roy, M., Courchesne-Loyer, A. Croteau, E., Tremblay, S. Castellano, A. Pifferi, F. Bocti, C. Paquet, N. Begdouri, H. Bentourkia, M. Turcotte, E. Allard, M. Barbeger-Gateau, P. Fulop, T. Rapoport, S. (2011). Brain fuel metabolism, aging, and Alzheimer's disease. *Nutrition* Vol. 27, No.1, pp. 3-20, ISSN 0899-9007.

D'Alton S.,George D. (2011) Changing perspectives on Alzheimer's Disease: Thinking outside the amyloid Box, *Journal of Alzheimer's Disease,* Vol. 24, (February 2011) pp. 1-11, ISSN 1384-2877.

Damci, T. Tatliagac, S. Osar, Z. Ilkova, H. (2003) Fenofibrate treatment is associated with better glycemic control and lower serum leptin and insulin levels in type 2 diabetic patients with hypertriglyceridemia. *Eur J Intern Med*, Vol.14: 357-360.

de la Monte, S.M. Tong, M. Lester-Coll, N. Plater, M. Jr. Wands, J.R. (2006) Therapeutics rescue of neurodegeneration in experimental type 3 diabetes: relevance to Alzheimer's disease. *Journal of Alzheimers Disease,* Vol. 10, No. 1, pp.89-109.

Dufouil, C. Richard, F. Fievet, N. Dartigues, J. F. Ritchie, K. Tzourio, C. Amouyel, P. Alperovitch, A. (2005) APOE genotype, cholesterol level, lipid-lowering treatment, and dementia: the Three-City Study. *Neurology* Vol. 64, pp.1531-8.

Ferrari, C. Frezzati, S. Romussi, M. Bertazzoni, A. Testori, G.P. Antonini, S. Paracchi, A. (1977) Effects of short-term clofibrate administration on glucose tolerance and insulin secretion in patients with chemical diabetes or hypertriglyceridemia. *Metabolism*, Vol 26, pp. 129-39.

Frisardi, V. Solfrizzi, V. Seripa, D. Capurso, C. Santamato, A. Sancarlo, D. Vendemiale, G. Pilotto, A. Panza, F. (2010) Metabolic-cognitive syndrome: A cross-talk between metabolic syndrome and Alzheimer's disease. *Ageing Research Reviews*, Vol. 9, No. 4 (October 2010) pp.399-417, ISSN 1568-1637.

Gibson, G.E. Starkov, A. Blass, J.P. Ratan, R.R, Beal, M.F. (2010) Cause and consequence: mitochondrial dysfunction initiates and propagates neuronal dysfunction, neural death and behavorial abnormalities in age-associated neurodegenerative diseases, Biochim Biophys Acta, Vol. 1802, pp. 122-34.

Goldenberg, I. Benderly, M. Goldbourt, U. (2008) Update on the use of fibrates: focus on bezafibrate. *Vascular Heath and risk management.* Vol. 4 No. 1 pp. 131-41

Guzman, M. Blazquez, C. (2001) Is there an astrocyte-neurone ketone body shuttle? TRENDS Endocrinology & Metabolism, Vol.12 No. 4 (May/June 2001) pp.169-73.

Haan, M. Wallace, R. (2004) Can dementia be prevented? Brain aging in a population-Based Context, Annu. Rev. Public Health, Vol. 25, pp. 1-24. ISSN 0163-7525.

Henderson, S. T. (2008). Ketone bodies as a therapeutic for Alzheimer's disease. *Neurotherapeutics*, Vol. 5, No. 3, pp. 470-480.

Idzior-Wallus, B, (2001) Fibrate influence on lipids and insulin resistance in patients with metabolic syndrome (In Polish) *Przegl Lek*, Vol. 58 pp. 924-27

Jonkers, I. J. de Man, F. H. van der Laarse, A. Frolich, M.. Gevers Leuven, J. A M. Kamper, A. Blauw G. J. Smelt, A. H. (2001) Bezafibrate reduces heart rate and blood pressure in patients with hypertriglyceridemia. *J Hypertens*, Vol. 19 pp. 749-55

Kashiwaya, Y. Takeshima, T. Nozomi, M. Kenji, N. Kieran, C. Veech, R.L. (2000).D-beta-hydroxybutyrate protects neurons in models of Alzheimer's and Parkinson's disease. *Proc Natl Acad Sci U S A*, Vol. 97 No. 10, (May 2000) pp. 5440-5444.

Kim, H. Haluzik, M. Asghar, Z. Yau, D. Joseph, J.W. Fernandez, A.M. Reitman, M.L. Yakar, S. Stannard, B. Heron-Milhavet,. Wheeler, M.B. Leroith, D. (2003) Peroxisome proliferator activated receptor-α agonist treatment in a transgenic model of type 2 diabetes reverses the lipotoxic state and improves glucose homeostasis. *Diabetes*, Vol. 52, pp. 1770-78.

Kobayashi, M. Shigeta, Y. Hirata, Y . Omori, Y. Sakamoto, N. Nambu, S. Baba, S. (1988) Improvement of glucose tolerance in NIDDM by clofibrate. Randomised double-blind study. *Diabetes Care*, Vol. 11 pp. 495-499.

König, B. Koch, A. Giggel, K. Dordschbal, B. Eder, K. Stangl, G. (2008) Monocarboxylate transporter (MCT)-1 is up-regulated by PPARα. Biochimica et Biophysica Acta, Vol. 1780, pp. 899-904. ISSN 0304-4165

Landreth, G. Jiang, Q. Mandrekar, S. Heneka, M. (2008) PPARγ agonists as therapeutics for the treatement of Alzheimer's disease, *Neurotherapeutic*, Vol. 5 No. 3, pp 481-89.

Leino, R.L. Gerhart, D.Z. Duelli, R. Enerson, B.E. Drewes L.R. (2001) Diet-induced ketosis increases monocarboxylate transporter (MCT1) levels in rat brain. *Neurochem Int* Vol. 38, pp. 519-27.

Murakami, K. Nambu, S. Koh, H. Kobayashi, M. Shigeta, Y. (1984) Clofibrate enhances affinity of insulin receptors in non-insulin dependent diabetes mellitus. *Br J Clin Pharmacol*, Vol. 17, pp. 89-91 et al. 1984

Owen, O.E. Morgan, H.G. Kemp, J.M. Sullivan, M. Herrera, G. Cahill, F. Jr. (1967) Brain metabolism during fastinf . J Clin Invest, Vol. 46, pp. 1589-95.

Page, K. A. Williamson, A. Yu, N. McNay, E.C. Dzuira, J. McCrimmon, R.J. Sherwin, R.S.(2009). Medium-chain fatty acids improve cognitive function in intensively treated type 1 diabetic patients and support in vitro synaptic transmission during acute hypoglycemia. *Diabetes*, Vol. 58 No. 5, pp. 1237-1244.

Pifferi, F. Tremblay, S. Croteau, E. Fortier, M, Tremblay-Mercier, J. Lecomte, R. Cunnane, S.C. (2011) Mild experimental ketosis increases brain uptake of 11C-acetoacetate and 18F-fluorodeoxyglucose: a dual-tracer PET imaging study in rats.*Nutr Neurosci*, Vol. 14, No. 2 (March 2011) pp. 51-8.

Peters, R. (2009). The prevention of dementia. Int. J. Geriatr. Psychiatry. Vol. 24 pp. 452-458.

Reger, M. A. Henderson S. T. Hale, C. Cholerton, B. Baker, L.D. Watson, G.S. Hyde, K. Chapman, D. Craft, S. (2004) Effects of beta-hydroxybutyrate on cognition in memory-impaired adults, *Neurobiol Aging*, Vol.25, No. 3, pp. 311-314.

Reiman, E. M. Chen, K. Alexander, G. E. Caselli, R.. Bandy J. D. Osborne, D. Saunders, A. M. Hardy, J. (2004) Functional brain abnormalities in young adults at genetic risk for late-onset Alzheimer's dementia. *Proc Natl Acad Sci U S A*, Vol. 101, pp. 284-9.

Rizos, E. Kostoula, A. Elisaf, M. Mikhailidis, D.P. (2002) Effect of ciprofibrate on C-reactive protein and fibrinogen levels. *Angiology*, Vol.53, pp. 273-277.

Rodriguez, E.G. Dodge, H.H. Birzescu, M.A. Stoehr, G.P. Ganguli, M. (2002) Use of lipid-lowering drugs in older adults with and without dementia: a community-based epidemiological study. *Journal of American Geriatrics Society*, Vol. 50, No.11 (November 2002) pp. 1852-6.

Rogers, R.L. Meyer, J.S. McClintic, K. Mortel, K.F. (1989) Reducing hypertriglyceridemia in elderly patients with cerebrovascular disease stabilizes or improves cognition and cerebral perfusion. *Angiology*, Vol. 40, pp. 260-9.

Sane, T. Knudsen, P. Vuorinen-Markkola, H. Yki-Jarvinen, H. Taskinen, M.R. (1995) Decreasing triglyceride by gemfibrozil therapy does not affect the glucoregulatory or antilipolytic effect of insulin in nondiabetic subjects with mild hypertriglyceridemia. *Metabolism*, Vol. 44, pp. 589-596.

Škrha, J. Šindelka, G. Haas, T. Hilgertová, J. Justaová, V. (1994) Relation between hypertriacylglycerolemia and the action of insulin in type 2 diabetes mellitus (in Czech). *Čas Lék Česk*, Vol. 133, pp. 496-499.

Snowdon, D.A. (1997) Aging and Alzheimer's disease: lessons from the Nun Study. *Gerontologist*, Vol. 37, No. 2, pp. 150-6.

Solfrizzi, V. Scafato, E. Capurso, C. D'Introno, A. Colacicco, A.M. Frisardi, V. Vendemiale, G. Baldereschi, M. Crepaldi, G. Di Carlo, A. Galluzzo, L. Gandin, C. Inzitari, D. Maggi, S. Capurso, A. Panza, F. for the Italian Longitudinal Study on Aging Working Group(2009). Metabolic syndrom, mild cognitive impairment, and progression to dementia, The Italian Longitudinal Study on Aging. *Neurobiol. Aging*, Vol. 12, 10.106/j.neurobiolaging.2009.12.012.

Steinberg, D. (2002) Atherogenesis in perspective: hypercholesterolemia and inflammation as partners in crime. *Nat Med*, Vol. 8, pp. 1211-7.

Sullivan, P. G. Rippy, N. A, Dorenbos, K. Concepcion, R. C. Agarwal, A. K. Rho, J. M. (2004) The ketogenic diet increases mitochondrial uncoupling protein levels and activity. *Ann Neurol* Vol. 55, pp. 576-80.

Tenenbaum, A. Motro, M. Fisman, E.Z. Tanne, D. Valentina, B. Behar, S. (2005) Bezafibrate for the secondary prevention of myocardial Infarction in patients with metabolic syndrome. *Arch Intern Med*, Vol. 165, pp. 1154-1160.

Tenenbaum, H. Behar, S. Boyko, V. Adler, Y. Fisman, EZ. Tanne, D. Lapidot, M. Schwammenthal, E. Feinberg, M. Matas, Z. Motro, M. Tenenbaum, A. (2007) Longterm effect of bezafibrate on pancreatic beta-cell function and insulin resistance in patients with diabetes. *Atherosclerosis*, Vol. 194 pp. 265-271.

Pineda-Torra, I. Gervois, P. Staels, B. (1999) Peroxisome proliferator-activated receptor alpha in metabolic disease, inflammation, atherosclerosis and aging. *Curr Opin Lipidol*, Vol. 10, No. 2, pp. 151-159.

Tremblay-Mercier, J., Tessier, D. Plourde, M. Fortier, M. Lorrain, D. Cunnane, S.C. (2010). Bezafibrate mildly stimulates ketogenesis and fatty acid metabolism in hypertriglyceridemic subjects. *J Pharmacol Exp Ther*, Vol. 334 No.1 pp. 341-346

Veech, R. L. Chance, B. Kashiwaya, Y. Lardy, H.A.Cahill, F.Jr. (2001). Ketone bodies, potential therapeutic uses. *IUBMB Life* Vol. 51, No. 4, pp. 241-47. ISSN 1521-6543.

Yong, Q.W. Thavintharan, S. Cheng, A, Chew, L.S. (1999) The effect of fenofibrate on insulin sensitivity and plasma lipids profile in non-diabetic males with low high density lipoprotein/dyslipidaemic syndrome. *Ann Acad Med Singapore.* Vol. 28, pp. 778-782.

Whitehouse P.J, George, D., (2008) *The Myth of Alzheimer's: What You Aren't Being Told About Today's Lost Dreaded Diagnosis*, (Solal) St Martin's press, ISBN 978-2-35327-080-4, New York, USA.

Whitelaw, D.C. Smith, J.M. Nattrass, M. (2002) Effects of gemfibrozil on insulin resistance to fat metabolism in subjects with type 2 diabetes and hypertriglyceridaemia. *Diabetes Obes Metab*, Vol. 4, pp. 187-194.

Zhu, X. Perry, G. Smith, M.A. (2005) Insulin signaling, diabetes mellitus, and risk of Alzheimer's disease: a population based study of the oldest old. *Int Psychogeriatr*, Vol. 14, pp. 239-48.

Part 2

Experimental Study

7

Modification of Interleukin-10 with Mannose-6-Phosphate Groups Yields a Liver-Specific Cytokine with Antifibrotic Activity in Rats

Heni Rachmawati[1,2], Adriana Mattos[2],
Catharina Reker-Smit[2], Klaas Poelstra[2] and Leonie Beljaars[2]
[1]*Pharmaceutics, Bandung Institute of Technology, Bandung*
[2]*University of Groningen, Dept. of Pharmacokinetics, Toxicology and Targeting,*
[1]*Indonesia*
[2]*The Netherlands*

1. Introduction

Cytokines and other biological compounds are considered as future drugs and they are of particular interest for the treatment of chronic diseases. These endogenous compounds, that normally mediate local cellular communications, are very promising candidates to generate new drugs because of their high potency (pM-nM concentrations) and their fundamental roles in pathological processes. However, the therapeutic application of cytokines is limited, because several problems are encountered with their application *in* vivo (Schooltink and Rose-John 2002; Standiford 2000; Vilcek and Feldmann 2004). For instance, some cytokines are efficiently degraded in plasma by various enzymes and cytokines are rapidly excreted by the kidneys. Consequently their residence time in the body and thus the exposure to the diseased cells is short (plasma half life is often minutes), which does not favour an optimal biological efficacy. Another major problem is the occurrence of side effects. Because cytokine receptors are ubiquitously expressed in all organs, unusual high plasma concentrations of the cytokine can lead to (unwanted) effects in various organs.

To overcome these problems, we use drug targeting techniques to selectively deliver the cytokine to a specific (diseased) cell (Allen and Cullis 2004; Beljaars, Meijer, Poelstra 2002). The challenge is to improve its distribution within the body and direct the cytokine to a cell of interest, while maintaining the biological activity of that particular cytokine after chemical modification. A conventional way to modify proteins is conjugation with poly-ethylene glycol (PEG) (Jevsevar, Kunstelj, Porekar 2010). The attachment of PEG moieties improves the pharmacokinetics. That is, PEG substitution prevents rapid renal elimination which results in compounds with prolonged plasma concentrations, thereby making a reduced number of doses possible. For instance, PEGasys (PEGylated interferon α2a), an example of a PEGylated cytokine that is now commonly used to treat patients infected with viral hepatitis, is dosed once a week while the unmodified interferon is dosed daily. This leads to an improvement in the compliance and quality of life in patients with chronic diseases. The side effects, however, are not diminished after PEGylation.

Our strategy of active drug targeting, in contrast to the abovementioned PEGylation approach, aims to improve pharmacokinetics and efficacy while simultaneously avoiding side-effects by cell-specific delivery of the cytokine to the diseased cell via receptor-mediated interaction. To that end, the cytokine is modified with homing devices that recognize receptors present on the diseased (target) cells. In the past, we designed sugars and receptor-recognizing peptides that interact with hepatic stellate cells (HSC) (Beljaars and others 1999; Beljaars and others 2000; Beljaars and others 2003). These cells play the central role in liver cirrhosis (Bataller and Brenner 2005; Friedman 2010; Schuppan and Afdhal 2008). Our newly designed homing devices displayed affinity for the mannose 6-phosphate/insulin-like growth factor (M6P/IGF) II receptor, platelet derived growth factor (PDGF)-β or collagen type VI receptors, which are all essential during stellate cell functioning in fibrogenesis, and upregulate in the diseased liver.

Currently, it is accepted that liver cirrhosis is a fibrotic disease that is reversible (Iredale 2007). However, to date, no drug is marketed that is able to reverse the fibrotic process in patients (Pinzani, Rombouts, Colagrande 2005). The only treatment that is applied to these patients deals with the treatment of complications and with eradication of the cause (for instance removal of the hepatitis virus in case of HCV-induced cirrhosis). However, fibrosis often progresses to end-stage liver failure leaving a liver transplantation as the only available option. Therefore, worldwide research focuses on the identification of compounds that are able to reverse the disease, but unfortunately many potential interventions fail in clinical trials (Pinzani, Rombouts, Colagrande 2005). We hypothesize that this failure may be due to an inadequate pharmacokinetic profile of the potential drugs or due to the occurrence of side-effects of these drugs preventing the administration of effective doses, which may be solved by applying drug targeting techniques.

The selective delivery of cytokines to the cells that control pathological processes is quite relevant. PEGylation of cytokines like interferon α, TNFα, and IL-2 has provided substantial benefits, but in that approach cytokines are not actively delivered to the site of action. In the present study, we will show an example of this second approach using the cytokine interleukin-10 (IL10). IL10 has potent immunosuppressive and anti-inflammatory effects (Di Marco and others 1999; Khan and others 2002; Kitching and others 2000; Oberholzer, Oberholzer, Moldawer 2002) and also direct antifibrotic properties in HSC (Cuzzocrea and others 2001; Demols and others 2002; Gloor and others 1998; Louis and others 1998; Louis and others 2003; Thompson and others 1998; Wang and others 1998). Several of these studies showed beneficial effects of IL10 therapies in animal models and clinical trials during various diseases. However, other studies demonstrated only a limited effect of IL10 or even showed disappointing results (Chadban and others 1997; Colombel and others 2001; Herfarth and Scholmerich 2002). This variable efficacy might be due to the low concentration of IL10 at the target sites. Recombinant IL10 is a low molecular weight protein that is rapidly cleared from the circulation through glomerular filtration. The plasma half-life of IL10 is only 2 min (Rachmawati and others 2004). The ultimate concentrations at the site of action therefore could be too low to result in clear effects. Dose escalation of systemically administered IL10 leads to adverse effects due to its inherent biological actions (Fedorak and others 2000; Schreiber and others 2000). In accordance with this, clinical studies reported beneficial effects of long-term IL10 therapy to treat HCV-associated liver fibrosis but this was accompanied by an immunosuppressive action, as noted in a flare-up of the viral burden, and low therapeutic efficacy (Nelson and others 2000)(Meijer and others

2001). Liver-selective delivery of this cytokine may prevent these clinical problems and create biological effects within relevant cells.

Upregulation of mannose-6-phosphate/IGF-II receptors during liver injury on HSC (de Bleser and others 1995) offers an excellent target for receptor-mediated antifibrotic drug delivery as shown with albumin substituted with mannose-6-phosphate groups (Beljaars and others 1999). We therefore modified IL10 with the sugar mannose-6-phosphate (M6P) to selectively deliver this cytokine to HSC in fibrotic livers (Rachmawati and others 2007). We showed that after modification of IL10 with mannose 6-phosphate (M6P) a compound was generated that binds to the M6P/IGF-II receptor which is highly present on activated HSC. Our chemically engineered cytokine, M6P-IL10, displayed good pharmacological activity in vitro in freshly isolated HSC. We now performed biodistribution studies of radiolabeled-M6P-modified IL10 using gamma-camera techniques to examine the active delivery of this compound to the diseased tissue. Furthermore, we studied the pharmacological activities of this conjugate in rats at an early stage of liver fibrosis and compared this to the effects of unmodified IL10.

2. Results

2.1 Synthesis of M6P-IL10

Mannose-6-phosphate-residues were coupled to the amino acid lysine in recombinant human IL10 as described (Rachmawati and others 2007). The product was first characterized by Western Blotting techniques using a rabbit polyclonal anti-IL10 antibody (Santa Cruz Biotechnology, USA). Western Blot analysis of unmodified IL10 yielded two bands corresponding to a molecular weight (MW) of 18.5 and 37 kD (fig.1) representing the monomeric and the homodimeric form of IL10 (Reineke and others 1998). The prepared conjugate M6P-IL10 revealed a shift in these bands: both bands had a higher MW (resp. approximately 20 and 40 kD) than unmodified IL10 indicating covalent binding of M6P to the cytokine.

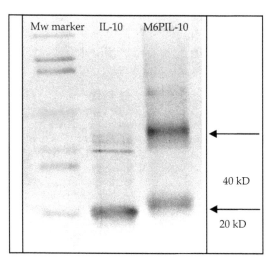

Fig. 1. Western blot analysis of M6P-IL10 and IL10. Note the increase in molecular weight of the monomeric (± 20 kD) and the homodimeric (± 40 kD) forms of M6P-IL10 compared with the monomeric and homodimeric forms of native IL10 (respectively, 18.5 kD and 37 kD).

2.2 Body distribution of IL10 and M6P-IL10

To visualize the body distribution of IL10 and M6P-IL10 with a gamma camera, both proteins were labeled with Iodine-123 (^{123}I). Fibrotic rats were monitored during the course of their disease by subjecting them to gamma camera analysis, just prior to BDL and one, two and three weeks after BDL (respectively, normal, BDL-1, BDL-2, and BDL-3, n=3). Anaesthetized rats were placed on a low-energy all-purpose collimator of a gamma-camera and received an intravenous tracer dose. The results are shown in figure 2. Already two min after iv injection of [123I]M6P-IL10, the gamma-camera detected high levels of radioactivity within the livers (white intensity) and low levels in the kidneys (yellow-red intensity). Hepatic levels of [123I]M6P-IL10 remained high for at least 30 min. The results of the distribution studies were similar in various stages of liver fibrosis (BDL-1, BDL- 2 and BDL-3). In contrast, native [123I]IL10 rapidly accumulated in the kidneys (white intensity) with low uptake in livers (fig.2a), which is in agreement with previous studies (Andersen and others 1999; Rachmawati and others 2004).

Subsequently, we quantitatively measured the distribution of [125I]IL10 and [125I]M6P-IL10 ten minutes after intravenous injection in rats with end-stage liver fibrosis (BDL-3 weeks). Native [125I]-IL10 accumulated in the kidneys in these rats (Fig 2b). Only, 15% and 30% of the dose was found in livers of normal and BDL-3 rats respectively. The rest was dispersed throughout the body or present in the blood. In contrast, [125I]M6P-IL10 accumulated for nearly 60% of the dose within the livers in BDL-3 rats. Uptake in kidneys was only 20%. Differences in blood-, liver- and kidney-concentrations between IL10 and M6P-IL10 were significant (p<0.05).

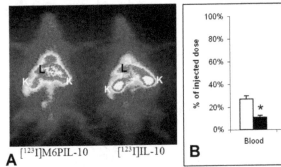 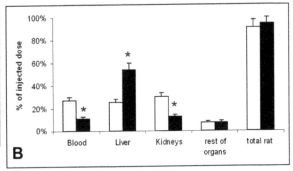

Fig. 2. Organ Distribution of M6P-IL10 and IL10. **A**: Gamma-camera images of [123I]IL10 and [123I]M6P-IL10 distribution in BDL-1 rats. Pictures show an overlay of recordings from t=20 to t=30 minutes after i.v. injection of radiolabeled proteins. The images show a high accumulation of M6P-IL10 in the liver (L) in contrast to IL10, which is mostly distributed to the kidneys (K). **B**: Quantitative measurement of organ uptake of [125I]-labeled IL10 (white bars) and M6P-IL10 (black bars) in BDL-3 rats 10 minutes after i.v. administration of the radiolabeled proteins. N = 3 per group (* p<0.05 compared with IL-10 distribution)

2.3 Identification of target receptors

(Modified) IL10 could not be detected within livers by immunohistochemistry, most likely due to the very low dose administered (2-2.5 µg). Therefore, several receptor antagonists were applied to identify the target receptors responsible for the uptake of the proteins in different organs in order to obtain information about the hepatocellular distribution. Rats were pre-treated with either succinylated human serum albumin (sucHSA) to block the scavenger receptor, or with mannose-6-phosphate-HSA, to block the M6P/IGFII receptor. These receptor antagonists (i.v. dose of 5 mg/kg) were administered 5 min. prior to the i.v. injection of a tracer amount of radiolabeled IL10 or M6P-IL10. Control animals received pre-treatment with unmodified HSA (5 mg/kg).

Kidney accumulation of [125I]IL10 or [125I]M6P-IL10 was not influenced by administration of any of the proteins (fig. 3). Uptake of [125I]IL10 in the livers was also not influenced by any of the proteins, but remained approximately 20% of the dose in all groups. However, liver uptake of M6P-IL10 was reduced from $54 \pm 6\%$ in rats receiving only M6P-IL10, to $29 \pm 4\%$ by sucHSA (p<0.05) and to $24 \pm 8\%$ by M6P-HSA pre-administration (p<0.05). Co-administration of both sucHSA and M6P-HSA did not have an additive effect ($24 \pm 5\%$ liver uptake). Unmodified HSA did not affect liver uptake of M6P-IL10 at all ($57 \pm 13\%$ liver uptake).

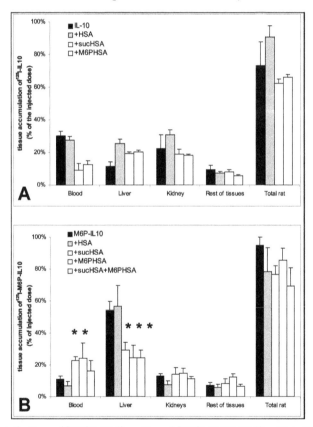

Fig. 3. Organ distribution of [125I]IL10 (fig. **A**) and [125I]M6P-IL10 (fig. **B**) in BDL-3 rats 10 min. after i.v. administration of the radiolabeled proteins. Five min. before administration of these proteins, HSA, sucHSA, M6PHSA or the combination of two proteins was administered to test receptor specificity. Note that sucHSA and M6PHSA influenced liver uptake and blood concentrations of M6P-IL10, whereas IL10 distribution was not affected by any of the proteins. N=4-6 per group. * =p<0.05 compared with HSA pre-administration.

2.4 Effects of IL10 and M6P-IL10 in vitro

The in vitro activities of IL10 and M6P-IL10 were studied in culture-activated primary HSC. The presence of IL10 receptors and M6P/IGFII-receptors on these cells was verified by immunohistochemical methods. No effect of IL10 or M6P-IL10 was found on HSC proliferation as assessed by Alamar blue assays (data not shown).

We also examined type I collagen deposition in cultures of HSC treated with IL10 or M6P-IL10 using immunostaining methods. Deposition of type I collagen was clearly detectable in HSC cultures at day-7 (fig 4A) and this staining was reduced in cultures treated for 24 hr with IL10 (Fig 4B) and in cultures treated with M6P-IL10 (fig 4C).

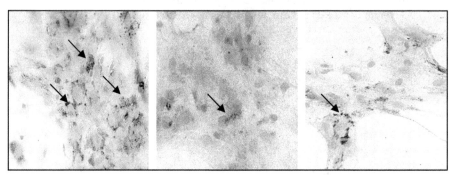

Fig. 4. Type I collagen deposition in cultures of primary isolated rat HSC's as detected with immunostaining methods. Collagen staining (using a goat polyclonal anti-collagen I antibody) is present on HSC's after 7 days in culture (**A**, arrows). Deposition of collagen is attenuated by 24 hr incubation with 12.5 ng/ml IL10 (**B**) or M6P-IL10 (**C**). Original magnification 200x.

2.5 Effects of IL10 and M6P-IL10 *in vivo*

2.5.1 Experimental design

Bile duct ligated rats were randomly divided into three groups: BDL rats received either vehicle (PBS, N = 5), or IL10 (N = 5) or M6P-IL10 (N = 5). Untreated normal rats (N = 3) served as reference group. Animals received a bolus iv dose (8 µg/kg/day) of (modified-) IL10 at day 4, 5 and 6 after BDL. At day 7, animals were sacrificed and samples of blood and various organs were harvested.

2.5.2 Effect of IL10 and M6P-IL10 on liver function

Plasma levels of markers reflecting liver injury and cholestasis in BDL-1 rats receiving IL-10 or M6PIL-10 were not significantly different from untreated BDL rats (table 1).

2.5.3 Effect of IL10 and M6P-IL10 on inflammatory parameters

To study the effects of IL10 and M6P-IL10 on inflammation, staining for reactive oxygen species (ROS)-production and IL10 receptor expression was performed. The number of 3,3'-diaminobenzidine (DAB)-positive cells in the liver was high around necrotic areas and in portal areas. DAB staining reflects ROS production (Poelstra and others 1990) by activated neutrophils, eosinophils and macrophages.

Parameters	PBS-treated rats	IL10-treated rats	M6PIL-10-treated rats
Alkaline Phosphatase (U/L)	493.8 ± 71.2	476.2 ± 53.8	450.6 ± 16.13
AST (U/L)	350.0 ± 166.6	354.0 ± 118.8	301.0 ± 109.64
ALT (U/L)	92.2 ± 27.44	90.2 ± 24.9	84.0 ± 17.0
Total bilirubin (μmol/L)	191.2 ± 43.13	231.6 ± 21.9	194.8 ± 68.6
GGT (U/L)	65.0 ± 56.0	74.0 ± 75.95	34.8 ± 23.34

Table 1. Plasma levels of markers reflecting liver injury and cholestasis in BDL-1 rats treated with PBS, IL10 or M6P-IL10. Values represent the mean ± SD of 5 rats per group.

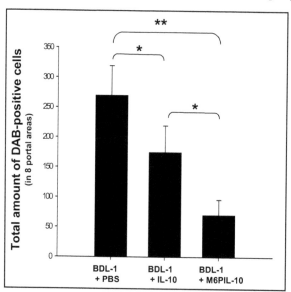

Fig. 5. Effect of IL-10- and M6PIL-10-treatment on the number of DAB-positive cells in livers of BDL-1 rats. Both treatments significantly reduced the number of DAB-positive cells in the portal areas compared with PBS-treated rats. *= p<0.05; **=p<0.01

IL10 and M6P-IL10 strongly attenuated the staining for DAB (Fig. 5). Quantitative evaluation of this staining by counting the number of positive cells/area showed that DAB staining was reduced by 35% in rats receiving IL10 (p<0.05 compared with untreated BDL-1 rats, Fig 5b), whereas the number of DAB-positive cells per area in M6P-IL10-treated rats was reduced by 74% compared with untreated rats (p<0.05). Thus, both IL10 and M6P-IL10 exerted anti-inflammatory effects within the liver and M6P-IL10 was superior in this respect.

Staining for IL10 receptors (with anti-IL-10 receptor IgG (Santa Cruz Biotech)) on liver sections of BDL-1 rats revealed occasional positive cells: some cells around the proliferating bile ducts and around hepatic arteries were positive. Based on the localization and the positivity for α-smooth muscle actin or HIS-48, these cells were identified as fibroblasts, HSC and neutrophils. In BDL-1 rats that received IL10, hepatic IL10 receptor expression was strongly reduced, in particular around the portal areas (fig.6). In contrast, in BDL-1 rats receiving M6P-IL10, IL10 receptor expression was still present.

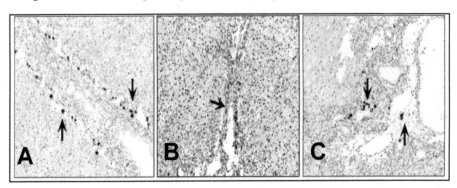

Fig. 6. Intrahepatic staining for IL10 receptor expression in fibrotic livers. In PBS-treated BDL-1 rats, positive cells were found around bile ducts (fig. **A,** arrows). In rats treated with IL10, only occasional IL10 receptor-positive cells were found (fig. **B**) whereas the portal areas contained many IL10 receptor positive cells in BDL-1 rats treated with M6P-IL10 (fig. **C**). Original magnification 100x.

2.5.4 Antifibrotic effects of IL10 and M6P-IL10

Characteristic for fibrosis is deposition of extracellular matrix in tissues. Collagen type I and III are the most important extracellular matrix proteins present in a fibrotic liver. Therefore, we assessed the effect of M6P-IL10 and IL10 administration on the deposition of collagen. First, we evaluated the deposition of fibrous tissue by histochemical staining with Sirius Red (figure 7A). This staining was strongly enhanced in BDL-1 rats compared with normal rats. The portal-to-portal bridging was already apparent in the untreated group at this time point. However, in IL10-treated rats, the portal-portal fibrous bridges were observed in only one out of five rats and bridging was not seen in any of the M6P-IL10-treated rats. The matrix deposition around portal areas was clearly reduced by the treatments compared to untreated group. This reduction was confirmed by immunostaining for collagen type III using goat anti-collagen III IgG (SouternBiotech, USA) antibodies. The strong staining seen in BDL-1 rats was reduced by IL10 and M6P-IL10 (fig. 7B).

With ImageJ software, the effects of IL10 and M6PIL10 on the deposition of fibrous tissue were quantified. In normal livers, 1.0 ± 0.45 % of the total liver area was positive for Sirius Red. This positive area increased to $4.6 \pm 1.0\%$ of the livers of BDL-1 rats ($p < 0.001$ compared with normal rats, Fig. 7C). In IL10-treated BDL-1 rats the Sirius Red-positive area per liver changed to 3.6 % ± 1.6 (not significant compared with untreated BDL-1 rats). In M6P-IL10-treated BDL-1 rats, Sirius Red-staining changed to 3.4 ± 1.1 % of liver area ($p < 0.05$ compared with untreated BDL-1 rats, Fig. 7C). The effect of IL10 and M6P-IL10 on the fibrotic process was also assessed by staging the lesions via a semiquantitative scoring system; the Histologic Activity Index-Knodell (Ishak and others 1995). Grading of the fibrotic lesions in these livers by the HAI-Knodell's index revealed a reduction of the fibrotic index from 3.2 ± 0.8 in untreated BDL-1 rats to 2.6 ± 0.9 and 2.2 ± 0.45 ($p < 0.05$) in rats receiving IL10 and M6P-IL10, respectively (fig. 7D).

Modification of Interleukin-10 with Mannose- 6-Phosphate Groups Yields a Liver-Specific Cytokine with
Antifibrotic Activity in Rats

151

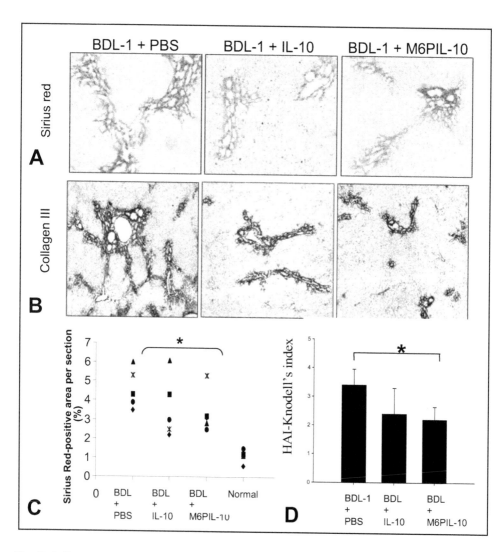

Fig. 7. Collagen deposition in BDL rats after treatment with M6P-IL-10 or IL-10. A.
Representative photomicrographs of Sirius Red (fig. **A**) and collagen type III staining (fig. **B**)
in livers of BDL-1 rats treated with PBS, IL-10 or M6PIL-10 (magnification 10x4). Figure **C**
depicts the quantitative analysis of the Sirius Red stainings in the livers of the different
groups as measured by Image J software. The individual values of each rat are shown in the
graph. Figure **D** shows the semiquantitative grading of the fibrotic process in BDL-1 rats
with the Histological Activity Index-Knodell method. N=5 per group, * = p<0.05 compared
with PBS-treated BDL rats.

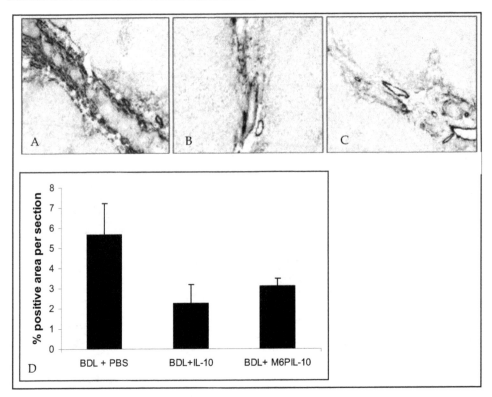

Fig. 8. Representative photomicrographs of immunohistochemical staining for α-smooth muscle actin (αSMA) in livers of BDL-1 rats treated with PBS (fig. **A**) or IL10 (fig. **B**) or M6P-IL10 (fig. **C**). Figure **D** depicts the quantitative analysis of the intrahepatic αSMA staining with Image J software (n=5 animals per group). *=p<0.05, Original magnification 100x.

Subsequently, we evaluated the in vivo effects of M6P-IL10 and IL10 on α-smooth muscle staining (α-SMA), that reflects the proportion of activated HSC and myofibroblasts. These cells are responsible for the production of collagen. One week after BDL, staining for α-SMA was highly increased around portal ducts and in fibrotic septa compared with normal rats. IL10 and M6P-IL10 clearly diminished this α-SMA staining (fig.8). Quantitative evaluation of this staining using ImageJ software (fig.8B), demonstrated a significant reduction by 54% ± 17% and 33% ± 19% after treatment with IL10 or M6P-IL10, respectively compared to PBS-treated BDL rats (p<0.05).

3. Conclusion/discussion

This study demonstrates that chemical modification of a cytokine, in our study IL10 modified with M6P groups, leads to a compound with improved biodistribution and pharmacological activity *in vivo* in a rat model of liver fibrosis. M6P is a homing device with high affinity for the M6P/IGF-II receptor which is upregulated on the cell membrane of HSCs during liver diseases (de Bleser and others 1995). Upregulation of this receptor on HSC during liver fibrosis yields

Modification of Interleukin-10 with Mannose- 6-Phosphate Groups Yields a Liver-Specific Cytokine with
Antifibrotic Activity in Rats

153

an excellent target for receptor-mediated drug delivery. The delivery of antifibrotic compounds to the major pathogenic cells in the liver by modification with M6P groups is a rational and new approach to treat this chronic disease (Schuppan and Popov 2009).

Chemical modification of a cytokine can influence the biological activity, in particular when essential amino acids necessary for interaction of the cytokine with its receptor are conjugated with homing devices or when the conformation of the protein is changed too much. Therefore, it is essential to test whether the prepared conjugate is pharmacologically active. In our study, we coupled several M6P groups to the lysine amino acids within the protein and some of these lysine-groups are present at the receptor-binding site of IL10 (Reineke and others 1998). Attachment of M6P-residues to these groups might therefore affect the biological activities of IL10. Studies on culture-activated primary HSC *in vitro* showed that M6P-IL10 reduced collagen deposition by these cells (fig 4) indicating that IL10-related activities are still intact in the modified cytokine. There was no effect of M6P-IL10 on HSC proliferation but native IL10 also did not affect growth of HSC. Previously, we demonstrated that M6P-IL10 was able to increase collagen degradation (by increasing the MMP13/TIMP ratio) in primary cultures of HSC (Rachmawati and others 2007). Based on its effects on collagen deposition, we conclude that M6P-IL10 is pharmacologically active within the target cell *in vitro*.

The key concept in active drug targeting is that the distribution within the body is confined to the diseased organ/cell-types. This will lead to more optimal effects and less side effects because uptake in other organs is avoided. In pharmacokinetic terms, this means that the Volume of Distribution (Vd) is decreased. The presented results of gamma-camera imaging studies and the biodistribution studies with radiolabeled IL10 and M6P-IL10 indicate a preferential homing of the modified cytokine to the fibrotic liver. The shift in biodistribution of IL10 from the kidney to the liver after coupling of M6P is in accordance with the high liver uptake of M6P modified proteins found in previous studies with HSA as the core protein (Beljaars and others 1999; van Beuge and others 2011). These studies showed uptake of M6PHSA within HSC. The cells responsible for the uptake of M6P-IL10 within the liver could not be directly identified due to the low amount of cytokines administered. Both proteins are only available in the microgram scale and immunohistochemical detection of proteins requires injection of milligrams per rat. Therefore, receptor antagonists were applied to identify the target receptors. These studies indicated that liver uptake of M6P-IL10 was receptor-mediated since the uptake was not attenuated by the control protein HSA whereas sucHSA and M6P-HSA, both ligands for receptors, significantly reduced its uptake. The fact that sucHSA and M6P-HSA both had an effect indicates that M6P-IL10 binds to at least two receptors: the scavenger receptor and the M6P/IGFII receptor, respectively. Involvement of the scavenger receptor, which recognizes strongly anionic compounds, can be explained by the negative charges introduced by phosphate groups (PO_4^{3-}). This was also found in another study in which liposomes were modified with M6P sugars (Adrian and others 2006). The combination of M6PHSA and sucHSA did not completely block the liver uptake which suggests the involvement of yet another receptor, possibly the IL10 receptor which is also present in the liver (fig 6). Based on the expression of M6P/IGF II receptors, scavenger receptors and IL10 receptors, the putative target cells for M6P-IL10 are HSC's, portal fibroblasts, endothelial cells, Kupffer cells and neutrophils within the liver. Antifibrotic effects of IL10 are anticipated in all these cells.

To test whether M6P-IL10 is effective *in vivo*, we now administered (modified-)IL10 to bile duct ligated rats after the initiation of the fibrotic process, i.e. from day 4 till day 7 after BDL. In this time frame, pro-inflammatory activity is high in the liver and fibrosis is initiated (39-43). In addition, M6P/IGF-II receptor expression on HSC is enhanced at day 4 (Greupink and others 2006), which ensures targeting to this receptor at this time point. During the first week after BDL, enhanced IL10 receptor expression was noted (fig 6), also providing a rationale for the start of treatment at day 4.

Treatment with IL-10 or M6P-IL10 had significant effects on the inflammatory activity within the liver. A reduction in the number of infiltrating cells as reflected by DAB-positive cells was noted. These data indicate that M6P-IL10 is pharmacologically active *in vivo*. Based on inflammatory cell influx, its effect may even be superior to native IL10. Of particular interest is the reduction in IL-10 receptor expression after treatment with IL10, but not after treatment with M6P-IL10. The down regulation of the target receptor during treatment is relevant for IL10-based therapies. This may contribute to the lack of effectiveness of such therapies (Chadban and others 1997; Colombel and others 2001; Herfarth and Scholmerich 2002).

Next to the anti-inflammatory effects, we evaluated the effects of M6P-IL10 on fibrogenesis *in vivo*. The target cell of IL10 is the (activated) HSC, the extracellular matrix producing hepatic cell, and therefore antifibrotic effects are primarily anticipated in HSC and the most important feature in this respect is collagen deposition. Our results showed a clear reduction in collagen deposition in these livers after treatment with M6P-IL10 (figure 7). This reduction was established with various methods. The lack of portal-to-portal bridging was evident in nearly all the livers of the cytokine-treated animals. In addition, IL10 and M6P-IL10 also significantly reduced αSMA staining which reflects a reduction in the activation of HSC in these livers. These results indicate that our modified IL10 is pharmacologically active *in vivo*.

Although cytokines are interesting compounds which may yield potent new drugs, so far only a relatively few are approved and clinically used. The number is still disappointing low regarding the large number of endogenous cytokines. The main reasons for this are the poor stability and poor pharmacokinetic profile of cytokines. To overcome these pharmacokinetic problems, we apply drug targeting techniques to selectively deliver the cytokine to a specific (diseased) cell. In the current study, we demonstrate the possibilities of this strategy with successful *in vivo* application of a modified IL10. Recently, we also reported on the cell-specific delivery of another very interesting cytokine with antifibrotic activities, that is interferon-gamma (IFNγ) (Bansal and others 2011). This study shows that HSC-targeted IFNγ, in contrast to unmodified IFNγ, blocked liver fibrogenesis in a chronic CCL4 mice model of liver fibrosis, by specifically acting on the key pathogenic cells within the liver. Furthermore, we clearly demonstrated that the targeted IFNγ was devoid of side effects. In addition, others show beneficial effects of a targeted cytokine by means of coupling receptor specific ligands to the cytokine (Curnis and others 2000; Curnis and others 2005; Fournier, Aigner, Schirrmacher 2011; Jazayeri and Carroll 2008; Nissim and others 2004) often focussing on the treatment of tumours. These approaches may lead to a more optimal use of cytokines for therapeutic purposes.

In summary, we demonstrated potent pharmacological effectivity of a novel liver-specific form of the cytokine IL10. After conjugation with M6P, the novel cytokine efficiently accumulates in the liver and attenuates the fibrotic process *in vivo*. Further dose-response

Modification of Interleukin-10 with Mannose- 6-Phosphate Groups Yields a Liver-Specific Cytokine with
Antifibrotic Activity in Rats

155

studies are required to examine whether M6P-IL10 is more effective than the native product and exerts less adverse effects. Furthermore, targeting of potentially interesting cytokines to the liver is promising and it may lead to the generation of a therapeutic antifibrotic compound which has not been realized so far.

4. Acknowledgment

We thank Dr. M.N. Lub-de Hooge, Mr. Hans Pol and Mr. Hans ter Veen (Department of Nuclear Medicine, University Medical Center Groningen, The Netherlands) for their radiolabelling of proteins and help during the gamma-camera studies.

5. References

Adrian JE, Poelstra K, Scherphof GL, Molema G, Meijer DK, Reker-Smit C, Morselt HW, Kamps JA. 2006. Interaction of targeted liposomes with primary cultured hepatic stellate cells: Involvement of multiple receptor systems. J Hepatol 44(3):560-7.

Allen TM and Cullis PR. 2004. Drug delivery systems: Entering the mainstream. Science 303(5665):1818-22.

Andersen SR, Lambrecht LJ, Swan SK, Cutler DL, Radwanski E, Affrime MB, Garaud JJ. 1999. Disposition of recombinant human interleukin-10 in subjects with various degrees of renal function. J Clin Pharmacol 39(10):1015-20.

Bansal R, Prakash J, Post E, Beljaars L, Schuppan D, Poelstra K. 2011. Novel engineered targeted interferon-gamma blocks hepatic fibrogenesis in mice. Hepatology 54(2):586-96.

Bataller R and Brenner DA. 2005. Liver fibrosis. J Clin Invest 115(2):209-18.

Beljaars L, Meijer DK, Poelstra K. 2002. Targeting hepatic stellate cells for cell-specific treatment of liver fibrosis. Front Biosci 7:e214-22.

Beljaars L, Weert B, Geerts A, Meijer DK, Poelstra K. 2003. The preferential homing of a platelet derived growth factor receptor-recognizing macromolecule to fibroblast-like cells in fibrotic tissue. Biochem Pharmacol 66(7):1307-17.

Beljaars L, Molema G, Schuppan D, Geerts A, De Bleser PJ, Weert B, Meijer DK, Poelstra K. 2000. Successful targeting to rat hepatic stellate cells using albumin modified with cyclic peptides that recognize the collagen type VI receptor. J Biol Chem 275(17):12743-51.

Beljaars L, Molema G, Weert B, Bonnema H, Olinga P, Groothuis GM, Meijer DK, Poelstra K. 1999. Albumin modified with mannose 6-phosphate: A potential carrier for selective delivery of antifibrotic drugs to rat and human hepatic stellate cells. Hepatology 29(5):1486-93.

Chadban SJ, Tesch GH, Lan HY, Atkins RC, Nikolic-Paterson DJ. 1997. Effect of interleukin-10 treatment on crescentic glomerulonephritis in rats. Kidney Int 51(6):1809-17.

Colombel JF, Rutgeerts P, Malchow H, Jacyna M, Nielsen OH, Rask-Madsen J, Van Deventer S, Ferguson A, Desreumaux P, Forbes A, et al. 2001. Interleukin 10 (tenovil) in the prevention of postoperative recurrence of crohn's disease. Gut 49(1):42-6.

Curnis F, Gasparri A, Sacchi A, Cattaneo A, Magni F, Corti A. 2005. Targeted delivery of IFNgamma to tumor vessels uncouples antitumor from counterregulatory mechanisms. Cancer Res 65(7):2906-13.

Curnis F, Sacchi A, Borgna L, Magni F, Gasparri A, Corti A. 2000. Enhancement of tumor necrosis factor alpha antitumor immunotherapeutic properties by targeted delivery to aminopeptidase N (CD13). Nat Biotechnol 18(11):1185-90.

Cuzzocrea S, Mazzon E, Dugo L, Serraino I, Britti D, De Maio M, Caputi AP. 2001. Absence of endogeneous interleukin-10 enhances the evolution of murine type-II collagen-induced arthritis. Eur Cytokine Netw 12(4):568-80.

de Bleser PJ, Jannes P, van Buul-Offers SC, Hoogerbrugge CM, van Schravendijk CF, Niki T, Rogiers V, van den Brande JL, Wisse E, Geerts A. 1995. Insulinlike growth factor-II/mannose 6-phosphate receptor is expressed on CCl4-exposed rat fat-storing cells and facilitates activation of latent transforming growth factor-beta in cocultures with sinusoidal endothelial cells. Hepatology 21(5):1429-37.

Demols A, Van Laethem JL, Quertinmont E, Degraef C, Delhaye M, Geerts A, Deviere J. 2002. Endogenous interleukin-10 modulates fibrosis and regeneration in experimental chronic pancreatitis. Am J Physiol Gastrointest Liver Physiol 282(6):G1105-12.

Di Marco R, Xiang M, Zaccone P, Leonardi C, Franco S, Meroni P, Nicoletti F. 1999. Concanavalin A-induced hepatitis in mice is prevented by interleukin (IL)-10 and exacerbated by endogenous IL-10 deficiency. Autoimmunity 31(2):75-83.

Fedorak RN, Gangl A, Elson CO, Rutgeerts P, Schreiber S, Wild G, Hanauer SB, Kilian A, Cohard M, LeBeaut A, et al. 2000. Recombinant human interleukin 10 in the treatment of patients with mild to moderately active crohn's disease. the interleukin 10 inflammatory bowel disease cooperative study group. Gastroenterology 119(6):1473-82.

Fournier P, Aigner M, Schirrmacher V. 2011. Targeting of IL-2 and GM-CSF immunocytokines to a tumor vaccine leads to increased anti-tumor activity. Int J Oncol 38(6):1719-29.

Friedman SL. 2010. Evolving challenges in hepatic fibrosis. Nat Rev Gastroenterol Hepatol 7(8):425-36.

Gloor B, Todd KE, Lane JS, Rigberg DA, Reber HA. 1998. Mechanism of increased lung injury after acute pancreatitis in IL-10 knockout mice. J Surg Res 80(1):110-4.

Greupink R, Bakker HI, van Goor H, de Borst MH, Beljaars L, Poelstra K. 2006. Mannose-6-phosphate/insulin-like growth factor-II receptors may represent a target for the selective delivery of mycophenolic acid to fibrogenic cells. Pharm Res 23(8):1827-34.

Herfarth H and Scholmerich J. 2002. IL-10 therapy in crohn's disease: At the crossroads. treatment of crohn's disease with the anti-inflammatory cytokine interleukin 10. Gut 50(2):146-7.

Iredale JP. 2007. Models of liver fibrosis: Exploring the dynamic nature of inflammation and repair in a solid organ. J Clin Invest 117(3):539-48.

Ishak K, Baptista A, Bianchi L, Callea F, De Groote J, Gudat F, Denk H, Desmet V, Korb G, MacSween RN. 1995. Histological grading and staging of chronic hepatitis. J Hepatol 22(6):696-9.

Jazayeri JA and Carroll GJ. 2008. Fc-based cytokines : Prospects for engineering superior therapeutics. BioDrugs 22(1):11-26.

Jevsevar S, Kunstelj M, Porekar VG. 2010. PEGylation of therapeutic proteins. Biotechnol J 5(1):113-28.

Modification of Interleukin-10 with Mannose- 6-Phosphate Groups Yields a Liver-Specific Cytokine with
Antifibrotic Activity in Rats

157

Khan AQ, Shen Y, Wu ZQ, Wynn TA, Snapper CM. 2002. Endogenous pro- and anti-inflammatory cytokines differentially regulate an in vivo humoral response to streptococcus pneumoniae. Infect Immun 70(2):749-61.

Kitching AR, Tipping PG, Timoshanko JR, Holdsworth SR. 2000. Endogenous interleukin-10 regulates Th1 responses that induce crescentic glomerulonephritis. Kidney Int 57(2):518-25.

Louis H, Le Moine O, Goldman M, Deviere J. 2003. Modulation of liver injury by interleukin-10. Acta Gastroenterol Belg 66(1):7-14.

Louis H, Van Laethem JL, Wu W, Quertinmont E, Degraef C, Van den Berg K, Demols A, Goldman M, Le Moine O, Geerts A, et al. 1998. Interleukin-10 controls neutrophilic infiltration, hepatocyte proliferation, and liver fibrosis induced by carbon tetrachloride in mice. Hepatology 28(6):1607-15.

Meijer DK, Beljaars L, Molema G, Poelstra K. 2001. Disease-induced drug targeting using novel peptide-ligand albumins. J Control Release 72(1-3):157-64.

Nelson DR, Lauwers GY, Lau JY, Davis GL. 2000. Interleukin 10 treatment reduces fibrosis in patients with chronic hepatitis C: A pilot trial of interferon nonresponders. Gastroenterology 118(4):655-60.

Nissim A, Gofur Y, Vessillier S, Adams G, Chernajovsky Y. 2004. Methods for targeting biologicals to specific disease sites. Trends Mol Med 10(6):269-74.

Oberholzer A, Oberholzer C, Moldawer LL. 2002. Interleukin-10: A complex role in the pathogenesis of sepsis syndromes and its potential as an anti-inflammatory drug. Crit Care Med 30(1 Supp):S58-63.

Pinzani M, Rombouts K, Colagrande S. 2005. Fibrosis in chronic liver diseases: Diagnosis and management. J Hepatol 42 Suppl(1):S22-36.

Poelstra K, Hardonk MJ, Koudstaal J, Bakker WW. 1990. Intraglomerular platelet aggregation and experimental glomerulonephritis. Kidney Int 37(6):1500-8.

Rachmawati H, Reker-Smit C, Lub-de Hooge MN, van Loenen-Weemaes A, Poelstra K, Beljaars L. 2007. Chemical modification of interleukin-10 with mannose 6-phosphate groups yields a liver-selective cytokine. Drug Metab Dispos 35(5): 814-21.

Rachmawati H, Beljaars L, Reker-Smit C, Van Loenen-Weemaes AM, Hagens WI, Meijer DK, Poelstra K. 2004. Pharmacokinetic and biodistribution profile of recombinant human interleukin-10 following intravenous administration in rats with extensive liver fibrosis. Pharm Res 21(11):2072-8.

Reineke U, Sabat R, Volk HD, Schneider-Mergener J. 1998. Mapping of the interleukin-10/interleukin-10 receptor combining site. Protein Sci 7(4):951-60.

Schooltink H and Rose-John S. 2002. Cytokines as therapeutic drugs. J Interferon Cytokine Res 22(5):505-16.

Schreiber S, Fedorak RN, Nielsen OH, Wild G, Williams CN, Nikolaus S, Jacyna M, Lashner BA, Gangl A, Rutgeerts P, et al. 2000. Safety and efficacy of recombinant human interleukin 10 in chronic active crohn's disease. crohn's disease IL-10 cooperative study group. Gastroenterology 119(6):1461-72.

Schuppan D and Popov Y. 2009. Rationale and targets for antifibrotic therapies. Gastroenterol Clin Biol 33(10-11):949-57.

Schuppan D and Afdhal NH. 2008. Liver cirrhosis. Lancet 371(9615):838-51.

Standiford TJ. 2000. Anti-inflammatory cytokines and cytokine antagonists. Curr Pharm Des 6(6):633-49.

Thompson K, Maltby J, Fallowfield J, McAulay M, Millward-Sadler H, Sheron N. 1998. Interleukin-10 expression and function in experimental murine liver inflammation and fibrosis. Hepatology 28(6):1597-606.

van Beuge MM, Prakash J, Lacombe M, Post E, Reker-Smit C, Beljaars L, Poelstra K. 2011. Increased liver uptake and reduced hepatic stellate cell activation with a cell-specific conjugate of the rho-kinase inhibitor Y27632. Pharm Res 28(8):2045-54.

Vilcek J and Feldmann M. 2004. Historical review: Cytokines as therapeutics and targets of therapeutics. Trends Pharmacol Sci 25(4):201-9.

Wang SC, Ohata M, Schrum L, Rippe RA, Tsukamoto H. 1998. Expression of interleukin-10 by in vitro and in vivo activated hepatic stellate c

8

The Influence of Cyclophosphamide on Immune Function of Murine Macrophages

Krzysztof Bryniarski
Jagiellonian University Medical College,
Department of Immunology, Krakow,
Poland

1. Introduction

1.1 The structure of cyclophosphamide (CY) and its active metabolites acrolein (ACR) and phosphoramide mustard (PM)

Cyclophosphamide (CY), an alkylating compound is commonly used as a cytoreductive agent in the treatment of cancer (blood, breast, ovary) because of its ability to interfere with DNA synthesis and its pharmacological action on dividing cells (Ben Efraim 2001). Its action is however more complex since it exerts a strong influence on the immune system. Studies on cyclophosphamide are conducted for a long time, but its effect on macrophages (Mf) was not yet definite, therefore this study was attempted.

CY is *in vitro* inactive by itself, and is converted *in vivo* into two ultimately biologically active alkylating metabolites: phosphoramide mustard (PM) and acrolein (ACR).The first step of that complicated pathway of CY metabolism occurs in the liver and results in the formation of derivative hydroperoxycyclophosphamide and then it is followed by several enzymatic reactions that format carbonamide, aldehyde and carboxylacide inactive structures or lead to non-enzymatic formation of phosphoramide mustard and acrolein, active metabolites of cyclophosphamide which were tested in our immune research. Instead of highly unstable phosphoramide mustard (PM), we used nitrogen mustard (NM, mechlorethamine) (see **Fig 1**.) which is structurally and functionally related to PM, previously shown *in vitro* and *in vivo* to have the same activity as CY (Bryniarski et al. 1996).

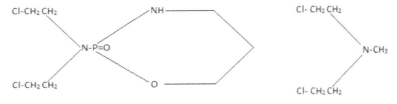

CYCLOPHOSPHAMIDE   MECHLORETHAMINE

Fig. 1. The chemical structure of cyclophosphamide and nitrogen mustard

2. Differences of CY dose treatment used in the treatment of malignant diseases and autoimmune diseases in comparison to immune regulation

Immunoregulatory function of CY is observed in doses 20-100 mg/kg in mice, which can be calculated in human treatment as below 2mg/kg (less than 100 mg/m^2). The higher doses of cyclophosphamide above 100mg/m^2 (2-3mg/kg) in humans mainly used in several pulses or as prolonged treatments are used in anticancer therapy of peripheral blood cancers and lymphoma (Audia et al. 2007; Vitolo et al. 2008) as well as in metastases of breast, ovarian and bronchial cancers (Snowden et al. 1997; Audia et al. 2007; Burger 2007) trophoblastic tumors (Cole et al. 2008), leiomyosarcoma (Durhan et al. 2009), pheochromocytoma (Adjalle et al. 2009), rhabdomyosarcoma (Breitfeld & Mayer 2005).

Much higher doses of CY (50mg/kg per 3 days) are proposed to be used in treatment of Graft Versus Host Disease (GVHD) after allogenic hematopoetic stem cells transplantation (alloHSCT) for treatment of hematologic malignancies (Luznik & Fuchs 2010). Post-transplantation CY promotes tolerance in alloreactive host and donor T cells leading to suppression of both graft rejection and GVHD after alloHSCT.

In autoimmune diseases like sclerosis multiplex (MS), lupus nephritis or immune mediated neuropathies, CY is the medicament used for pulsed first treatment as well for the retreatment in several doses mainly higher than 100 up to 1600 mg/m^2. It is proved that CY treatment seems to give better therapeutic effect in patients in earlier stages of MS where inflammation predominates over degenerative processes in the central nervous system (CNS). There is no evidence of efficacy in primary progressive MS or later stages of secondary progressive MS. In these high doses of CY therapy, patients show low pro-inflammatory cytokine secretion which activates anti-inflammatory cytokine secretion, what is suggested in an elegant review by Weiner and Cohen as one of curative effects in MS neurodegenerative disease (Weiner & Cohen 2002). That high dose treatment can express quite a different suppressor effect on the immune system mediated by B and T lymphocytes that mediate two branches of humoral and cellular immune responses. High doses of CY used for the treatment of malignant or autoimmune diseases express more toxic effects on the immune system by elimination of different currently activated subpopulations of immune cells and lead to inhibition of inflammatory reactions which diminish the formation of degenerative lesions.

Cyclophosphamide is commonly used in multiagent chemotherapy rather than intravenous (i.v.) monotherapy for treatment of malignancies, therefore its dose can be relatively lesser than in case of single use (because of the effect of summarizing or multiplying of drug activity and toxicity). It also must be taken into consideration what kind of regulatory therapeutic effect is desired – the activating effect based on elimination of natural suppression in case of low doses treatment, or suppressor effect on the immune cells, maintained mainly by cytotoxic effect which appears in case of treatment with high doses of CY. It is estimated that the therapeutic dose of endoxan equals about 25-50% of toxic dose. The control of unwanted and unexpected toxic effects must be also taken into consideration in case of establishing any kind of CY therapy. Between the most frequent unwanted toxic effects observed in case of CY treatment is gonadal disfunction observed in man in a lower cumulative dose in man (60 g/m^2) less expressed in female (Vitolo et al. 2008). Moreover, apart from alopecia and nausea, the other toxic effects are infections and hemorrhagic cystitis. There is also an increased risk of cancer and bladder toxicity which appears in the cumulative life-time dose exceeding 80-100 g (which is about 50 doses of 1000 mg/m² during life-time) (Weinar & Cohen 2002) .

3. Immunoregulatory activities of cyclophosphamide treatment – The evidence performed in mice by the low dose cyclophosphamide treated macrophages

Macrophages (Mf) carry out the fundamental protective function of phagocyting and killing invading organisms and release a vast number of factors involved in host defense and inflammation. Moreover they play a critical role in the induction, regulation and expression of both cellular and humoral responses. These highly diversified functions are accompanied by heterogeneous morphology and biochemical and phenotypical characteristics.

3.1 Methods for estimation of macrophage activity in innate and in adaptive humoral and cellular immune responses

My experimental studies were aimed at the establishing the influence of low dose of CY treatment (20-50 mg/kg) on the macrophages (Mf) – the important cells involved in an innate and humoral or cellular adaptive immune responses in mice. The innate immune response was measured by both the capacity of reactive oxygen intermediates production and secretion by phagocytic activating macrophages and by the ability of production of proinflammatory cytokines (IL-1β, IL-6 and TNF-α) (Marcinkiewicz et al. 1994). The ability of cyclophosphamide treated Mf (MfCY) to secrete regulatory cytokine (proinflammatory IL-12 and inhibitory TGF-β and IL-10) was also tested in their supernatant over the Mf culture and was estimated by ELISA (total concentration) (Bryniarski 2004 & 2009), or in bioassays which utilize proliferation effect of particular cytokine by cytokine-dependent cell lines and measures exclusively bioactive form of particular cytokine (Marcinkiewicz et al. 1994 & Bryniarski et al. 1996). The cell surface markers of tested Mf were estimated cytofluorimetrically in FACS (Szczepanik et al. 1993 & Bryniarski et al. 2009), but the phenotypical differences between functionally differentiated macrophages were estimated by measuring the pattern of esterase activity (Czajkowska et al. 1995).

The induction of cellular response was tested in contact hypersensitivity against TNP/PCL hapten (Szczepanik et al. 1993, Bryniarski et al. 2004) which activates CD4 Th1 subpopulation of lymphocytes and macrophages and is classified by Pichler as a classical type IVa delayed type hypersensitivity (Lerch & Pichler 2004; Posadas & Pichler 2007). Humoral activity against corpuscular antigen was tested in plaque forming assay (PFA) from Mf pulsed with sheep red blood cells and cultured 4 days in the presence of naïve B cells. The antigen presenting activity was estimated as a number of plaque forming cells PFC/10⁶ splenocytes (Bryniarski et al. 2004).

3.2 Treatment of donors of macrophages with low dose of CY uncovers the subpopulation of peritoneal macrophages that induce CHS response in mice

Application of hapten on the skin is a classical way to immunize for contact sensitivity reaction, but animals can also be sensitized by subcutaneous injection of hapten substituted peritoneal macrophages. However, if haptenated macrophages are injected i.v. a long-lasting unresponsiveness ensues, in which the activity of Th1 immune effector lymphocytes is obliterated by simultaneously recruited CD8+suppressor cells. When subsequently skin sensitized, such animals have significantly diminished CHS reactions. Moreover this state of unresponsiveness can be adoptively transferred to naïve syngeneic animals by lymphoid cells.

The CHS reaction to trinitrophenyl (TNP/PCL) hapten is activated by CD4 Th1 lymphocytes which recognize TNP/PCL hapten on the surface of MHC class II expressed by hapten-labeled macrophages. After 5 days the sensitized recipients of TNP-Mf are able to reduce the CHS reaction when challenged by applying a very low dose of the same hapten (TNP/PCL) on the ear skin. The CHS reaction develops 24 h after challenge (with hapten) as ear swelling CHS response and is measured with the engineering micrometer and expressed in units of ear swelling (Szczepanik et al. 1993). When the donors of macrophages are injected intravenously (i.v.) with low dose of cyclophosphamide (20-100mg/kg) a day before cell harvesting, then the cells are labeled with hapten and injected i.v. into naïve recipients instead of unresponsiveness strong contact hypersensitivity develops 24 h after the challenge with the same hapten. Moreover it was shown that in vivo CY treatment activates strong functional diversification of macrophage subpopulations in mice. Thus result of in vivo CY treatment, hapten-conjugated Mf (TNP-MfCY) when injected i.v. into naïve recipients TNP-MfCY activate strong contact hypersensitivity (CHS) reaction against hapten, instead of unresponsiveness induced by TNP-Mf mediated by CD8+ T suppressor lymphocytes, which inhibit hapten specific CHS response (**Fig. 2**).

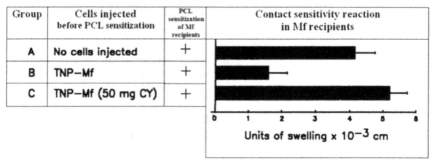

Group	Cells injected before PCL sensitization	PCL sensitization of Mf recipients	Contact sensitivity reaction in Mf recipients
A	No cells injected	+	
B	TNP—Mf	+	
C	TNP—Mf (50 mg CY)	+	

CBA/J mice were injected i.v. with 1 x 10⁶ TNP-Mf from donors treated (group C) or untreated (group B) with CY. Seven days later these animals and a group of naïve mice (group A) were skin sensitized with PCL and tested for contact hypersensitivity (CHS) after additional 4 days. Statistical significance group B ve groups A & C p<0.002

Fig. 2. Peritoneal macrophages from cyclophosphamide-treated mice do not induce suppressor cells.

It was shown by us that CY sensitive subpopulation of peritoneal macrophages responsible for induction of suppressor cells has higher density when separated in discontinuous gradient of Ficoll than population activating CHS response. Moreover it has also strong adherent and higher phagocyting properties and has high expression of FcγRI and FcγRII (33-44%) in comparison to the low density cell fraction, which is CY resistant. The latest fraction of cells is weakly phagocytic and adherent, has less FcγR (22-26%). It is widely known that antigen presenting cells (APC) are macrophages, dendritic cells and B lymphocytes. First two populations can phagocyte, but last is inactive in this activity. For two reasons it seems unlikely that previously described light fraction of cells are contaminated with dendritic cells.

First almost all of them labeled with macrophage specific F4/80 antibody, second, as shown previously by Steinman and Cohn peritoneal exudate cells induced by thioglycolate, although contaminated by several cell types do not contain dendritic cells (Szczepanik et al. 1993). Both subpopulations of tested macrophages express no significant differences in Mac-1 (30-50%) and Mac-3 (33-46%) markers and no differences were found between CY-treated and untreated mice in a surface expression of I-A (7-14%) and I-E (3-6%) antigens. We were not able to associate the differences in surface markers expression in both populations of macrophages with variety of their bioactivity and immune function (Szczepanik et al. 1993). We also found that Mf CY express slightly higher percentage of molecules important in the stimulation of phagocytosis (CD14 and CD23) and molecules basic for activation of antigen-presenting immune response (CD80/CD86 and MHC class II) in comparison to control oil-induced peritoneal macrophages. Results are shown in **Table 1**.

Macrophages	CD23/Mac3	CD80/Mac3	CD86/Mac3	CD14/Mac3	DR/Mac3
Mf	62.0	50.0	51.6	59.3	45.4
Mf CY [50mg/kg]	73.7	68.4	71.6	71.7	59.0

Oil-induced macrophages were labeled for direct immunofluorescence with monoclonal antibodies specific against specific macrophage antigen (Mac3-FITC) and cell surface markers (CD23-PE, CD80-PE, CD86-PE, CD14-PE, MHCII DR-PE). Results are expressed as a percent of double positive cells. The measurement was performed on the FASC Cytoron-Absolute.

Table 1. Expression of selected surface markers on macrophages isolated from oil-induced peritoneal cavity from donors treated or not treated with cyclophosphamide in dose 50 mg/kg.

In following experiment we have shown (Bryniarski et al. 2009) that cyclophosphamide in vivo as well as its both tested metabolic products in vitro - acrolein (ACR) and mechloretamine (NM) (nitrogen mustard – an analogue of phosphoramide mustard) make TNP-substituted Mf (TNP-Mf) immunogenic for the induction of CHS response. The results are shown in **Table 2**.

Group	Mice injected with	CHS response [U x 10-2 mm] ± SD
A	TNP-Mf	0.2 ± 0.84
B	TNP-Mf CY	4.8 ± 0.68
C	TNP-Mf ACR	5.3 ± 1.12
D	TNP-Mf NM	5.2 ± 0.66
E	TNP-Mf ACR & NM	5.5 ± 0.90

The following abbreviations are used: TNP-Mf - TNP substituted Mf from control mice; TNP-Mf CY - Mf from mice treated with CY (50 mg/kg); TNP-Mf ACR – normal Mf treated in vitro with 10^{-7} M ACR; TNP-Mf NM - normal Mf treated in vitro with 10^{-7} M ACR; TNP-Mf ACR & NM - Mf treated with both metabolites.

CBA/J mice were injected i.v. with 1×10^6 TNP-substituted Mf . Seven days after TNP-Mf injection the mice were tested for CHS reaction which is expressed in units x 10^{-2} mm ± SD. The negative values (ear swelling in control, unimmunized mice) were substracted from experimental values. The statistical significance (a posteriori Bonferroni test): Group A vs. Groups B, C, D, E $p < 0.001$. Each group consisted of five mice.

Table 2. Immunognecity of oil-induced peritoneal macrophages untreated or treated in vivo with 50 mg/kg CY or in vitro with acrolein (ACR) or mechloretamine (NM).

3.3 The phenotypical differences between functionally differentiated macrophages estimation of activity IL-6 and a heterogeneity of α- and β- naphtyl acetate esterase isoenzymes

Some differences were shown when a population of different immune functions were tested by unspecific esterase activity, which is regarded to play a role in intracellular processing and trafficking of antigen (Czajkowska et al. 1995). In these experimental works we tested two different, but phenotypically indistinguishable macrophage clones 59 and 63 obtained from Martin Dorf and coworkers from Harvard University, Boston, MA. Both are adherent and phagocytic, produce IL-1 and IL-6 and constitutively express a number of identical cell surface markers, including Ia. However they differ functionally and while clone 59 presents antigen to Th1 lymphocytes, clone 63 induces suppressor T lymphocytes. These obvious functional differences in antigen presenting capacities between the seemingly phenotypically identical cell lines were identified by us in testing them for activity of nonspecific α- and β- naphtyl acetate esterase isoenzymes and secretion of IL-6 in case of cell lines stimulated with mechloretamine (NM)– the alkylating agent relating to cyclophosphamide. The isoenzymatic patterns of α-esterase express strong differences in line 59 treated with MN in comparison to background non-activated cells. In line 59, NM treatment increases the heterogeneity and activity of esterase in both pH 7.5 and pH 5.8. In contrast to line 59 no differences in the isoenzymatic pattern of α–esterase in NM-treated and untreated 63 line cells were found. The β-esterase activity was also tested but no significant differences were found between untreated and MN-treated cell lines.

The results in **Table 3** show that CHS inducing clone 59 produces little IL-6 and NM does not activate its production in comparison to basal activity. In contrary clone 63 is a high producer of IL-6 and stimulated by NM.

Groups	Clone 59 IL-6 [ng/mL] X ± SD	Clone 63 IL-6 [ng/mL] X ± SD
Mf	62 ± 9.6	111 ± 9.3
Mf & NM 10^{-6} M	27 ± 4.3	358 ± 3.1
Mf & NM 10^{-8} M	35 ± 4.7	226 ± 1.5
Mf & NM 10^{-10} M	21 ± 5.5	209 ± 2.1

2×10^7 Mf were treated with NM at concentrations from 10^{-10} to 10^{-6} M for 40 min at 0^0C then thoroughly washed out from NM with phosphate buffered saline (PBS). Cells cultured in RPMI 1640 medium supplemented with 5% fetal calf serum (FCS) at concentration 10^6 Mf per mL in 24 wells flat bottom plates at 37^0C at 5% CO_2. The concentration of IL-6 was estimated in bioassay with B9 cell line with (data not shown, but all results were estimated less than 2ng/mL) or without mAb anti-IL-6 and expressed in ng/mL.

Table 3. The production of IL-6 by Mf cell line 59 and 63 treated with different concentration of nitrogen mustard

Our experiments show that two macrophage lines differ in isoenzyme patterns such that α and β esterases of line 59 which induces immunity, are more heterogeneous than esterase of line 63, which induces suppression. Both cell lines, when non activated with NM however produce comparable amounts of IL-6 (Czajkowska et al. 1995). We have shown previously the peritoneal macrophages (Bryniarski et al. 1996), like line 63 cells, when tagged with the antigen, induce T suppressor cells, however, when treated with NM, a pharmacological derivative of cyclophosphamide, produce high amounts of IL-6, also change their functional (suppressive) properties to activation the hapten specific CHS immune response (Bryniarski et al. 2009).

It was also shown that NM, changed the isoenzyme pattern in line 59, which was accompanied by somewhat decreased production of IL-6, while esterases of line 63 were not affected by NM, which however activated the production of IL-6. NM, like other alkylating factors, binds covalently and non-selectively to variety of molecules including amino acids, proteins and DNA. Since the Mf were incubated with NM at 0^0C the possibility of its intracellular penetration was negligible and we presume that under such condition NM binds mainly to cell surface proteins. We suggested that the translation of intracellular membrane signal acts in a different way, which can result in a different production of IL-6 by line 59 and 63 cells and their isoenzyme patterns after NM stimulation (Czajkowska et al. 1995).

3.4 Proinflammatory cytokine secretion by functionally different subpopulation of Mf treated with CY or its derivatives ACR or NM

CY influence on the cytokine releasing activity by the functionally different subpopulation of macrophages was examined by Marcinkiewicz and Bryniarski (Marcinkiewicz et al. 1994 and Bryniarski et al. 1996 & 2009). They have shown that low dose of CY treatment activates Mf to production and secretion of mainly IL-6 while simultaneously diminish TNF-α and IL-1β production (Marcinkiewicz et al. 1994). The strong activation of IL-6 production was observed in case of peritoneal macrophage stimulation with mechloretamine (NM) the analogue of nitrogen mustard (Bryniarski et al. 1996). This is a common phenomenon which is observed in NM-treated oil-induced and thioglycolate peritoneal macrophages obtained from different mouse strains (CBA/J, Balb c, C57/BL6 and SWISS) and tested in bioassay with IL-6 dependent B9 cells as well as in IL-6 ELISA assay (Bryniarski et al. 1996 & 2009).

3.4.1 Production of cytokines by control Mf or Mf from animals treated *in vivo* with CY or Mf treated *in vitro* by its metabolites

Control Mf or Mf from CY-treated animals (50 mg/kg) or Mf incubated *in vitro* with ACR (10^{-7} M) or NM (10^{-6} M) were cultured for 24 or 48 h in RPMI 1640 medium and the production of five different cytokines was measured in the resultant supernatants by ELISA. These results are shown in **Table 4**. Mf from CY treated animals (Group B) and Mf treated *in vitro* with NM (Group D) showed an increased production of pro-inflammatory IL-6 and IL-12, and a decreased production of anti-inflammatory IL-10 and TGF-β cytokines compared to the control group (Group A). Mf treated with ACR (Group C) manufactured more IL-6 and less TGF-β than control cells (Group A), but the production of IL-12 remained unchanged. Treatment with CY or its derivatives did not influence TNF-α production although in Group B, there it was somewhat lower than in the control group.

Cell cultured		Cytokine production [pg/ml]				
		TNF-α	IL-6	IL-10	IL-12	TGF-β
A	Mf	250 ± 5	283 ± 7	61 ± 3	213 ± 3	109 ± 2
B	Mf CY [50 mg/kg]	182 ± 4	467 ± 4	22 ± 4	455 ± 14	50 ± 4
C	Mf ACR [10^{-6} M]	287 ± 21	982 ± 25	33 ± 2	167 ± 10	33 ± 3
D	Mf NM [10^{-7} M]	245 ± 30	1500 ± 100	47 ± 4	460 ± 28	59 ± 17

Five $\times 10^5$ control Mf or cells from cyclophosphamide-treated animals (Mf CY) or Mf treated with acrolein (Mf ACR) or nitrogen mustard (Mf NM) *in vitro* (for details see legend to Table 3) were cultured in 1 ml of RPMI 1640 medium supplemented with 5% FCS for 24h (TNF-α and IL-6) or 48h (other cytokines) and concentrations of cytokines were measured by ELISA assays. Table 2 shows the results of one representative experiment out of three as the mean of three estimations ± SD.

Table 4. Cytokine production by macrophages (Mf) from naïve mice, or animals treated with cyclophosphamide (CY) *in vivo* or acrolein (Mf ACR) or nitrogen mustard (Mf NM) *in vitro*.

3.4.2 High tolerogenicity of TNP-Mf *in vivo* can be reversed by administration into recipients of anti-IL-10 and/or anti-TGF-β mAbs

Since inefficient immunogenicity of administered intravenously control TNP-Mf as compared with CY-treated cells may be due to the different cytokine sets that they produce, we injected these cells into recipients that simultaneously received an *i.v.* injection of 500 µg of anti-IL-10, anti-TGF-β or a mixture of both antibodies. The CHS reaction was measured 7 days later. **Figure 3** shows that TNP-Mf

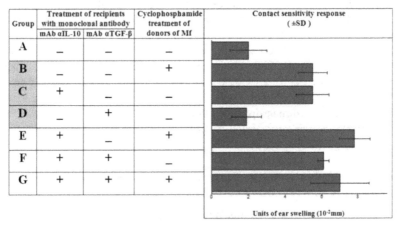

CBA/J mice were injected i.v. with 1×10^6 TNP substituted Mf (groups A, C, D and F) or TNP-Mf CY (groups B, E, G). In the groups C and E the mice simultaneously received i.v. 500 µg of anti-IL-10 mAb and in group D, 500 µg anti-TGFβ mAb, and in groups F & G both mAbs were given. Seven days later the CHS response was measured (see legend to Table 2). Statistiacally significant (a posteriori Bonferroni test) Group A ve groups B, C and F p<0.002; group A ve groups E and G p<0.001; Group B ve groups C, F and G →NS; group B ve D p<0.02

Fig. 3. Tolerance induced by intravenous injection of TNP-Mf can be reversed by simultaneous administration of anti-IL-10 and/or anti-TGF-β mAbs. Comparison with in vivo CY treatment (50 mg/kg) of TNP-Mf (TNP-Mf CY) combined with administration with mAbs anti-IL10 or/and anti-TGF-β.

obtained from naïve donors were non-immunogenic (Group A) but from CY-treated donors (Group B) induced CHS response, while animals treated with anti-IL-10 alone (Group C & E) or together with anti-TGF-β (Group F & G) from both donors produced a significant CHS reaction. Anti-TGF-β alone (Group D) had no influence on the level of the CS reaction.

3.5 Production of the reactive oxygen intermediates by Mf CY or macrophages treated with low doses of ACR or NM

The testing of innate immune response mediated by macrophages can be estimated by reactive oxygen intermediates (ROI's) production. We use the luminol-dependent chemiluminescence as a measure of activity in Mf stimulated by opsonized zymosan particles. **Figure 4** shows that Mf from animals treated with 20 or 50 mg/kg of CY produce a significantly increased level of ROI's while the dose of 100 mg/kg remains without effect and 200 mg/kg diminished the production of ROI's below the control level. A marked increase of ROI's level was induced by in vitro incubation Mf in a low concentration of NM (10^{-7} or 10^{-6} M) while 10^{-5} M had a slightly inhibitory effect. ACR at concentration 10^{-7} M and 10^{-6} M had no effect when compared with control Mf, whereas 10^{-5} M was inhibitory.

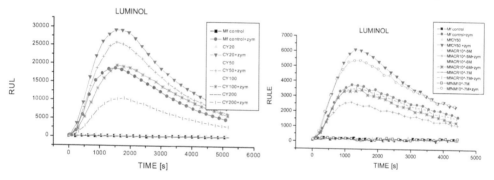

Production of reactive oxygen intermediates (ROI's) by macrophages is dependent upon the dose of cyclophosphamide (CY) used to treat donors. The highest activity is observed with doses 20-50 mg/kg. The higher dose of CY (200 mg/kg) decreases ROI's production by Mf in comparison with control cells (Mf). The low concentration of nitrogen mustard (NM) used to treat Mf increases the production of ROI's to a similar level as in vivo treatment of Mf–donors with CY (50 mg/kg). Treatment by 10^{-5}M NM was slightly inhibitory (results not shown). Treatment of Mf with acrolein (ACR) (10^{-5}-10^{-7} M) reduces the secretion of ROI's in a dose dependent manner in comparison to the control group (Mf). Zym – zymosan

Fig. 4. Influence of in vivo treatment with cyclophosphamide (CY) and in vitro treatment with nitrogen mustard or acrolein on the production of reactive oxygen intermediates (ROI's)by murine peritoneal Mf.

3.6 Testicular macrophages (TMf) and their immune response in the reaction with CY

Residual testicular macrophages (TMf) that are present in interstitial tissue of male gonads are regarded as essential cells for male reproductive function involved in the regulation of hormonal balance in the testis. TMf by released products and also directly by cell-to-cell contacts participate in the process of steroidogenesis by Leydig cells. They also influence the behavior of Sertoli cells by releasing mediators and regulate spermatogenesis in testis.

Apart from that function TMf play an important role in their functional contribution of anatomical blood-testis barrier formed by Sertoli cells (Bryniarski et al 2004).

3.6.1 Induction of contact hypersensitivity by TMf and effect of CY-treatment

Similarly to peritoneal macrophages testicular macrophages can be purified by glass adherence or fractionation on discontinuous gradient (Bryniarski 2004). Results in **Table 5** show that TNP substituted TMf (TNP-TMf) when injected i.v. into naïve recipient induce unresponsiveness since the following PCL skin sensitization fail to induce CHS reaction (group B), but TNP-TMf obtained from donors treated with low dose of CY under the seen conditions express strong CHS reaction comparable with control mice actively immunized with PCL (group C ve group A).

Groups	Cells injected i.v. before PCL sensitization	PCL sensitization	CHS reaction in TMf recipients in units of swelling x 10^{-2} mm
A	No cells injected	+	8.2 ± 1.25
B	TNP-TMf	+	2.5 ± 0.80
C	TNP-TMf (50 mg CY)	+	7.5 ± 1.54

Purified TMf obtained from CY-untreated (group B) or CY-treated donors (group B) when substituted with TNP hapten (TNP-TMf) were injected i.v. into mice. Seven days later all TMf recipients and naïve mice (group A) were skin sensitized with 5% PCL and 4 days later challenged on ear skin with 0.4% PCL. 24 h later CHS ear swelling response was measured with engineers micrometer and results expressed in units of swelling x 10^{-2} mm. Statistics: group A ve group B $p<0.001$, group B ve group C $p<0.01$.

Table 5. Testicular macrophages (TMf) from cyclophosphamide-treated mice do not induce suppressor cells in contrast to non-CY treated donors.

Our further experiments show that the tolerogenic activity of TNP-TMf is mediated by the high cytokine secretory activity mainly TGF-β. This cytokine is a very basic tool for functional strategy of TMf within testis and generates the state of organ as immune privileged site.

The methods used by us for obtaining enriched populations of TMf form mixture of testicular interstitial cells lead to separation of TMf into two functionally different cellular fractions – low density (fractions between interfaces of Percoll gradient 21/27 – 33/39) and high density (over 39/45). Low density fraction produces significantly more TGF–β than heavier cells and are CY-sensitive, while high density cells are not (Bryniarski et al. 2004). Our later experiments show that elimination of TGF-β activity by injection of anti-TGF-β mAb, but not anti-IL-10 mAb completely removed unresponsiveness obtained in TNP-TMf recipients after i.v. injection. The other adequate results implementing experiments with anti-TGF-β mAbs are shown in our paper (Bryniarski 2004).

Our experiment with TMf shows that injected intravenously induced CHS response in recipients pre-treated with CY. We found them also actively presenting corpuscular antigen (SRBC) in humoral response (Bryniarski et al. 2004). Again the low density subpopulation of TMf failed to induce CHS when injected i.v. into recipients, but in fact induced the state of tolerance in which subsequent skin application of hapten did not lead to development of contact sensitization. More interestingly, pretreatment of TMf donors with CY made the whole TMf population immunogenic. The mechanisms of action of CY are not cleared, but it has been argued that CY metabolites bind to sulfhydryl groups on antigen presenting cells (APC) changing their function (Bryniarski et al. 2004).

4. Discussion

Our results show that cyclophosphamide in vivo and both its metabolic highly reactive alkylating products -$\alpha\beta$-unsaturated aldehyde acrolein (ACR) and nitrogen mustard a derivative of phosphoramide mustard second metabolic agent formed in CY metabolism, activate TNP substituted Mf that leads to activation of CHS reaction mediated by Mf and hapten specific Th1 lymphocytes. We are tempted to suggest that this activity is mediated by the net of different proinflammatory (TNF-α, IL-1β, IL-6) and suppressory (IL-10 and TGF-β) cytokines secreted by Mf which can uncovering TNP-specific immunization activated by TNP substituted Mf and change their potential from inhibition of unresponsiveness (untreated Mf) into Mf immunogenicity (treated with CY or with CY metabolites).

4.1 CY and its action on CHS

Low dose of CY activates mainly of subpopulation of oil- or thioglycolate- induced peritoneal macrophages which are able to present hapten and subsequently activate trigger of Th1 mediated immune CHS response and diminishes the bioactivity of high density subpopulation of macrophages. That subpopulation induces specific immunologic unresponsiveness as a result of activating a network excess of efferent suppressor cells and mainly cooperates with T suppressor CD8$^+$ hapten specific cells (Treg) and mediates the hapten specific tolerance. (Szczepanik et al. 1993; Marcinkiewicz et al. 1994, Bryniarski et al. 2004 & 2009). The question arises as to how treatment with ACR or NM converts tolerogenic Mf into immunogenic Mf. One possibility is that these CY metabolites disrupt the function of the Mf subpopulation that induces Treg cells. Alternatively they can enhance the activity of Mf subpopulation responsible for the induction of Th1 cells that mediates CHS reaction. Finally these two possibilities are not mutually exclusive and the increased production of IL-12 and IL-6, and the simultaneously decreased production of anti-inflammatory IL-10 and TGF-β cytokines, make these later assumptions most likely.

4.2 CY regulates cytokine network released by Mf

One of the most strongly expressed of CY and their derivatives treatment of macrophages is the activation of IL-6 production (Bryniarski 1996, 2009) . Our results do not address directly the questions by which mechanisms NM modifies the macrophages to produce more IL-6. IL-6 gene expression can be induced by a variety of physiological (cytokines, growth factor, bacterial products) and non-physiological stimuli (certain toxins, medicaments, prostaglandin E1), by at least three different signals pathways (diacygloglycerol, cAMP- and Ca^{2+}- activated pathways). At the DNA level three functional promoter domains were described in conserved region of IL-6 promoter (MRE, NF-IL6 and NFκB). Exactly how transduction pathways are assigned seems unknown with the possible exception of protein kinase C signal which seems to focus on MRE region (Bryniarski et al. 1996). Since NM binds to both DNA and proteins, it could stimulate IL-6 production directly by alkylating any domain of promoter region, or indirectly, by the alkylation of cell surfaces or by both mechanisms simultaneously.

IL-6 is one of the major mediators of the immune response, with pleotropic and sometimes opposed effects on many different targets. It has been shown for instance that IL-6 enhances the cytotoxic activity of NK cells, thus may potentially augment the host defenses and contribute to anti-tumor effects of alkylating agents. Nonetheless, in case of the IL-6 dependent tumours like myelomas or plasma cell leukemias increased IL-6 level could be deleterious. The increased production of IL-6 may be responsible for observed paradoxical effects of CY which under certain conditions enhances, rather than suppresses both the humoral and cell mediated immune responses (Bryniarski et al.1996).

Apart from the influence of CY and its metabolites on the IL-6 production the inhibition of IL-10 and TGF-β production by macrophages was also observed. The results presented above in Table 4 and Fig.3 clearly suggest that the state of tolerance or unresponsiveness observed after TNP-Mf i.v. injection seems to be mediated by the network of pro- and anti-inflammatory cytokines secreted from macrophages and also tentatively delivered by natural regulatory cells. It is highly unlikely that low concentration of cytokine metabolites (10^{-7} and 10^{-6}M) have a direct cytotoxic effect on the Treg-inducing Mf since the cell viability remains unchanged during 24 h culture. Our interpretation is also supported by finding that shifting the balance between pro- and anti-inflammatory cytokines allows for deliberate manipulation of the outgoing response. IL-10 and TGF-β, which are anti-inflammatory cytokines, inhibit the activity of Th1 cells and Mf and down-regulate their function. As shown in Figure 3, administration of anti-IL-10 and/or anti-TGF-β mAbs into animals which received non-immunogenic TNP-Mf restores their immune potential although to different degrees. It indicates that the key suppressive cytokine is IL-10, a finding that is supported by other groups (Bryniarski et al. 2009). In a symmetrical situation, as we have shown previously, administration of anti-IL-12 antibodies inhibits the function of immunogenic TNP-Mf *in vivo* (Bryniarski et al. 2009). The increased production of IL-12 and IL-6 by macrophages indicates that the cell surface signal delivered by ACR or NM activates the transcription factor NF-κB required for the release of inflammatory cytokines (Bryniarski et al. 2009). As reported by other groups, ACR, when allowed free access to the interior of the cell, can either block or enhance the activity of NF-κB in alveolar macrophages depending on the design of cell treatment (Bryniarski et al. 2009).

4.3 CY modulates oxygen radicals formation by macrophages

Our results indicate that CY upregulates not only the specific immune response, by converting non-immunogenic (tolerogenic) Mf into antigen-presenting cells but also positively influences a typical parameter of innate immunity – production of oxygen radicals. In up-regulating the immune function of Mf, ACR and NM had much the same effect. This was however not the case with regard to the production of ROI's by these cells. Using the low concentrations of metabolites, NM was highly stimulatory while ACR did not influence the formation of oxygen radicals above the level observed in control Mf (high concentration of both metabolites were inhibitory). One possibility is that the ACR and NM bind to different targets on the cell surface. NADPH oxidase catalyzing the generation of ROI is composed of several cytosolic and membrane-bound proteins which, after the cell receives a proper signal (e.g. phagocytosis), translocate to form an active enzyme. We propose a possible explanation that under our experimental conditions, ACR, in contrast to NM, does not bind efficiently to important docking proteins to trigger the increased production of ROI. Conflicting results regarding ROI production were also published by other groups. Some reports describe the inhibitory activity of ACR, and others indicate an increased production of radicals. In effect, one can conclude that experimental conditions were the key (Bryniarski at al. 2009).

Our experimental data showed that untreated and in vivo CY treated populations of peritoneal macrophages produce the similar level of nitrogen oxide (Marcinkiewicz et al. 1994) which does not allow to speculate on its function in the immune regulatory system mediated by macrophage stimulated with CY.

4.4 Immunomodulation in chemotherapy with low doses of CY

Our data show that chemotherapy by CY or its products may activate the immune system by modulating cytokine networks and activation of Mf. This may lead to an enhancement of antigen-specific cell mediated immunity but also to activation of mechanisms of innate immunity mediated by Mf, like the production of ROI. Additionally, in animal models derivatives of different mustards led to decreased secretion of IL-10 and TGF-β by tumor cells and to their elimination. These and other similar experiments in humans support the notion that, at a correct dosage, CY and its metabolites can be a promising accessory tool in anti-tumor therapy.

The mechanism of CY influences macrophage immune function in as was shown previously in case of peritoneal Mf and TMf and seems to be the effect of network of different related factors. The analysis shows as the most important the influence of CY on the secretory activity of Mf which is the inhibition of IL-10 (in case of peritoneal Mf) and TGF-β (mainly in case of TMf) with parallel activation of proinflammatory cytokines secretion mainly IL-6, and to a lesser degree IL-12. Both cytokine signals lead to activation of antigen presentation in Mf. The other important factor mediated by CY treatment is an influence on the activation of a cell surface markers expression responsible for uptaking antigen into APC (FcγR I, FcγRII, CD23 – FcϵRII/III) and their following presentation to T lymphocytes subpopulations (CD80/CD86, MHC class II, CD14-LPS receptor).

4.5 Influence of CY on testicular macrophages

Although our experiments indicate that in the testis – immune privileged organ – some subpopulations of Mf are potentially able to present antigen if they would sneak through the blood-testis barrier, they also suggest how this potential activity is under control of other Mf and Sertoli cells. Our previous observations have shown that TMf are poor producers of oxygen radicals and nitric oxide both involved in the mechanisms of natural immunity which may be an evolutionary adaptation to diminish the risk of DNA mutations during spermatogenesis. Additionally we showed that specific immune responses controlled by the male gonads minimize the risk of development of autoimmune reactions and are potentially deleterious to testicular functions (Bryniarski 2004). Testicular Mf are good producers of TGF-β, which allows them to play an important functional population of testicular interstitial tissue cells that preserves state of tolerance in testes an immune privilege organs.

That state of tolerance eliminates the cellular immune response from the testis and in consequence makes an extremely dangerous the viral infection as well as in malignances taking place in testis. CY treatment often change TMf activity from unresponsiveness into actively antigen presenting cells which in consequence help to undertake anticancer response but also often can leads to activation an autoimmune response and immunological infertility as a consequences of chemotherapy.

5. Conclusions

The influence of CY on Mf can be summarized as a sum of several different mechanisms mediated by macrophages such as secretion of a specific pattern of cytokines and enhances expression of cell surface markers that can stimulate antigen presenting function by macrophages and last not least production of ROI's. On the other side there are several observations that low dose CY treatment has a direct influence of the different regulatory cells in immune system. One of them is a negative activation of CD8+ T lymphocytes leading to elimination of their effector mediators - suppressor cytokines secretion mainly TGF-β and IL-10, which negatively regulate the cellular immune response, but do not express any negative effect of humoral response. That state of abrogation of unresponsiveness is also observed experimentally when the TNP-substituted Mf obtained from oil-induced donors are injected into CY treated recipients of cells (see **Figure 5**) group C. In that case instead of unresponsiveness expressed by control group (group A) strong CHS response appears 24 h after challenge. This phenomenon clearly shows the influence of CY on the suppressor network of T reg cells. This also clearly shows that CY-manipulation leads to manifold effects in which manifold can be described as wiped out or misdirected. In the literature there are two papers suggesting depletion activity of CY on Treg CD4 CD25 T lymphocytes and Treg CD4 CD25 FoxP3+ lymphocytes (Ghiringhelli et al. 2004 & Zhao et al. 2010)

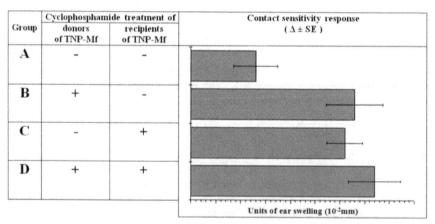

Group	Cyclophosphamide treatment of		Contact sensitivity response ($\Delta \pm SE$)
	donors of TNP-Mf	recipients of TNP-Mf	
A	-	-	
B	+	-	
C	-	+	
D	+	+	

Units of ear swelling (10^{-2}mm)

1×10^6 TNP substituted Mf (groups A and C) or TNP-Mf CY (groups B and D) were injected i.v. into naive (groups A and B) or treated with low dose of CY CBA/J mice. Seven days later the CHS response was measured (see legend to Table 2). Statistical significance (a posteriori Bonferroni test) Group A ve groups B, C and D p<0.001.

Fig. 5. Alleviation of suppression of contact sensitivity response induced by low dose treatment with cyclophosphamide applied either to macrophage donors or recipients.

A single administration of low dose of CY (50 mg/kg) into either donors or recipients restores the ability of Mf to induce significant CS reaction as a result of: i.) elimination of suppressive properties of Mf; ii.) and/or depletion of population of regulatory T cells in recipients or iii.) elimination of their suppressive activities. In vitro studies with metabolites of CY in contrast to studies in vivo allow identifying the factors which express direct action on selected populations of cells in contrary to experimental research in vivo which is able to identify parallel with direct also indirect effects of cyclophosphamide action on other than macrophages cell populations (T reg cells) that may change and modulate the activity of macrophages and their influence on the immune response. We propose the schemes which summarize the influence of low doses of CY on the immune response in mice (**Figures 6a-6c**).

Figure 6 a-c. The network of the CY influence on the macrophage and regulatory T cells in mice.

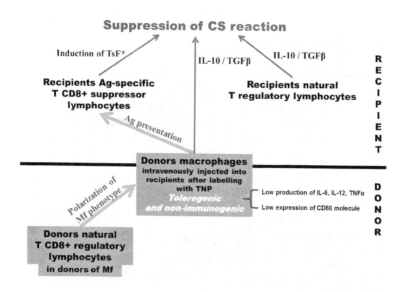

* Induction of T suppressor factor (see the reference by Bryniarski et al. 2-nd European Congress of Immunology Berlin 2009)

Fig. 6.a. Activation of unresponsiveness in recipients after i.v. injection of TNP substituted Mf – lack of CHS reaction.

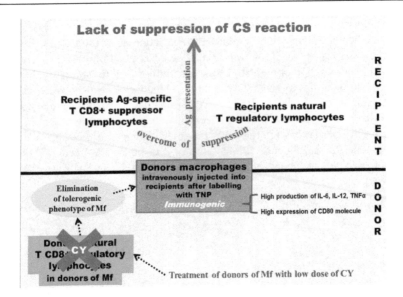

Fig. 6.b. The network of the CY influence on the macrophage and regulatory cells in mice. The i.v. injection into naïve recipient of TNP substituted Mf harvested from CY treated donors results in a state of high CHS reaction 24 h after challenge.

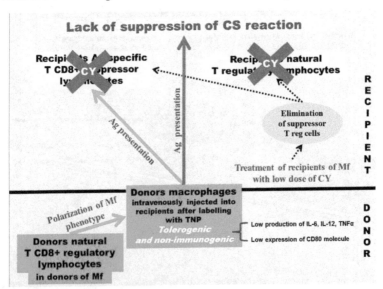

Fig. 6.c. The network of the CY influence on the macrophage and regulatory cells in mice. The i.v. injection of TNP substituted Mf harvested from naïve donors into recipients previously treated with low dose of CY results in expression of high CHS reaction 24 h after challenge with PCL hapten. The activation of CHS is the effect of blocking of natural reg T cells or antigen specific Ts cells.

6. Acknowledgments

The work is supported by grant No K/ZDS/001429 to KB. The author expresses gratitude to Ms. Katarzyna Nazimek M.Sc. for precious help in preparing the Figures and Tables.

7. References

Adjalle, R. Plouin, P. F. Pacak, K. & Lehnert, H. (2009). Treatment of malignant pheochromocytoma. *Horm Metabol Res.* Vol. 41, pp. 687-696.

Audia, S. Nicolas, A. Cathelin, D Larmonier N, Ferrand C, Foucher P, Fanton A, Bergoin E, Maynadie M, Arnould L, Bateman A, Lorcerie B, Solary E, Chauffert B, Bonnotte B.(2007). Increase of CD4+CD25high regulatory T cells in the peripheral blood of patient with metastatic carcinoma: a phase I clinical trial using cyclophosphamide and immunotherapy to eliminate CD4+CD25+ T lymphocytes. *Clinical and Experimental Immunology.* Vol. 150, pp. 532-30.

Ben-Efraim, S. (2001). Immunomodulating anticancer alkylating drugs targets and mechanisms of activity. Curr Drug Targ Vol. 2, pp. 197-212.

Breitfeld, P. P. & Meyer, W. H. (2005). Rhabdomyosarcoma: New windows of opportunity. *The Oncologist.* Vol. 10, pp. 518-527.

Bryniarski, K. Ptak, M. & Ptak, W. (1996). The in vivo and in vitro effects of an alkylating agent, mechlormethamine, on IL-6 production in mice and the role of macrophages. *Immunopharmacology.* Vol. 34, pp. 73-78.

Bryniarski, K. Szczepanik, M. Maresz, K. Ptak, M. & Ptak, W. (2004). Subpopulations of mouse testicular macrophages and their immunoregulatory function. *American Journal of Reproductive Immunology.* Vol. 52, pp. 27-35.

Bryniarski, K. Szczepanik, M. Ptak, M. Zemelka, M. & Ptak, W. (2009). Influence of cyclophosphamide and its metabolic products on the activity of peritoneal macrophages in mice. *Pharmacological Reports.* Vol. 61, pp. 550-557.

Bryniarski, K. Ptak, M. Sikora, E. Szczepanik, M. Guerrier-Takada, C. Altman, S. Askenase, P.W. Ptak, W. (2009) Role of low molecular weight RNA in contact sensitivity response. Medimond International Proceedings ECI Berlin 2009 pp 183-186.

Burger, R. A. (2007). Experience with Bevacizumab in the management of epithelial ovarian cells. *Journal of Clinical Oncology.* Vol. 25 (20) Jul.10, pp. 2902-2908.

Cole, M. E. Broaddus, R. Thaker, P. Lauden, C. & Freedman, R. S. (2008). Placenta – side of trophoblastic tumors: case of resistant pulmonary metastasis. *Nature, Clinical Practice, Oncology.* Vol. 5, (3), pp. 171-175.

Czajkowska, B. Ptak, M. Bobek, M. Bryniarski, K. & Szczepanik, M. (1995). Different isoenzyme patterns of nonspecific esterases and the level of IL-6 production as markers of macrophage functions. *Folia Histologica et Biologica* Vol. 33, (2), pp. 111-115.

Durhan, N. Singh, S. Singh Kadin, Y. Durhan, V. Rajotia & N. Sangwen N. (2009). Primary leiomyosarcoma of broad ligament: case report and review of literature. *Arch Gynocol Obstet.* Vol. 279, pp. 705-708.

Ghiringhelli, F. Larmounier, N. Schmidt, E. Parcellier, A. Cathelin, D. Garrido, C. Chauffert, B. Solary, E. Bonnotte, B. & Martin F. (2004). CD4+CD25+ regulatory T cells suppress tumor immunity but are sensitive to cyclophosphamide which allows immunotherapy of established tumors to be curative. *European Journal of Immunology.* Vol. 34 pp.336-344.

Lerch,M. & Pichler, W. J. (2004). The immunological and clinical spectrum of delayed drug-induced exanthems. *Current Opinion in in Allergy and Clinical Immunology.* Vol. 4, pp. 411-419.

Luznik, L. & Fusch, E. J. (2010). High-dose post-transplantation cyclophosphamide to promote graft-host tolerance after allogenic hematopoetic stem cell transplantation. *Immunological Research.* Vol. 47 (1-3), pp. 65-77.

Marcinkiewicz, J. Bryniarski, K. & Ptak, W. (1994). Cyclophosphamide uncovers two separate macrophage subpopulations with opposite immunogenic potential and different patterns of monokine production. *Cytokine.* Vol. 6 (5), pp. 472-477.

Posadas, S. J. & Pichler, W. J. (2007). Delayed drug hypersensitivity reactions – new concepts. *Clinical and Experimental Allergy.* Vol. 37, pp. 989-999.

Snowden, J. A. Angel, C. A. Winfield, D. A. Pringle, J. H. West, K. P. (1997). Angiotropic lymphoma: report of a case with histiocytic features. *Journal of Clinical Pathology* Vol. 50, pp. 67-70.

Suzuki, R. (2010). Treatment of advanced NK/T cell lymphoma: Nasal type and aggressive NK-cell leukemia. *Int J Hematol.* Vol. 92, pp. 697-701.

Szczepanik, M. Bryniarski, K. Pryjma, J. & Ptak, W. (1993). Distinct population of antigen-presenting macrophages are required for induction of effector and regulatory cells in contact sensitivity response in mice. *Journal of Leukocyte Biology* Vol. 53 (3), pp. 320-326.

Vitolo, V. Ferreri, A. J. M. & Zucca, E. (2008). Primary testicular lymphoma. *Critical Review in Oncology/Hematology.*Vol.65, pp. 183-189.

Weiner, H. L. and Cohen, J. A. (2002). Treatment of multiple sclerosis with cyclophosphamide: critical review of clinical and immunologic effects. *Multiple Sclerosis.* Vol. 8, pp. 142 –154.

Zhao, J. Cao, Y. Lei, Z. Yang, Z. Zhang, B. & Huang B. (2010). Selective depletion of CD4+CD25+FoxP3+ regulatory T cells by low-dose cyclophosphamide is explained by reduced intracellular ATP levels. *Cancer Research.* Vol. 70, (12), pp. 4850-4858.

Part 3

Pharmacogenetic

9

Pharmacogenetics: The Scientific Basis

Bosun Banjoko

Obafemi Awolowo University, Ile-Ife,
Nigeria

1. Introduction

The history of genetic variations in drug responses can be traced to the 1950s with the observations that muscle relaxant suxamethonium chloride and drugs metabolized by N-acetyl transferase exhibit differences in response in patients. One in 3500 caucasians was found to possess the less efficient variant of the enzyme, butyryl chlolinesterase that metabolizes suxamethonium chloride; an anaesthetic agent.As a consequence, the drug's effect is prolonged with slower recovery from surgical paralysis.

The term pharmacogenetics evolved from the combination of two areas of study namely pharmacology and genetics. Pharmacology is the study of how drugs work in the body and genetics is the study of how characteristics that result from the action of genes acting together are inherited and how they function in the cells of the body . Therefore, pharmacogenetics refers to genetic differences in metabolic pathways which can affect individual responses to drugs both in terms of therapy and adverse effects. Pharmacogenetics helps our understanding of why some individuals respond to drugs and others do not and why some require higher or lower doses to achieve optimal therapeutic responses.

In addition, pharmacogenetic information helps the physician to identify those patients who will respond favourably to therapy or develop side effects.

A recent offshoot of pharmacogenetics, termed pharmacogenomics is the study of drug response in the context of the entire genome. Pharmacogenomics facilitates information on variations in all the genes in a group of individuals simultaneously to determine the basis of variants in drug response. It is therefore not uncommon to find the two being used interchangeably.However for the purpose of this chapter, pharmacogenetics will be the focus.

Individual variation in response to drug ranges from failure to respond to drug therapy to drug to drug interactions when several drugs are taken simultaneously. The clinical consequences range from patients' discomfort through serious clinical illness to the occasional fatality. Approximately 7% of patients are affected by adverse drug reactions, increasing the overall hospital costs by 19% and drug costs by 15%. Some 0.3% of adverse drug reactions have fatal outcome (Topic 2010).

1.1 Individual variation in drug effects

Variation in drug metabolism and drug response among individuals of the same body weight and on the same drug dose can be due to temporary causes such as transient enzyme inhibition, induction or permanent causes such as genetic mutation, gene deletion or amplification. (Shenfield 2004).

Genetic variability is known to affect drug absorption, drug metabolism and drug interactions with receptors. These therefore form the basis for slow or rapid drug absorption, poor, efficient or ultrarapid drug metabolism and poor or efficient receptor interactions.

A genetic mutation frequency exceeding 10% of a population is considered a genetic polymorphism (Meyer 2000). Genetic polymorphism based on drug metabolizing ability is related to four phenotypic classes. The phenotype of extensive or normal drug metabolizers (EM) is characteristic of the normal population .Individuals are either homozygous or heterozygous for wild type allele. Those individuals who are heterozygous for the wild type allele may have intermediate metabolizer phenotype (IM) and may require lower than average drug dose for optimal therapeutic response. Those individuals with mutation or deletion of both alleles for the determinant of phenotypic response can be classified as poor metabolizers (PM) and therefore prone to accumulation of drug substrates in their systems with attendant effects. The fourth class, termed the ultrarapid metabolizers (UM) possess enhanced drug metabolism capabilities due to gene amplification and are prone to drug failure because drug concentrations at normal doses are expected to be too low for therapeutic effects (Meyer 2000, Davies 2006).

There are ethnical and racial differences in the frequency of variant alleles and up to 10 – 20% of patients belong to the risk groups. (Evans 1986, Banjoko & Akinlade 2010).

1.2 Mechanism of genetic polymorphism

Pharmacogenetic polymorphism can manifest at the pharmacokinetic and pharmacodynamics levels. The pharmacokinetic level deals with gene polymorphism that modify concentrations of drugs and its metabolites at the site of their molecular action (polymorphism of drug metabolizing enzymes, drug transporters) whereas the pharmacodynamics level deal with polymorphism of action not related to its concentration (receptors, ion channels). Genetic variations are the result of multiple mechanism such as insertion, deletion, variable tandem repeats and microsatellites but the most frequent polymorphism are point mutation or single nucleotide polymorphism (SNPS). Some of the polymorphism are without consequences but others cause synthesis of altered proteins, truncated proteins, unstable proteins or proteins at the level of expression.

Genotype is the detailed gene structure of an individual whereas the more commonly measured phenotype is the outcome of metabolism of a drug in an individual. Since genotype is the result of interactions between genetic make up and the environment, it is not always concordant with phenotype.

1.3 Consequences of pharmacogenetics

The underpinning factors for the growing importance of pharmacogenetics are the necessity to prevent adverse drug reaction, obtain maximum benefits from drug therapy and reduce therapeutic failure.

Adverse drug reactions are thought to kill many hospitalized patients worldwide. In the US alone, the estimate of deaths attributable to drug reactions is about 100,000 annually and it is believed that many of these reactions are due to genetic variations. Thus many deaths are avoidable if genetic testing or genomic information of patients are available and utilized prior to therapy.

Pharmacogenetics will therefore permit gene profiling to answer questions about drug responses and promote the design of better and safer drugs. In addition, individualized dosing has the potential of better therapeutic outcome. Therefore pharmacogenetics is expected to revolutionise drug dosing and therapy .However, there are still many challenges to overcome. These include cost implications, standardization , quality control of testing, and relevance of biomarkers and tests. Nevertheless, the advent of pharmacogenetics and establishment of guidelines by regulatory bodies like Food and Drugs Administration (FDA) European Medicines Agency (EMEA) and American Association of Clinical Chemists (AACC) are expected to impact individualized dosing of many drugs.

1.4 Confounding issues in pharmacogenetics

The understanding that drug response may be multifactoral helps us to recognize the importance of examining more than the classical "single gene-single protein concept which gave birth to pharmacogenomics. In addition, there are more evidences that modifications besides outright mutation of genes, for example, methylation of promoter region by epigenetic factor impact gene expression and drug responses. Moreover, genotype is not the only determinant of phenotype. For example, individuals whose genotypes falls extensive metabolizers via CYP2D6 can display a phenotype that would characterize them as poor metabolizers if they are co-administered low doses of quinidine which is a potent inhibitor of CYP2D6 . Therefore, differences in phenotype does not necessarily translate into difference in pharmacologic response between subjects. In the same fashion, mutation of the genes may not necessarily translate into effect on drug metabolism (Henningson et al 2005).

Because of significant racial differences in genetic composition, it is important that caution is exercised in the interpretation of genetic testing. For example different genotypes may give rise to the same phenotype.In addition, there are varieties of mutations in NAT2 that give rise to slow acetylator status.

Furthermore the historical use of wild-type alleles and mutant alleles may not necessarily hold true for all the races hence the migration to the term reference and mutant alleles.

2. Basic genetics

Genetics is the study concerned with hereditary and variation. One of the most fundamental properties of all living organisms is the ability to reproduce. All organisms therefore inherit the genetic information specifying their structure and function from their parents. In the same manner, all cells arise from pre – existing cells, so the genetic material must be replicated and passed from a parent to progeny cell at each cell division. The hereditary molecules that are transmitted from one generation to the next i.e. inherited are called genes. These molecules (genes) reside in the deoxyribonucleic acid (DNA) that exist within all cells. The DNA in conjunction with a protein matrix forms nucleoprotein and become organized into structures called chromosomes located in the nucleus or nuclear region of cells. The genes contains coded information for the synthesis of proteins and some ribonucleic acids (RNA). Occasionally, a change may occur spontaneously in some part of the DNA. This change is called mutation and may result in an alteration of the code designated for a particular function resulting in production of a defective protein.

A mutation may lead to a change in the physical appearance of an individual or change in some other measurable attributes of the organism called a character or trait. Through the process of mutation, a gene may be changed into two or more alternative forms called alleles. Each gene occupies a specific position on the chromosomes called the gene locus. All allelic forms of a gene therefore are found at corresponding positions on genetically similar (homologous) chromosomes.

All the genes on a chromosomes are said to be linked to one another and to belong to the same linkage group. Since a gene can be changed to alternative forms by the process of mutation, a large number of alleles are theoretically possible in a population of individuals. Whenever more than two alleles are identified at a gene locus in a population, such is described as multiple allele series.

Genetic information is stored and transmitted in the four letter alphabet and language of DNA (A,C,G,T) and ultimately expressed in the twenty letter alphabet of proteins. Protein biosynthesis is called translation because it involves the biochemical translation of information between languages.

A capital letter is commonly used to designate the allele that is dominant to other alleles in the series. For example letter "R" for a character is dominant over 'r' which is an allele that is recessive to all others in the series .Intermediate in their degree of dominance between the two extremes are usually assigned the lower case letter with superscript which in this example is r*. Many genes may contribute to a single character or trait (polygenic traits) or traits exhibiting continuous variation. In addition, each gene may have multiple phenotypic effects (pleiotropy).

Each character is controlled by a pair of genes. The progeny or offspring are therefore hybrids of the parents, inheriting a pair of gene, one each from each parent. For example for trait for tallness being represented by letter T, possible genetic composition are TT, Tt, and tt whereby T allele is dominant over t. It is expected that an offspring with tt genetic composition will be short while those with TT or Tt will be tall.

The genetic composition of a trait is referred to as the genotype and the physical appearance corresponding to the genotype, in this example tallness is called the phenotype.With different generations of offsprings i.e. the filial generations, different genotypes and corresponding phenotypes are obtainable.

The originator of the classical principles of genetics is Macgregor Mendel who made public the result of his study of peas breeding in 1865. Mendel studied the inheritance of a number of well defined traits in the pea such as seed colour and was able to deduce general rules for their transmission. He was the first to observe that each trait was determined by a pair of inherited factors later termed the genes. Mendel's findings provided the template for determination of genotypes and phenotypes of different genetic diseases of humans, animals and plants and notable examples include: sickle cell disease, albinism and thalassaemias.

By 1900, Mendel's laws of inheritance were well established and are thus stated:

Law of segregation: Each parent possesses 2 copies of a unit of inheritance (now called the gene) for each trait. However, only one of these two genes (an allele) is transmitted through a gamete to the offspring.

Law of independent assortment: says segregation of one gene pair occurs independently of any other gene pair.

2.1 Chromosomes, genes and inheritance

Chromosomes are known to be carrier of genes. Most cells of higher plants and animals are diploid. i.e. they contain two copies of each chromosome. Formation of the germ cells; the sperm and egg involves a unique type of cell division termed meiosis. In this process, only one member of each chromosome pair is transmitted to each progeny cell. Therefore, the sperm and egg are haploid containing only one copy of each chromosome. The fusion of these two haploid cells at fertilization result in a new diploid organism; the offspring which consists of one member of each chromosome pair. Behaviour of chromosome pairs is directly related to their genes indicating a strong relationship between genes and chromosomes.

Genetic alterations i.e. mutation which is the basis of genetic diseases was first identified in the experiment with *Drosophilia melanogaster* (the fruit fly) in the early 1900. Mutations in drosophila was observed to involve such phenotypes like eye colour and wing shape. Experimented evidences revealed that the genes governing these traits are inherited independently of each other, suggesting that these genes are located on different chromosomes that segregate independently during meiosis. Other genes are inheritable as paired characteristics and such are said to be linked to each other by virtue of being located on the same chromosome. The frequency of recombination between two linked genes depends on distance between them on the chromosomes. In addition, genes that are close to each other recombine less frequently than do genes further apart. Thus the differences with which the different genes recombine can be used to determine their relative position on the chromosome allowing the construction of a genetic map.

2.2 Genes, proteins and enzymes

Genes act by determining the structure of proteins which are responsible for directing cell metabolism through the activities of enzymes. Many genes encode enzymes that are important for catalysing biological synthesis (anabolic) and degradation (catabolic reactions) within a cell. These reactions grouped together into a series of reactions are called biochemical pathways and commence with the enzymes acting on their corresponding substrate.

The first indication linking genes and enzymes can be traced to 1909 when it was observed that patients suffering from phenylketonuria were suspected to have a genetic defect in the metabolism of the amino acid for phenylalanine.This line of thought was supported by the experiment of George Beadle and Edward Tatum in 1941 with the fungus; *Neurospora cassa*. Using mutant strains of the organism, they observed that each mutant required specific nutritional supplement such as a particular aminoacid for growth.Furthermore, the requirement for a specific nutritional supplement correlates with the failure of the mutant to synthesize that particular compound. Thus each mutant resulted in a deficiency in a specific metabolic pathway. Since metabolic pathways are known to be controlled by enzymes, these findings gave rise to the one – gene – one enzyme hypothesis which by implication means that each gene specified the structure of a single enzyme. However, the revelation that genes not only codes for proteins and enzymes but tRNAs resulted in this hypothesis being modified to one – gene – one – polypeptide concept.

Transfer RNA's (tRNAs) serve as adaptations between aminoacids and messenger RNA (mRNA) during translation. Prior to its use in protein synthesis, each aminoacid is attached by a specific enzyme to its appropriate tRNA. Base pairing between a recognition sequence in each tRNA and a complimentary sequence on the mRNA then directs the attached aminoacid to its correct position on the mRNA template.

2.3 Genetic polymorphism

Genetic polymorphism can be defined as differences in DNA sequence among individuals, groups or population. Genetic mutation can create genetic variance in a population and this can manifest in different ways. Somatic cell mutation can create a genetic variation in a cell population which may induce cancer and tumour when such mutation takes place in repressor genes controlling cell cycles such as p53 gene. On the other hand,germ line cell mutation can cause genetic diseases such as sickle cell disease, thalassemia, Parkinson's disease as well as defect of biochemical pathway that influence drug – receptor interaction with attendant deleterious effects on patients. Point mutation such as a single base nucleotide substitution (SNP) are common particularly with adverse drug reactions. Mutation that occurs in germ line cell would be inherited by the progeny and these mutated genes can spread in a population through the fertilization process. Mutations that occur in coding frame of DNA region that are responsible for synthesis of specific products could give rise to genetic disease. Similarly, mutation that affects enzymes responsible for biotransformation of drugs particularly C450 gene family and pharmacokinetic and pharmacodynamic gene functions can result in adverse drug reactions or drug inefficacy. These reasons make phamacogenetics an important area of study.

3. Basic pharmacology

Pharmacology is the study that deals with interaction of endogenously administered chemical molecules termed drugs with living systems. It involves such studies like (i) Pharmacokinetics (ii) Pharmacodynamics (iii) Toxicology

i. **Pharmacokinetics** : Pharmacokinetics is the quantitative study of drug movement from administration throughout out the body till excretion. All pharmacokinetic processes involve transport of the drug across cell membrane,. absorption, distribution and excretion

ii. **Pharmacodynamics**: Pharmacodynamics coined from two Greek words pharmacon; drugs and dynamis: power, involves the physiological and biochemical effect of drugs and their mechanism of action at organ, systemic, subcellular and macromolecular levels. The pharmacodynamic process describes all those matters concerned with the pharmacological action of a drug, whether they be determinants of the therapeutic effect or of the toxic effect.

iii. **Toxicology:** This is the study of poisonous effects of drugs and other chemicals. Although a speciality on it's own, it is nevertheless still considered under pharmacology with regards to adverse drug effects.

3.1 Principles of drug actions

There are eight main drug actions and these are:

Stimulation: Through direct receptor agonism and downstream effect e.g. adrenaline stimulates heart, pilocarpine stimuates salivary glands. However, excessive stimulation is often followed by depression of that function e.g. high dose of picrotoxin, a CNS stimulant, produces convulsions followed by coma and respiratory depression.

Depression: Through direct receptor agonism and down stream effect e.g. barbiturates depress CNS while quinines depresses the heart. The action of this mechanism is selective.

Blocking/Antagonizing action: The drugs binds the receptor but does not activate it.

Stabilizing action: In this case, the drugs seem to act neither as a stimulant nor as a depressant but to stabilize general receptor activation like buprenorphine in opioid dependence or aripiprazole in schizophrenia.

Replacement: Refers to the use of natural metabolites including hormones and vitamins in deficiency stages e.g. levodopa in Parkinsonism, insulin in diabetes mellitus, iron in anemia and oestrogen replacement in women of menopausal age.

Direct beneficial chemical reaction: As in use of antioxidants like Vitamins C,E and B-carotene for free radical scavenging

Cytotoxic action: Selective cytotoxic action for parasite, bacterial or cancer cells, attenuating them without significantly affecting the host cells e.g. use of antibiotics like penicillin, zidovudin and cyclophosphamide

Irritation: A none selective often noxious effect applicable to less specialized cells, for example the epithelial, connective tissue cells). Mild irritation may stimulate associated function e.g. bitters increase salivary and gastric secretions which results in increased blood flow to the site. However, strong irritation may result in inflammation, corrosion, necrosis and morphological damage with resultant diminution or loss of function. Therefore caution should be exercised in the administration because of tendency of excessive ingestion.

4. Metabolism of drug and other xenobiotics

Metabolism of drugs and other xenobiotics involves activities that modify the chemical structure of the substances which are foreign to the body's internal mileu. These reactions often act to detoxify poisonous compounds; however in some cases, the intermediate metabolite can themselves be toxic

The purpose of biotransformation is to convert lypophilic compounds to hydrophilic ones which will facilitate their excretion. The consequences of biotransformation is changes in pharmacokinetic characteristics.

Xenobiotics metabolism can be divided into three phases. In phase 1, enzymes such as cytochrome p450 oxidases introduce an active or polar group into the xenobiotics. These modified compounds are then conjugated to polar compounds in phase II reactions. The main enzyme that catalyses the reactions in phase II is glutathione S-transferase since it acts on a wide range of substrates.

The final phase; phase III may involve further metabolism of conjugates of phase II reactions like the processing of glutathione conjugates to acetylcysteine (mercapturic acic) conjugates before being recognized by efflux transporters and pumped out of the cells (Boyland & Chassaud 1969, Thomalley 1990)

Peculiar to all organisms is the possession of cell membranes which serve as hydrophobic permeability barriers to control access to their internal environment. Polar compounds cannot diffuse across these cell membranes, and the uptake of useful molecules is mediated through transport proteins that specifically select substrates from the extracellular mixture. The implication of this structure is that most hydrophilic molecules cannot enter the cells since they need to be recognized by specific transporters (Mizuno et al 2003).

The detoxification of reactive by-products is via a different mechanism. Because these species are derived from normal cellular constituents, they usually share the same polar characteristics therefore, specific designated enzymes can metabolize them. A notable example of these specific detoxification system is the glyoxalase system which catalyses the removal of the reactive aldehyde, methylglyoxal (Thormalley 1990) and the various antioxidant systems that eliminate reactive oxygen species (Sies 1997).

4.1 Phase I reactions

In Phase I reactions, a variety of enzymes act to introduce reactive and polar groups into their substrates. This is basically a functionalization reaction. One of the most common modifications in this phase is hydroxylation, a reaction catalysed by the cytochrome P-450 dependent mixed function oxidase system. These enzymes complexes act to incorporate an atom of oxygen into nonactivated hydrocarbons, which can result in either the introduction of hydroxyl groups, or Nitrogen, Oxygen.and Sulphate- dealkylation of substrates (Schlichting et al 2000).Of all the enzymes involved in drug metabolism, the cytochrome P450.(CYP450) is regarded as the most important because many drugs are substrates for the enzymes of the group. In all, CYP3A4, CYP2D6, CYP2C9, CYP219, CYP2B6 and CYP1A2 subtypes play the most critical role and account for more than 90% of drugs metabolized by CYP 450 enzymes (Evans & Relling 1999). These enzymes have proven genetic polymorphism with associated drug responses (Hiratsuka et al 2002, Wong et al 2005, McAlpine et al 2011) and racial variations (Meyer 2004 & Suarez – Kurtz 2005).

Phenotypes of P450 are divided into four groups and these are; the extensive metabolizers (EM)who show low metabolic activities, the poor metabolisers(PM)who carry gene alterations on both alleles which are inherited in an autosomal manner, the intermediate metabolizers (IM) with metabolic capacity in between those of PM and EM and finally the ultra rapid metabolizers (UM)who show higher metabolic capacity than the EM. (Murphy 2001, Hiratsuka et al 2005). Genetic variations have been observed particularly with CYP 2D6, CYP2C9 and CYP2C19 genotypes (Ingelman – Sundberg 1999, Hiratsuka 2006). With regards to CYP2D6,five to ten percent of caucasians are poor metabolizers and have little enzyme activities. In addition, there is a distinct racial diversity in the frequency of the classes. Examples of CYP450 catalyzed drug metabolic reactions include

i.   **Hydroxylation**: S-mephenytoin CYP3A4 4-OH-S-mephenytoin
ii. **Epoxidation:** Carbamazepine CYP3A4/5 10,11 Epoxide
iii. **Oxygenation**: Amines CYP 2D6 Hydroxylamines
iv. **O-dealkylation**: Dextromethorphan CYP2D6 Dextrophan
v.   **N-demethylation**: Caffeine CYP2E1 Theobromine
vi. **N-demethylation:** Caffeine CYP1A2 Paraxanthine
vii. **N-demethylation** Caffeine CYP2E1 Theophylline
viii. **Oxidative Group Transfer**: Parathion CYP2B6 Paraoxon
ix. **Dehydrogenation:** Acetaminophen CYP2E1 N-Aacetyl benzoquinoneimine
x.   **Ester Cleavage**: Loratidine CYP3A4, CYP2D6 Desacetylated Loratidine
xi. **Reduction**: Paraquat FLAVOPROTEIN REDUCTASE paraquat radicals

4.1.1 Non P450 enzyme catalysis

Besides the CYP 450 enzymes, other enzymes that participate in drug biotransformations include; monoamineoxidases, peroxidases, lactoperoxidases myeloperoxidases, prostaglandin-H-synthetase and flavin-containing monooxygenases.(FMO).Examples of the reactions they catalyse include:

i.   **Hydrolysis:** hydrolysis of peptide bond of Insulin
ii. **Reduction**: Chloral Hydrate ALC. DEHYDROGENASE Trichloroethanol
iii. **Oxidoreduction**: Alcohol ALC.DEHYDROGENASE Aldehyde

4.2 Phase II reactions

In phase II reactions, the activated xenobiotic metabolites are conjugated with charged species such as glutathione (GSH), sulfate, glycine or glycuronic acid and increased risk of early renal complications in type 2 diabetes mellitus (Banjoko & Akinlade 2010). These reactions are catalysed by substrate specific transferases which in total can metabolize almost any hydrophobic compound that contains nucleophilic or electrophilic group.

One of the most important of this group is the glutathione S-transferase (GSTs). The addition of large anionic groups such as glutathione detoxifies reactive electrophiles and produces more polar metabolites that cannot diffuse across membranes and may therefore be actively transported.

4.2.1 Glutathione conjugation

Glutathione is a tripeptide of glycine, cysteine and glutamic acid formed by the action of glutamylcysteine synthetase (glutathione synthetase).The enzyme glutathione transferase catalyses the conjugation of modified xenobiotic with glutathione. A large number of drugs are conjugated by glutathione during metabolism. Inhibitors of the enzyme include Buthione – S – Sulfoxine. Two types of reactions are common with glutathione. The first is displacement of halogen, sulfate, sulfonate or phosphonitro group. The second is the addition of glutathione to activated double bond or strained ring system. Some of the conjugation reactions include:

i.   N – acetylbenzoquinoneimine, an activated metabolic of acetaminophen.
ii.   O – demethylation of organophosphates
iii. Activation of trinitroglycine to oxidized glutathione (GSSG) dinitroglycerine and Nitric oxide (NO) a vasodilator.

Distinct cytosolic and microsomal glutathione -S transferases have been identified. In all, four classes of soluble glutathione S transferase are known to exist. The enzyme also exhibit genetic polymorphism and overexpression of the enzyme leads to e.g. resistance of insects to DDT, corn to atrazine and cancer cells to chemotherapy. The enzyme also participates in reduction of hydroperoxides and prostaglandin metabolism. Inducers of the enzyme include 3-methylcholanthrene, phenobarbital, corticosteroids and antioxidants. GST exhibit specie specificity; for example, aflatoxin B_1 is not carcinogenic in mice because it conjugates with glutathione very rapidly in them. Conjugates are excreted intact in bile or converted to mercapturic acid in kidney and excreted in urine in a reaction catalysed by glutamyl transpeptidase an aminopeptidase

4.2.2 Uridyl Diphosphate Glucuronyl transferase (UDPG transferase)

The reaction of UDP Glucuronyl transferase results in the formation of O-, N-, S and C-glucuronides. Six forms of this enzyme have been identified in the liver. The cofactor for its reaction is UDP – glucuronic acid. Inducers include phenobarbital, indoles, 3 methyl cholanthrene and cigarette smoke. Some of its substrate are dextrophan, methalidone, morphine, p-nitrophenol, valproic acid, non steroidal anti-inflamatory drugs, bilirubin and steroid hormones. In Criggler Najjar syndrome; a severe form of bilirubinaemia, the enzyme is inactive hence inducers have no effect. However, in Gilbert's syndrome; a mild form of hyperbilirubinaemia, phenobarbital can increase the rate of bilirubin glucuronidation to normal functions . Other substrates of the enzymes include, morphine and chloramphenicol. Conjugates of UDPG transferase are excreted in bile and urine. An S-glucuronidase from the gut microflora cleaves the glucuronic acid, the glycone formed can be reabsorbed to undergo enterohepatic cycling. Other associated reactions include metabolic activation of 2, 6 dinitrotoluene by S-glucuronidase; whereby the latter removes glucuronic acid from N-glucuronide. The nitrogroup is then reduced by microbial N-reductase and the resultant hepatocarcinogen may be reabsorbed.

4.2.3 Sulfation

The sulfation process is catalysed by sulfotransferases which are widely distributed in the body. The co-factor for their reaction is 3^1 phosphoadenosine 5 phosphosulfate (PAPS). Their conjugation result in highly water soluble sulfate esters which are eliminated in urine and bile. Examples of substances for sulfation include phenols, catecholamines and hydroxylamines. Sulfation is a high affinity, low capacity pathway which is limited by low PAPS level. Acetaminophen is a drug that undergoes both sulfation and glucuronidation. At low doses, sulfation predominates but at high doses glucuronidation predominates. Four sulfotransferases in human liver cytosol have been identified to date. Aryl sulfatases in gut microflora remove sulfate groups in a sort of enterohepatic recycling. Sulfation decreases pharmacologic and toxic activities but can also cause activation of chemically unstable groups to carcinogens, for example hydroxylamine.

4.2.4 Methylation

This is a common minor pathway of xenobiotic biotransformation which generally decreases water solubility. Enzymes that catalyse the reactions are called methyltransferases and the co-factor is S-adenosylmethionine (SAM). In methylation, a methyl group (CH_3) is transferred to O, N, S or C molecule   on the substrates which include phenols, catecholamines and heavy metals like Hg, As and Se. There are several methyltransferases in human tissues examples of which are phenol – O – methyltransferases, catechol – O – methyltransferase, O-methyl transferase and S-methyl transferase. Genetic polymorpohism has been observed in thiopurine metabolism in a reaction catalysed by a member of this group of enzymes. High activity allele causes increased toxicity and low activity allele causes decreased efficacy.

4.2.5 Acetylation

This is the major route of biotransformation of aromatic amines and hydrazines. The reaction is catalysed by N – acetyl transferases (NAT) enzyme and the co factor acetyl-coenzyme-A. The process generally causes a decrease in water solubility. Substrates of the enzyme include sulfanilamide, isoniazid, dapsone and caffeine. In humans three phenotypic forms have been identified and these are slow, intermediate and rapid acetylators (Evans 1999, Murphy 2001). Various mutations of the enzyme result in decreased enzyme activity or stability. Like every other entity exhibiting genetic polymorphism, there are various ethnic and tribal variations. For example, 70% of slow acetylator status was observed in Middle Eastern population, 50% in Caucasians and 25% in Asians (Hiratsuka 2006, Evans and Relling 1989). Drug toxicities in slow acetylators include nerve damage from dapsone and bladder cancer in cigarette smokers due to increased levels of hydroxylamines (Ohno and Yamaguchi 2000, Evans 1999, Hiratsuka et al 2006).

4.2.6 Amino acid conjugation

This is an alternative pathway to glucuronidation. Amino acid conjugation operate with two principles. The first is that carboxylic group (COOH) group of a substrate is conjugated with an amino (NH_2) group of glycine, serine, glutamine requiring co enzyme-A activation. Notable example is the conjugation of benzoic acid with glycine to form hippuric acid. Benzoic acid is commonly used as a preservative in carbonated drinks. Alternatively aromatic NH_2 or NHOH conjugate with COOH of serine proteins requiring ATP activation. This metabolic pathway demonstrate specie specificity in accepting amino acid. For example, in mammals, benzoic acid is conjugated by glycine whereas for the same substrate in birds, ornithine acts. Dogs and cats utilize taurine to conjugate bile acids while other non human primates utilize glutamine for conjugation. Metabolic activation of serine or proline results in N-esters of hydroxylamine which are unstable and may degrade to reactive electrophile.

4.2.7 Ribonucleoside/nucleoside synthesis

This pathway is important for the activation of many purine and pyrimidine antimetabolites used in cancer chemotherapy

4.3 Phase III reactions

Phase III reactions can be described as a stage of further modification and excretion. Although many authors do not regard this phase as a distinct phase, current knowledge of efflux transporters tend to support the categorization. A common example is the processing of glutathione conjugates to acetylcysteine (mercapturic acid) conjugates (Boyland and Chassaud 1969). In this scenario, glutamate and glycine residing in the glutathione molecule are removed by gamma-glutamyltranspeptidase and dipeptidases. Finally, the cysteine residue in the conjugate is acetylated .The conjugates and their metabolites can then be excreted from cells in phase III of their metabolism with anionic groups acting as affinity taps for a variety of membrane transporters of the multidrug resistance protein (MRP) family (Homolya et al 2003). These proteins are members of the family of ATP-binding cassette transporters and can facilitate the ATP dependent transport of a large varieties of hydrophobic ions (Konig et al 1999) and thus act to remove phase II products to the extracellular medium, where they may be further metabolized and excreted (Commandeur et al 1995).

Since the discovery of permeability glycoprotein (P – glycoprotein) complex; an initial member of the ATP binding cassette (ABC) family of drug transporters by Juliano and Ling in 1976, (Juliano and Ling 1976) research into this group of proteins has been gaining wide interests. Some of the membrane transporters confer on the cells the ability to be resistant not only to the selective agent but also to a broad spectrum of structurally and functionally distinct antibiotics and alkaloids.This phenotypic character is referred to as multiple drug resistance (MDR). The MDR genotype/phenotype relationship is complex with over 18 ABC genes associated with human disease (Dean and Annilo 2005).

In addition to the ABC transporters, other important drug/xenobiotic transporters include the organic cation transporters of the SLC 22A super family and the organic anion transporting peptides of the SLC21 superfamily (Hagenbuch 2010). It is expected that with the growing interests in this phase of drug metabolism, investigations on the transcriptional regulatory control of this important transport system in target organs such as the liver, kidney and central nervous system will become intense in the next few decades (Omiecinski 2011).

5. Target genes of pharmacogenetics

About 20 kinds of enzymes are involved in metabolism of drugs. The cytochrome enzyme (CYP450) is regarded as the most important enzyme in drug metabolism. About 15 types of this group have been identified in human beings where they catalyse the biotransformation of many xenobiotics. Other enzymes include thiopurine methyl transferase (TMPT) which metabolizes 6- mercaptopurine and azathioprine, uridyl diphosphate glucuronyl transferase (UDGT) responsible for the conjugation of bilirubin, N – acetyltransferase (NAT2) responsible for metabolism of sulpha containing drugs and caffeine, catachol – o – methyl transferase (COMT) responsible for the metabolism of levodopa and dihydropyrimidine dehydrogenase (DPD) a rate limiting enzyme for the metabolism of 5 – florouracil (5 FU). Genetic polymorphism has been identified in many of these enzymes with varying degrees of drug response (Evans & Relling 1999, Furuta et al 2001, McAlpine et al 2001,Suzuki et al 2011) Of all the enzymes involved in drug metabolism, the cytochrome P450.(CYP450) is regarded as the most important because many drugs are substrates for the enzyme of the group. CYP3A4, CYP2D6, CYP2C9, CYP219, CYP2B6 and CYP1A2 play the most critical role and account for more than 90% of drugs metabolized by P450 (Evans & Relling 1999). These enzymes have proven genetic polymorphism with associated drug responses (Hiratsuka et al 2002, Wong et al 2005, McAlpine et al 2011) and racial variations (Meyer 2004 & Suarez – Kurtz 2005). As discussed earlier, genetic polymorphism can manifest at both pharmacokinetic and pharmacodynamic levels whereby many genetic variants of respective enzymes, membrane transporters, receptors and ion channels have been dectected (Wiesler et al 2008, Phipps – Green et al 2010 & Bouamar et al 2011)

5.1 Pharmacokinetic related genes

5.1.1 Genes of phase i reaction enzymes

Genetic variations have been observed particularly with CYP2D6, CYP2C9 aand CYP2C19 genotypes (Ingelman – Sundberg 1999, Hiratsuka 2006) and therefore will be further elucidated.

i.   **CYP2D6:** With regards to this CYP subtype, 5 – 10% of Caucasians are poor metabolizers and have little enzyme activity and there is a distinct racial diversity in the frequency of the classes. About 50 genetic polymorphisms of CYP2D6 have been reported. The popular ones are CYP2D6*3, CYP2D6*4 and CYP2D6*5. More than 90% of PMs in Caucasians are ascribable to these three genetic polymorphism (Daly et al 1996,& Suzuki et al 2011). In blacks, the common variant is CYP2D*17 (Evans 1989)

ii. **CYP2C9:** is involved in the metabolism of an epileptic agent; phenytoin and an anticoagulant; warfarin. To date, 12 CYP2C9 variants have been reported. For example in cases with phenytoin, oral clearance decreased to one quarter in subjects with homozygous polymorphism for CYP2CP*3 (Kidd et al 1999 , Scodo et al 2002, Linder et al 2009). Many studies focused on CYP2C9 polymorphism to link variability with warfarin therapy. However only about 10% of dosage variation can be attributed to CYP2C9 polymorphism. It is thought that environmental and genetic factors can influence warfarin response therefore dosage is individualized based on sex, age, vitatmin K intake, and disease states. Warfarin dosing can be challenging because of its narrow therapeutic index and the serious risk of bleeding in overdosage. Warfarin exerts its anticoagulant effects by inhibiting hepatic vitamin K epoxide reductase; an enzyme involved in the vitamin K epoxide reductase complex sub unit 1 (VKORC1). The gene that encodes this enzyme has been identified and is believed to contribute to the variability in warfarin response (Scodo et al 2002, Aquilante et al 2006, Linder et al 2009, Guengerich 2001).

iii. **The CYP2C19:** enzyme metabolizes many drugs including the proton pump inhibitor; citalopram (lelexa) diazepam (valium) and imipramine (toranil). More than 16 variants of CYP2C19 associated with deficient, reduced, normal or increased activity have been identified. The most common genotypic variants for poor metabolizers are CYP2C19*2 and CYP2C19*3. The CYP2C19*17 variant is associated with ultrarapid metabolizers and seems to be common in Swedes (18%), Ethiopians (18%) and Chinese (4%). (Sum et al 2006). The proton pump inhibitor omeprazole (prilosec) is primarily metabolized by CYP2C19 to its inactive metabolite 5 – hydroxyl-omeprazole. Individuals who are CYP2C19 poor metabolizers can have five fold higher blood concentrations of omeprazole and experience superior acid suppression and higher cure rate than the rest of the population. Conversely, blood concentrations of omeprazole are predicted to be 40% lower in ultrarapid metabolizers than the rest of the population and are therefore at risk of therapeutic failure. (Sum et al 2006)

5.1.2 Genes of phase II reaction enzymes

N – Acetyl Transferase: Activities of human hepatic drug metabolizing enzymes was earlier been recognized as a cause of inter – individual variation in the metabolism of drugs. Therefore acetylation of many drugs like isoniazid caffeine, nitrozepam and sulphonamide exhibit genetic polymorphism. The N – acetyl transferase (NAT) enzyme is controlled by two genes, (NAT 1) and (NAT 2) of which NAT2 A and B are responsible for clinically significant metabolic polymorphism. (Heiss 1988, Grant et al 1990). Three phenotypes have been recognized with activities of NAT2 and these are rapid acetylator (RA), intermediate acetylator (IA) and slow acetylator (SA) status (Cranswick 2005). The frequency of slow acetylator in Caucasians and Negro populations is 50% and 10% in Oriental groups. (.Evans D.A 1989) Slow acetylator phenotype is preponderant among different Arab populations irrespective of geographical location of the country. (Woolhouse et al 1997, At- Moussa et al 2002 & Desoky et al 2005). Three genetic polymorphisms NAT2*5, NAT2*6, NAT2*7 but not NAT2*4 (wild type allele) are responsible for almost all SAs in the Japanese (Huang et al 2002) Drug induced hepatitis caused by isoniazid occurs often in SA than RA (Ohno et al 2000) and Type II diabetes SA may be predisposed to progression to renal complications than their RA counterparts (Banjoko & Akinlade 2010).

Thiopurine - S –Methyl Transferase (TPMT: Catalyses the S – Methylation of the thiopurine agents, azathioprine, mercaptopurine and thiogleamine. These agents are commonly used for a diverse range of medical indications including leukaemia, rheumatic diseases and organ transplant. The principal cytotoxic mechanism of these agents is mediated via incorporation of thioguanine nucleotides (TGN) into DNA. Thiopurines are inactive prodrugs that require metabolism to thioguanine nucleotides to exert cytotoxicity. This activation is catalyzed by a multienzyme pathway which include hypoxanthine phosphoribosyl transeferase (HPRT), oxidation by xanthine oxidase (XO) or methylation by TPMT. During metabolism, hypoxanthine-guanine phosphoribosyl transferase (HPGRT) converts 6-mercaptopurine to cytotoxic6-thioguanine nucleotide analogues, while thiopurine methyl transferase (TPMT) inactivates 6-mercaptopurine through methylation to form 6 –methylmercaptopurine. However, TMPT is the major pathway and it is highly variable and polymorphic. More than 12 TPMT alleles have been identified. The most common ones are TPMT*2, TPMT*3A, TPMT*3C, with all three associated with lower enzyme activity attributable to enhanced rates of proteolysis of the variant proteins (Donnan et al 2011, Haghuid et al 2011, Guengerich 2001). Caucasian infant patients with acute myeloid leukaemia carrying TPMT*2, TPMT*3A, TPMT*3B, TPMT*3C showed significantly higher concentrations of the thiopurine intermediate metabolite 6-mercaptopurine in their red cells that requires dose reduction or termination of thiopurine administration due to adverse effects such as myelosuppression (Relling et al 1999, Tavadia et al 2001).

Dihydro Pyrimidine Dehydrogenase (DPD): Dihydro pyrimidine dehydrogenase (DPD) is a rate limiting enzyme for the metabolism of the anti cancer drug; 5 fluorouracil (5FU). With DPD being responsible for over 50% of its biotransformation. Other substrates for DPD are carmofur, tegafur and doxifluridine. The gene encoding for DPD is DPDY and about 13 genetic variants have been reported (McLeod et al 1998, Collie – Duguid et al 2000). The genetic variant that is responsible for decreased DPD activity has been reported to be DPYD*2 with a polymorphism at the splicing recognition site. (Wei at al 1996) Administration of 5 – FU to the patients with decreased enzyme activity results in adverse effects such as leukocytopenia, stomatitis, diarrhea, nausea and vomiting (Etienne et al 1994)

Glutathione – S – Tranferase (GST): GSTs and the human genes encoding these enzymes are highly polymorphic with about 50% and 25% of most populations having a mutation or complete deletion of these gene respectively rendering them deficient or lacking the enzyme. Major racial and ethnic differences exist and GST M and GST T1 are the major genes. Other GSTs include GST P1 and GST*A which are also subject to genetic polymorphism and have been implicated in resistance to anti cancer drugs. High GST activity has been associated with decreased risk of haematologic relapse, central nervous system response and improved prednisolone response. (Commandeur et.al 1995) Inherited GST – P1 allele encoding for the 11e 105 Val. amino acid substitution, has been associated with improved overall breast cancer survival compared with patients who have at least one wild type GST P1 allele. Conversely in patients with acute myeloid leukaemia treated with high doses of combination therapy, the homozygous GST – T1 deletion is associated with a higher risk of toxic death during remission. (Arruda et. al 2001)

Uridyl Diphosphate Glucuronyl Transferase (UGT): The UDP – glucuronyl transferase (UGT) belongs to a super family of membrane bound proteins localized in the endoplamic reticulum and are responsible for glucuronidation of many xenobiotics and endobiotics. The UGT genes have been classified into families and sub families based on evolutionary divergence with all known human UGT's being in the UGT1A 2A and 2B sub families. (Mackenzie et al 1997, Randominska – Pandya et al 1999, Tukey & Strassburg 2000). To date, polymorphism in UGTA1 have been more studied extensively and seem to have clinical significance. The anticancer drug irinotecan is metabolized by the enzyme and polymorphism resembling condition seen in Gilbert's syndrome characterised by total lack of UGT enzyme due to deletion of the gene which leads to fifty fold reduction in irinotecan metabolism and such patients can be at risk of toxicity (Huang et al 2002 Desai et al 2003).

5.1.3 Phase III reactions: Transporter genes

Membrane transporters as mentioned earlier are heavily involved in drug clearance and alter drug disposition by actively transporting drugs between organs and tissues. Therefore polymorphisms in the genes encoding these proteins may have significant effects on the absorption, distribution, metabolism and excretion of xenobiotics and may alter the pharmacodynamics of these agents. Uptake transporters are required for the uptake of some drugs into the cell whereas efflux transporters are responsible for pumping some drugs out of cells or preventing them from ever getting in. Transporters are also thought to be involved in drug – drug reactions.

The most important families of the transporters include (i) ATP binding cassette (ABC) family whose genes include important members like the multi drug resistance gene also classified as ABCB 1 i.e. (ABCB1/MDR1), ABCC1, ABCC2, uric acid transporter (ABCG2), breast cancer resistance protein BCRP also classified ABCG2 i.e. (BCRP/ABCG2).(ii) The solute transporter superfamily (SLC) which include the organic anion transport polypeptide

(SLC 21/OATP), organic cation transporter SLC 22 OCT), zwitterion/cation transporter (OCTNs), folate transporter(SLC19A1), neurotransmitter transporter(SLC6,SLC17,&SLC18)and serotonin transporter (5HTT).Genetic polymorphism in drug transporter genes have increasingly been recognized as a possible mechanism accounting for variation in drug response because these transporters play important roles in the gastrointestinal absorption, biliary and renal elimination and distribution to target sites of their substrates. (Meier et al 2007, Shu et al 2007, Choi & Song 2008)

5.1.3.1 The ABC family genes

ABCB1: Refers to ATP binding cassette (ABC) sub family B member 1, or MDR 1 also designated cluster of differentiation (CD243) is the permeability glycoprotein (P – glycoprotein).ABC genes are divided into seven distinct sub families (ABC1, MDR/TAP, MRP, ALD, OABP, CaCW 20 andWhite). Members of the MDR/TAP sub- family are involved in multi drug resistance. The protein encoded by this gene is an ATP dependent drug efflux pump of xenobiotics with broad substrate specificity. It is responsible for decreased drug accumulation in multi drug resistant cells and often mediates the development of resistance to cancer cells (Viguie 1998). This protein also function as a transporter in the blood brain barrier (Viguie 1998, Phipps – Green et al 2010). It likely evolved as a defense mechanism against harmful substances. Some of the functions of protein encoded by ABCB 1 gene include regulation of distribution and bioavailability of drugs, removal of metabolites and xenobiotics from cells into urine, bile and intestinal lumen, transport of compounds out of the brain across the blood – brain barrier, digoxin uptake, prevention of invermectin entry into the central nervous system and protection of hamatopoietic cells from toxins (Dean 2002.) Mutation of ABCB1 gene will therefore result in disruption of these functions. The activity of the transporter can be determined by both membrane ATPase and cellular calcein assays. Drug resistance had been observed in M89T, L662R, R669 and S1141T variants of the gene and decreased drug efficacy in W1108R variant. In addition, genetic variation in ABCB1 has been associated with both toxicity and drug response in 5Fluoro-uracil (Gonzalez – Haba et al 2011) and pacilitaxel therapy (Henningson et al 2011).

ABCC 1 genes: Multidrug resistant protein 1 (MRP1) an ATP bounding cassette transporter encoded by ABCC 1 gene is expressed in many tissues and function as an efflux transporter for glutathione, glycine and sulphate conjugates as well as unconjugated substrates. An evaluation of single nucleotide polymorphism (SNP) revealed 7 mutations in the gene (Colombo et al 2005) while in a Japanese study, 86 genetic variants were identified (Fukushina – Uesaka et al 2007). Mutations in ABC transporters cause or contribute to many different Mendelian and complex disorders including adrenoleukodystrophy, cystic fibrosis and retinal degeneration (Dean & Annilo 2005). There has been no evidence of clinical significance in studies of the variants. (Colombo et al 2005, Pauli Magrus & Kroetz 2005 & Fukushina -Uesaka 2007).

ABCC2 gene: ABBCC2 genes codes for the ABCC2 or MRP2 protein. (MRP2) is an export pump expressed at tissue barriers. Genetic variants 24 e>T, 1249Ca>A and 3972 > T had been observed and are thought to cause inter individual differences of bioavailability of various endogenous and exogenous compounds (Colombo et al 2005, Laechelt et al 2011). About 27 other variants have also been detected (Colombo et al 2005). A haplotype dependent influence on transport capacity of ABCC2 had been observed but seems to be mainly based on post transcriptional modifications rather than transport rates (Laechelt et al 2011).

TheABCG2 gene encodes an inhibitor of breast cancer resistance protein (BCRP) (ABCG2) protein, another member of the ABC transporter. The protein confers protection against the development of breast cancers. Evaluation of single nucleotide polymorphism identified 16 variants (Morisaki et al 2005, Colombo et al 2005). Genetic polymorphism in ABCG2 might alter the transport activity of some drugs causing therapy in drugs like irinotecan, to cause severe myelosuppression (Choi et al 2009, Hampras et al 2010). A polymorphism, C421A observed in human placenta is not a genetic variant acting in cis but is considered to influence the translational efficiency (Kobayeshi et al 2005). Another genetic variant (ABCG2) (rs 2231142, Q141K) encoding a uric acid transporter is associated with gout in diverse populations (Phipps – Green et al 2010)

5.1.3.2 Solute Carrier Superfamily: (SLC) Genes

The solute carrier (SLC) superfamily of transporters consists of more than 300 members subdivided into 47 families. They are expressed in most tissues but primarily in liver, lungs, kidney and intestine.

i.   **OATP/SLC21:** Organic anion transporter facilitates movement of anion across the cell membrane.OATP1B and OATP1B3 are human hepatocyte transporters that mediate the uptake of various endogenous and exogenous substrates. Genetic variation was observed in the SLCO1B1 and SLCO1B3 genes which encode OATP1B1 and OATP1B3 proteins. Forty nine (49) and 41 nucleotide sequence variants leading to 10 and 9 in SLCO1B1 and SLCO1B3 genes respectively were identified (Bowin   et al 2010). Furthermore, in OATPC (SLC21A6) and OATP3 (SLC22A8) genes, polymorphism did not appear to be associated with changes in renal and tubular secretory clearance in the latter but the former was associated with differences in the disposition kinetics of pravastin. Individualswith the OATP – C*15 allele (ASP 130 Ala 174) had a reduced total and non renal clearance compared with those of OATPC*15 allele (ASP130Val 174) (Nishizato Y et al 2003).

ii. **SLC 19A1 (Folate Transporter)member 1:** The SLC19A1 are the proteins responsible for the transport of folate. Transport of folate into the mammalian cells can occur via receptor mediated (folate receptor 1) or carrier mediated (SLC19A1) mechanism. Methotrexate is an antifolate chemotherapeutic agent that is actively transported by the carrier mediated uptake system. Individuals carrying a specific polymorphism of SLC19A1 gene ï.e (C80GG) have lower levels of folate. (Whetsine 2003, Matherly et al 2007) and those carrying the C80AA genotype treated with methrotrexate have higher levels of this antifolate chemotherapeutic agent. This underpins requirements for personalized dosing with the drug based on patients genotype

iii. **OCT/SLC22:** Most solute carrier transporters are localized at either the basolateral or apical plasma membrane of polarized cells but some are also expressed in mitochondria and other organelles (Wojtal et al 2009). The genes encoding the three organic cation transporter isoforms OCT1, OCT2 and OCT 3 are clustered together on the long arm of chromosome 8 in humans and carry out functions of transport of small organic cations with different molecular structures independent of sodium gradient. These organic cation substrate include drugs like metformin, procainamide and cimetidine as well as endogenous compounds like dopamine and norepinephrine and toxic substances like tetraethylammonium bromide (TEA) (Kang et al 2007).

5.2 Pharmacodynamic related genes

i.   **Receptors:** Many receptors are involved with several signaling pathways. Example of which is epidermal growth factor receptor(EGFR). This receptor has been implicated in the oncogenesis and progression of several solid tumours thereby being identified as a suitable target for anticancer treatment. Polymorphism has been observed in the development of cancer on dinucleotide repeats in intron 1 of the EGFR gene and this has correlated with EGFR expression with therapeutic implication for treatment with tyrosinase kinase inhibitor. A higher proportion of Asians do overexpress EGFR that may influence their responses to tyrosine kinase inhibitor (Tan et al 2004).

G-protein Coupled Receptors (GPCR): Over 50% of all drug targets have G-protein coupled receptors (GPCR). Genes of GPR has more coding regions than non – GPCR genes making them more important for pharmacological investigations.

GABAA Receptor Mutation in GABAA receptor ion channel may be a reason for the diminished protection of anti epileptic drugs.

Insulin Receptor(INSR): The receptor is important in the management of diabetes mellitus patients and mutation of the gene encoding the receptor will result in poor response particularly in type 2 diabetes.Mutation of the gene has also been suspected to contribute to genetic susceptibility to the polycystic ovarian syndrome(Siega et al2002)

B2 Receptor: B2 agonist; albuterol (Proventil) is used to control acute attacks of asthma and are prescribed as needed .Patients with β_2 receptor arginine genotype experience poor asthma control with frequent symptoms and a decreasing scores of poor exploratory volume compared with those with glycine genotype (Cowburn et al 1998, de Maat et al 1999). Seventeen (17%) of whites and 20% of blacks carry the arginine genotype (Wechsler et al 2005)

ii. **Ion Channels:** Many genes encode for different ion channels including those of the central nervous system which include KCNJ10, KCNJ3, CLCN2, GABRA1, SCN1B and SCN1A. Some polymorphism of this channel has been linked to idiopathic generalized epilepsy (Lucarini et al 2007)

The 5-HT3 receptor is a ligand-gated ion channel composed of five subunits. To date, five different human subunits are known; 5-HT3A-E, which are encoded by the serotonin receptor genes HTR3A, HTR3B, HTR3C, HTR3D and HTR3E, respectively. Functional receptors are pentameric complexes of diverse composition. Different receptor subtypes seem to be involved in chemotheraphy-induced nausea and vomiting (CINV), irritable bowel syndrome and psychiatric disorders. 5-HTR3A and HTR3B polymorphisms may also contribute to the etiology of psychiatric disorders and serve as predictors in CINV and in the medical treatment of psychiatric patients. (Niesler et al 2008).

iii. **Enzymes:** Polymorphism of pharmacokinetic enzymes no doubt influence the pharmacodynamics of drugs. However there are few enzymes that influence drugs at the point of actions one of these enzymes is the tyrosine kinase which modulate receptor activities. Therefore polymorphism in tyrosine kinase gene will affect drugs at the target point.

Another important enzyme of drug target is vitamin K epoxide reductase complex subunit 1(VKORC1). This enzyme is the drug target for warfarin an anticoagulant with a narrow therapeutic window and with serious consequences of bleeding in the event of an overdose. Variation in maintenance dose of warfarin is largely attributable to genetic variants in the genes that encode the drug target VKORC1 the major metabolizing enzyme. The two genetic polymorphisms explain 30 – 40% of the total variation in those on therapy.

Angiotensin converting enzyme (ACE) genes encode for ACE, a target for ACE inhibitors which improves symptom and survival in cases of heart failure. Genetic polymorphism is suspected to be causing greater effects of the drug in Europeans than Afro-Americans. Pre-treatment genetic screening is therefore apt to improve therapy

iv. **Neurotransmitter Transporters:** Neurotransmitter transporters namely SLC6, SLC17 and SLC18 families are primarily expressed in the neurons of the central and peripheral nervous system. These transporters are the sites of action of various drugs of abuse e.g cocaine, amphetamine and other clinically approved drugs like desipramine, reserpine, benztropine and tiagabine. Genetic variation in the SLC6, SLC17 and SLC18 encoding genes may result in altered expression and function of these proteins. In particular, antidepressants and antiepileptic drugs target these neurotransmitters as part of their primary mechanism of action. Therefore genetic variations may affect the efficacy of such drugs.

6. Pharmacogenetic testing

A genetic test is the analysis of human DNA, RNA chromosomes, proteins or certain metabolites in order to detect alterations related to a heritable disorder. This can be accomplished by directly examining the DNA or RNA that makes up a gene (Direct testing), looking at markers co-inherited with a disease causing gene (linkage testing), assaying certain metabolites (biochemical testing), or examining the chromosomes (cytogenetic testing). Although genetic testing shares some features common with other kinds of laboratory testing, it is however unique in many ways and therefore requires special consideration .Pharmacogenetic testing can therefore be defined as utilization of aforementioned genetic biomarkers related to drug metabolism and effects. A biomarker can be described as a characteristic that is objectively measured and evaluated as an indicator of normal biological processes to a therapeutic intervention (EMEA 2006)

Methods of Pharmacogenetic testing depends on the biomarker to be assessed. These vary from simple spectrophotometric estimation of metabolites to DNA sequences, use of PCR and DNA probes, enzymes linked immunosorbent assay, cell culture, gel electrophoresis high performance liquid chromatography and DNA hybridization techniques. It is not uncommon to use combined techniques to study clinical relevance of pharmacogenetic testing.

Because information on pharmacogenetics is still evolving, there is a necessity for guidelines to be adopted for ethical reasons, economic considerations and patient benefit. Overall, the quest for pharmacogenetic information is likely to grow. As a matter of fact some drugs already carry labels addressing such.

6.1 European medicines agency guideline for pharmacogenetic testing

The guidelines for European Medicines Agency (EMEA) was desighned by the Agency's committee for Human Medicinal Products (CHMP). The rationale for this guidelines include standardization, data analysis, interpretation, evaluation of clinical relevance, ethical consideration and setting the stage for technical, scientific and regulatory issues. The guidelines addresses the following among other issues.

i.   Chosen design and rationale
ii.   the population selected for pharmacogenetic studies (i.e. species, age, gender and other variable related to the phenotype e.g. for human exposure ethnic group)
      *In the target population or relevant animal model
      *In the study population e.g. matched groups (responders/non responders, presence/absence of adverse events)
iii. The population size selected for PG studies and a discussion on the power to detect an association in appropriate
iv.   Predictive values (positive and negative) of the PG biomarkers as per clinical   trials experience
v.   Assumptions on clinical utility e.g. benefit In using predictive pharmacogenetics testing versus other predictive biomarkers, use of a pharmacogenetic biomarker as a segregation marker or as a stratification tool for a subpopulation in a general matching population.

6.2 Pharmacogenetic testing and clinical benefits

The overall purpose of PG testing is clinical benefits. Pharmacogenetic testing have resulted in some clinical benefit so far, some of which can be life saving. It was observed that roughly about 106,000 deaths and 2.2 million serious events caused by adverse drug reactions were reported yearly (Lazarom 1998) and 5 – 7% of hospital admissions in US and Europe lead to the withdrawal of 4% of new medicines with attendant financial loss. Since such drugs were linked to metabolizing enzymes with known polymorphism,prudence dictates suggestion of pharmacogenetic testing in indicated instances Pharmacogenetics testing is expectedly becoming commonly required particularly with drugs with low therapeutic window (Phillips et al 2001). However, the decision to use pharmacogenetic testing will be influenced by the relative costs of genotyping technologies and the cost of providing a treatment to a patient with an incompatible genotype.

Notable clinical benefits of pharmacogenetic testing have been observed in NAT2 genotyping for isoniazid treatment (Hiratsuka et al 2002, Weishilboum et al 2003, Gardiner and Begg 2006) andCYP2C19 genotyping for omeprazole treatment (Desta et al 2002).

Others are TPMT genotyping for 6-mercaptopurine and azathioprine treatment (Relling et al 1999, Gardener and Begg 2006) mtDNA A155G genotyping for aminoglycoside treatment (Cortopassi and Hatchin 1994, Usami et al 1999) CYP 2D6 genotyping for codeine treatment (Bradford 2002) Hepatitis C genotype for pegylated interferon – alpha – 2a or pegylated – interferon – alpha – 2b treatment. (Ingelman – Sundberg et al 2009, Thomas et al 2009) and Dihydropyrimidine dehydrogenese (DPI) testing for 5-fluoro-Uracil (5FU) treatment (Gionzalez and Fernandez –Salguero, 1995, McMurrough et al 1996, Wei et al 1996, Van Kuilenburg et al 1998).

There are currently requirements of pharmacogenetic testing of specific drugs before they can be prescribed and these include cetuximab, trastuzumab, maraviroc and dasatinib. In December 2007, the FDA recommended testing for HLA-B* 1502 allele in patients with Asian ancestry before initiating carbamazepine therapy because of high risk of developing carbamazepine induced Steven's Johnson syndrome (SSS) or toxic epidermal necrolysis.

Pharmacogenetic testing is also recommended for patients treated with warfarin, thiopurine, valproic acid, irinotecan, abacavir or rasburicase.

Currently, drug labels contain information on pharmacogenetic tests which are classified as test required, test recommended and for information only.

7. Conclusion

With the application of molecular biology methods and completion of the human genome projects and establishment of guidelines for pharmacogenetics practices and applications, it is expected that the interwoven field of pharnmacogenetics and pharmacogenomics will revoluntionise personalized medicine. Furthermore the field of predictive medicine is expected to receive a boost from pharmacogenetic information with attendant reduction in morbidity and mortality particularly from adverse drug reactions and therapeutic failure. With more intense researches and genotyping profiling, the challenges of standardization and interpretation of pharmacogenetic testing are apt to be overcome. It is worthy of note that currently some drug labels carry information on pharmacogenetic testing and requirements for therapeutic use. The promise of pharmacogenetics is therefore improvement of the overall health being of the patients.

8. References

Ait Moussa L, Khassouni CE, Hue B, Jana M, Begand B, Soulaymani R (2002). Determination of the acetylator phenotype in Moroccan tuberculosis patients using isoniazid as metabolic probe *Critical Care Medicine 30 (2) 107 – 14*

Arruda VR, Lima CS, Grignoll CR, de Melo MB, Lorrand-Metze I, Alberto FL, Saad ST & Costa FF (2001) Increased risk of acute myeloid leukaemia in individuals with glutathione-S-transferase MU1(GST M1 and theca 19GST T10 gene defects *.European Journal of Haematology 66(6) 383-8*

Aquilante CL, Langace TY, Lopez Lm (2006) Influence of coagulation factor, vitamin K epoxide reductase complex subuniit 1 and cytochrome P4502C9 gene polymorphisms on warfarin dose requirements. *Clinical Pharmacology and Therapeutics 79 (4):291 – 302*

Banjoko, S.O. &Akinlade K.S. (2010) Acetylation Pharmacogenetics and renal function in diabetes mellitus patients. *Indian Journal of Clinical Biochemistry, 25(3) 289*

Boivin A A, Cardinal H, Barama A, Pichelte V, Hebert M J, Rocher M (2010) Organic Anion Transporting Polypeptide 1B1 (OATP1B1) and OATP1B3. genetic variability and haplotype analysis of the white Canadians. *Drug Metabolism and Pharmacokinetics 25 (5): 508 – 515*

Boyland E,& Chassaud LF, (1969) The role of glutathione and glutathione S transferase in mercapturic acid synthesis. *Advances in Enzymology Related Area of Molecular Biology 32 (1) : 173 – 219*

Choi MK, Song IS (2008) Organic cation transporters and their pharmacokinetic and pharmacodynamic consequences *Drug Metabolism and Pharmacokinetics* 23: 243 – 253

Collie – Dughid ES, Etienne MC, Milano G,& Mc Leod HL. (2000) Known variant of DPYD alleles do not explain DPD deficiency in cancer patients *Pharmacogenetics10:217 – 23*

Colombo S, Soranzo N, Rolger M, Sprenger R Bleiber G, Furrer H, Buclin T. Goldstein DB, Descoslerd L, Telenti A & Swiss HIV cohort (2005). Influence of ABCB1, ABCC 2 and ABCG 2 haplotypes on the cellular exposure of nelfinavir in vitro. *Pharmacogenetics & Genomics 15(9)599-60*

Commandeur JN, Stintes GT, and Vermeulen NP (1995) Enzymes and transport systems involved in the formation and disposition of glutathione S – conjugates. Role in bioactivation and detoxication mechanisms of xenobiotics *Pharmacology Review 47 (2) : 271 – 330*

Cowburn AS, Sladek, Soja J et al 5(1998) Overexpression of leukotriene C4 synthase in bronchial biopsies from patients with aspirin-intolerant asthma..*Journal of Clinical Investigations,101(4):834-836*

Cranswick N. and Mulholland K. (2005) Isoniazid treatment of Children. can genetic help guide treatment? *Archives of Diseases in Children 90:551 – 3*

Daly AK, Brockmoller J, Body F (1996) Nomenclature for human CYP2D6 alleles. *Pharmacogenetics 1996, 6: 193 – 201.*

Dasai AA, Innocent F, and Ratain MJ (2003) UGT pharmacogenomics. implications for cancer risk and cancer therapeutics. *Pharmacogenetics 13:517 – 523.*

de Maat MP, Jukema JW, Ye S et al (1999) Effect of the stromelysin-1 promoter on efficacy of provastatin in coronary atherosclerosis and restenosis *American Journal of Cardiology 83 (6): 852-856*

Dean M and Annilo T (2005) Evolution of the ATP – Binding Cassette (ABC) transporter superfamily in vertebrates. *Annual Review of Genomics and Human Genetics 6: 123 – 1.42*

Desta Z, Zhas X, Shin JG, Flockhart DA (2002) Clinical significance of the cytochrome P450 2C19 genetic polymorphism. *Clinical Pharmacokinetics 41 : 913 – 58*

Donnan JR, Ungar WS, Matthews M and Rahman PV Systematic review of thiopurine methyl transferase genotype and enzymatic testing strategies. *Therapeutic Drug Monitoring 33 (2): 192*

El. Desoky ES, Abdel Salam YM, Salama RH, El Akkah MA, Atansova S, Von Ahsen N (2005) NAT 2*5/*5 genotype (351T<C) is a potential risk factor for schistosomiasis associated bladder cancer in Egyptians. *Therapeutic Drug Monitoring 27(3) 297 – 304.*

Etienne MC, Lagrange JL, Dassonville O. (1994) Population study of dihydropyrimidine dehydrogenase in cancer patients. *Journal of Clinical Oncology 12:2248 – 53*

EuropeanMedicinesAgency(EmeA)(2006)*DocRefEMEA/CHMP/PGXWP/2027/2004*

Evans DA (1989) N – acetyl transferase, *Pharmacology and therapeutics, 42:157 – 234*

Evans WE (2004) Pharmacogenetics of thiopurine S – methyl transerase and thiopurine. *Therapeutic drug monitoring 26:186 – 9*

Evans WE, Relling MV (1999) Phrmacogenomics translating functional genomics into rational therapeutics *Science: 286 : 487 – 91*

Fukushima-Uesaka H, Saito Y, Tohkin M, Maekura K, Hasegawa R, Kawamoto M, Kamatani N(2007).Genetic variation and haplotype structures of the ABC transporter gene ABCC1 in a Japanese population.*Drug Metabolism & Pharmacokinetics, Feb 22(1):48-60*

Gardener SJ, Begg EJ (2006) Pharmacogenetics, drug-metabolizing enzymes and clinical practice. *Pharmacocology Review 58 (3): 521 – 90*

Gonzalez-Haba E, Garcia MI, Corte Joso L, Lopez –Lillo C, Barrue N, Garcia –Alfonsop, Alvarez S, Jimenez JL, Martin ML, Munoz-Fernandez MA, Sanjurjo M and Lopez-Fernandez LA (2011)ABCB 1 Polymorphism in fluoropyrimidine treatment. *Pharmacogenomics 11(12);1715-1723*

Goldstein DB, Tate SK, Sisodiya SM pharmacogenetics goes genomic (2003) *Nature Review of Genetics, 4: 937-4*

Grant DM (1990) Morike K, Eichelbaum M, Mayer V.A Acetylation Pharmacogenetics, the slow acetylators pharmacogenetics, the slow acetylators phenotypes is caused by decrease or absent arylamine N – acetyl transferase in human live. *Journal of Clinical Investigations .85(3):968-72*

Guengerkich FB (2001) Common and uncommon cytochrome p450 reactions related to metabolism and chemical toxicity. *Chemical Research &Toxicology 14 (6) 611 – 50*

Hagenbuch B (2010) Drug uptake systems in liver and kidney a historic perspective. *Clinical Pharmacology and Therapeutics 87 (1) 39 – 47.*

Haglund S, Vikingssons Soderman J, Huidorf U, Granno G, Donelius M, Coulthard S, Peterson C & Aliner S (2011) The role of Inosine 5^1 – Monophosphate Dehydrogenase in Thiopurine metabolism in patient with Inflammatory Bowel Disease. *Therapeutic Drug Monitoring 32(2):192-199*

Hampras S S, Sucheston L, Weiss Joli, Baer MR, Zirpoli G, Singh PK, Wetzler M, Chennamaneni R, Blanco JG, Ann Ford L, Moysich KB, (2010) Genetic Polymorphisms of ATP – binding cassette (ABC) proteins, overall survival and drug toxicity in patients with acute myeloid Leukaemia *International Journal of Molecular Epidemiology and Genetics 1 (3): 201-207*

Hanene C, Jihene I, Jamel A, Kamel A & Agnestl (2007) Association of polymorphism with genes of GST with asthma in Tunisian Children. *Mediators of Inflammation Dol:10.1155/2007/19567*

Henningson A, Marsh S, Loos WJ, Karlsson MO, Garba A, mross K, Mielke S, Vigano L, Locatelli A, Verweij, Sparreboom A, McLeod HL (2005)Associate of CYP2C8, CYP3A4, CYP3A5 and ABCBI polymorphism with the pharmacogenetic of paclitroxel in Clinical Cancer research Nov. 22: 8097 – 104ABCBI polymorphism in Fluoro pyramidine – Treated Patient .*Pharmacogenomics (2011) 11 (12) 1715 – 1723*

Hiratsuka M, Agatsuma Y, Omori F et al (2002) Allele and genotype frequencies of CYP2B6 and CYP3A5 in the Japanese population. *European Journal of Clinical Pharmacology* 58 : 417 – 21

Hiratsuka M, Kishikawa Y, Takekuma Y (2002) genotyping of the N-acetyl transferase-2polymorphism in the prediction of adverse drug reactions to isoniazid in Japanese patients. *Drug metabolism &Pharmacokinetics* 17:357-361

Hiratsuka M, sasaki T, Mizugaki M (2006) Genetic testing for Pharmacogenetics and its clinical application in drug therapy *Clinical Chimica Acta* 363 177 – 185

Huang Y, Galijatoric A, Nguyen N, Geske D, Beaton D, Green J (2002) Identification and Functional Characterization of UDP – glycuronyl transfeerase UGT1A8*1, UGT1A8*2, UGT1A8*3. *Pharmacogenetics* 12:287 – 297.

Huang, YS, Cher, HD, SUWJ (2002) Polymorphism of the N – acetyl transferase 2 gene as a susceptibility risk factor for anti tuberculosis drug induced hepatitis. *Hepatology 35:* 839 – 83

Ingelman – Sundberg M, Rodrighmez – Antona C, McHutchinson JG, Goldstein DB (2009) Genetic variation in IL28B predicts hepatitis C treatment induced viral clearance – *Nature 461 (7262) 399 – 401*

Juliano RL and Ling V (1976) A surface glycoprotein modulating drug permeability in Chinese hamster ovary cell mutants. *Biochemical & BiophysicaActa, 465 (1) 15 – 62.*

Kang HJ, Song I S, Shin H J, Kim WY, Lee CH, Shim JC, Zhou H H, Lee S S, Shin J. G (2007) Identification and Functional Characterization of genetic variant of human organic cation transporters in a Korean population. *Drug metabolism and Disposition 35: 667 – 675*

Kimura M, Leiri I, Mamiya K, Urae A, Hignchi S. Genetic polymorphism of cyto chrome P450s CYP2C19 and CYP2C9 in a Japanese population. *Therapeutic Drug Monitoring 20: 243 – 7.*

Klotz V (2007) The role of Pharmacogenetics in the metabolism of antiepileptic drugs: Pharcomacokinectic and therapeutic implications. *Clinical Pharmacokinetics* 46 (4): 27 – 9

Konig J, Nies AT, Cui Y, Leier I, Keppler D (1999) conjugate export pump of the multidrug resistance protein (MRP) family: localization substrate specificity and MRP 2 – mediated drug resistance. *Biochemica and BiophysicaActa* 1461 (2) 377

Kroetz DL, Yee SW, Griacomini KM (2010) The Pharmacogenetics of membrane transport project : research at the interface of genomics and transporter pharmacology *Clinical Pharmacology.& Therapeutics* 87: 109 – 116

Kweon YS, Lee HK, Lee CT, Lee KU, Pae CU (2005) Association of the serotonin transporter gene polymorphism with Korean male alcoholics *Journal of Psychiatry Research Jul, : 39 (4) : 371 – 376*

Laechelt S, Turrini SL, Ruehmkorf A, Siegmind W, Cascorbi I and Haenisehi S. (2011) Impact of ABCC2 haplotypes on transcriptional and post transcriptional gene regulation and function.*The Pharmacogenetics Journal* 11,23-34

Linder MW, Homme MB, Reynolds KK, Gage BF, Eby C, Silverstrov Natalia and Valdes R Jr (2009) Interactive Modeling for ongoing utility of Pharmacogenetic

Diagnostic Testing. Application for Wanfarin Therapy *Clinical chemistry 55 (10) 1861 – 1868*

Mackenzie P1, Owens IS, Burchell B, Brock KW, Bairoeh A, Belanger A (1997). The UDP glyceronyl transferase gene super family: recommended nomenclature update based on evolutionary divergence *Pharmacogenetics 7:255 – 259.*

Matherly L H, Hou Z, Deng Y (2007) Human reduced folate carrier: translation of basic biology to cancer. *Cancer Metastasis Review 26 (1): 111 - 12*

Mc Leod HL, Collie – Dugiud ES, Vreken P. et al (1998) Nomenclature for human DPYD alleles. *Pharmacogenetic 8:455 – 9*

McAlpine DE, Biernacka JM, Mrazdek D.A., O'Kane DJ, Stevens S.R, Longman LJ, coverson VI Bhagia J and Moyer TP (2011) Effect of cytochrome P450 Enzyme Polymorphism on Pharmacokinetics of venlafaxine *Therapeutic Drug Monitoring 33 (1) 14 – 20*

Mcleod HL (2005) Pharmacogenetic analysis of clinically relevant genetic polymorphism *Clinical Infectious Diseases, 41 suppl, 7:5449 – 52*

Meyer UA (2004) Pharmacogenetics: Five decades of therapeutic ;lessons from genetic diversity *Nature Review of Genetics 5: 669 – 676*

Meyer VA (2000) Pharmacogenetics and adverse drug reacgtions. *Lancet, 356: 1667-71*

Meier Y, Eloranta JJ, Darimont J, Ismair MG, Hiller C, Fried M, Kullak – Vblick GA, Varricka Sr (2007) Regional distribution of solute carrier MRNA expression along the human intestinal tract. *Drug metabolism and Disposition 35: 590 – 594.*

Morisaki K, Robey RW, Ozregy Laceka C, Honjo Y, Polgar O, Steadinain K, Sarkadi B, Bates SE (2005) Single Nucleotide Polymorphism modify the transporter activity of ABCG 2 *Cancer Chemotherapy and Pharmacology April 19 : 1 – 2*

Murphy PJ (2001) Xenobiotic mechanism a look from the past to future. *Drug Metabolism and Disposition 29 (6): 779 – 80*

Niesler B, Kapeller J, Hammer C and Rappold G (2008) Serotonin type 3 receptor genes: HTR 3A, B, C, D E, *Pharmacogenomics May (9) 5: 501 – 504*

Nilsson KW, Sjberg RL, Damberg M, Alm PO, Ohrvi KJ, Leppert J, lundstrom L, Oreland L (2005) Role of the serotonim transporter gene and family function in adolescent alcohol consumption. *Alcohol Clinical and Experimental Research. Apr 29 (4): 564 – 70*

Nishizato Y, Leiri I, Suzuki H, Kinura M, Kawabata K, Hirota K et al (2003) Polymorphism of OATP – C (SLC 21A6) and OAT3 (SLC22AB) genes. Consequences for Pravastin pharmacokinetics .*Clinical Pharmacology and Therapeutics June 73 (6): 554 –*

Ohno M, Yamaguchi I, (2000) slow N-acetyl transferase 2 genotype affects the incidence of isoniazid and rimfapicin induced hepatoroxity. *International Journal of Tuberculosis and lime Diseases 4: 256 – 61*

Omiecinski CJ, Vanden Heuvel JP, Perdew GH and Peters JM (2011) Xerobiotic Metabolism, disposition and regulation by receptors: from biochemical phenomenon to predictors of major toxicities. *Toxicological Science 120 (51) 549 – 575.*

Phillips KA, Veenstra DI, Oren E, Lee JK, Sadee W (2001) Potential role of Pharmacogenetics in reducing adverse drug reactions: a systemic review. *Journal of American Medical Association 286 (18) 2270 –*

Phipps Green A, Hollis Moffa HJE, Dalbeth N, merriman ME, Topless R, Gow PJ, Harrison AA, Highton J, Jones PBB, Stamp LK, Merrkiman TR (2010) A strong role for the ABCG2 gene in susceptibility to gout in New Zealand, Pacific island and Caucasian, but not Maori, case and control sample sets. *Human Molecular Genetics 19 (24): 4813 – 4819*

Radominska – Pandya, Zemik PJ, Little JM (1999) Structural and Functional Studies of UDP. glucuronyl transferases, *Drug Metabolism Review 31:817 – 899*

Roepke TK and Abbot GW (2006) Pharmacogenetics and cardiac ion channels. *Vascular Pharmacology Feb. 44 (2) 90 – 160*

Sakata T, Anzal N, Shis HJ, Noshire R, Hirata T, Yokoyama H, Kanai Y, Endou H (2004) Novel single nucleolide polymorphisms of organic Cation transporter 1 (SLC 22A 1) affecting transport functions. *Biochemistry and Biophysics Research Communication 313: 789 – 793*

Scordo MG, Pengo V, Spina E, Da2). Influence of CYP2C9 and CyP2C19 genetic polymorphism on warfarin maintenance dose and metabolic clearance. *Clinical Pharmacology and Therapeutics 72: 702 – 10*

Shar GM, Hammer EJ, Zhu H et al (2002) Maternal periconceptional vitamin use genetic variation of infant reduced folate carrier (ASOG) and risks of spina bifida: *America Journal of Medical Genetics 108 (1): 1 – 6*

Shenfield GM, (2004) Genetic polymorphosis, drug metabolism and drug concentrations, *Clinical Biochemistry Review; Nov 203 -6*

Shin J, Kayser SR, Langace T, (2009) Pharmacogenetics: from discovery to patient care pharmacogenetic test information on drug labels *American Journal of Health Systems Pharmacy 66 (7) : 66 – 637*

Shord SS (2010) Pharmacogenomic: A testing issue. *FDA Perspective on pharmacogenetic testing. PSWC 2010 New or Leans.*

Shu Y, Sheardown SA, Brown C, Owen RP, Zhang S, Castro RA, Lanculescu AG, Yive L, Lo JC, Bachard EG, Brett CM, Giacomini KM (2007) Effect of genetic variation in the organic cation transporter 1 (OCT 1) on metformin action. *Journal of Clinical Investigation 117: 1422 -1431*

Sies H (1997) Oxidative stress,oxidants and antioxidants. *Experimental Physiology 82 (2): 291 – 5*

Soldner A, Christians V, Susanto M, Wacher VJ, Silver man JA, benet LZ (1999) Grape fruit juice activates P-glucoprotein mediated drug transport *Pharmacology Research April 16 (4) 478 – 85.*

Steiner W (2010) Pharmacogenetics and psychoactive drug therapy: ready for the patient *Therapeutic Drug Monitoring 32 (4) 381 – 386*

Suarez – Kurtz G (2005) Pharmacogenomics in admixed population. Trends in *Pha.rmacological Science 26: 196 – 201*

Suzuki T, Mihara K, Nakemura A, Naga G, Kogenwa S, Nemoto K, Ohia I, Arakaki H, Uno T & Kondo T (2011) Effect of the CYP 206 10 Allele on the steady state plasma concentrations of Arupiprazole and its active metabolite dehydroaripiprazole, in Japanese Patients with Schizophrenia. *Therapeutic Drug Monitoring 33 (1) 21 – 24*

Taradia SM, Mydlarski PR, Reis MD et al (2000) screening for azathioprine toxicity: a pharmaco economic analysis based on a target case .*Journal of American Academy of Dermatology* 42:628 – 32

Thomalley PJ (1990) The glyoxalase s.ystem: new developments towards functional characterizations of a metabolic pathway fundamental to biological life. *Biochemistry Journal* 269 (1) : 1 – 11

Thomas DL, Thio CL, Martin MP, QiY, Ge D, O' Hiigin C, Kidd J, Kidd K, Khakoo S.I., Alexander G, Goedert JJ, Kurk GD, Donfield SM, Rosen HR, Tobler LH, Busch MP, McHwchison JG, Goldstein DB, Carrington M (2009) Genetic Variation in Il 28 B and spontaneous clearance of Hepatitis C. virus. *Nature 461 (7265): 798 – 801*

Tukey RH and Strassburg CP. (2000) Human UDP – Glucuronyltransferases: metabolism, expression and disease *Annual Review of Pharmacology and Toxicology 40: 581 – 616*

Tzevetkov MV, Vormfelde SV, Balen D, Meineke I, Schmidt T, Sehrt D, Sabolic I, Koepsell H, Brockmoller (2009) The effects of genetic polymorphism in the organic cation transporters OCT1; OCT2 and OCT 3 on the renal clearance of metformin. *Clinical Pharmacology and Therapeutics 66: 299 – 306*

Usami S, Abe, S, Shinkawa H, Inouse Y, Yamaguchu T (1999) Rapid mass screening method and counselling for the 1555A-G mitochondrial mutation *Journal of Human Genetics 44: 304 – 7*

Wechsler M E and Israel E. (2005) How pharmacogenomics will play a role in the management of asthma. *American Journal of Respiratory and Critical Medicine 172(1): 12-18.*

Weishilboum RC, Francis S, Weinshilboum (2003) Inheritance in drug response. *New England Journal of medicine 348 (6): 529 – 37*

Weix, Mc Leod Hc, Mc Murrough J, Caonzalez FJ, Fernandez – Salguero P. (1996) Molecular basis of the human dihydropyrimidine dehydrogenase deficiency and 5 fluorouracil toxicity. *Journal of Clinical Investigations* 98:610 – 5

Wherstine JR, Gifford AJ, Witt t et al (2002) single nucleotide polymorphism in the human reduced folate carrier : characterization of a high frequency G/A variant at position 80 and transport properties of the His (27) and Arg (27) carriers. *Clinical Cancer Research 7 (11) : 3416 – 22*

Whetstine JR, Flatley RM, Mattherly LH (2002) The human reduced folate carrier gene is ubiquitously and differentially expressed in normal human tissues, identification of seven non-coding exons and characterization of a novel promoter *Biochemistry Journal 367 (3) : 629 – 40*

Wojtal KA, Eloranta JJ, Hruz P, Gutmann H, Drewe J, Staumann A, Beglinger C, Fried M, Kullak-Ublick GA, Varricka SR (2009) Challenges in mRNA express ion levels in solute carrier transporters in inflammatory bowel disease patients. *Drug Metabolism and Disposition 37 : 1871 – 1877*

Wong M, Balleine RL, Collins M, Liddle C, Clarke CL, Caumey H (2004) CYP 3A5 genotype abd midazotam clearance in Australian patients receiving chemotherapy. *Clinical Pharmacology & Therapeutics 75 : 529 – 38*

Wool house WM, Qureshi MM, Bastaki SMA, Patel M, Abchilrazzaq, Y, Bayoumi RAL (1997). Polymorphic N – acetyltranseferase (NAT2) genotyping of Emiratis *Pharmacogenetics 7:73 – 82*

Yamaka Y, Hamada A, Nakashima R, Yuki M, Hirayama C, Kawaguchi T and Saito H (2011) Association of genetic polynmorphism in the influx transporter SLCOIB3 and the efflux transporter ABCB1 with Imatinib pharmacokinetics in patients with chronic myeloid leukaemia .*Therapeutic Drug Monitoring 33(2):244-250* .

Zhou Q, Kibat C, Cheung YB, Tan EH, Ang P, Balran C (2004) Pharmacogenetics of epidermal growth factor receptor (EGFR) gene in Chinese, Malay and Indian populations.*Journal of Clinical Oncology: ASCO Annual Meeting Proceedings (Post meeting Edition) 22 (145) : 3014*

10

Pharmacogenetics –
A Treatment Strategy for Alcoholism

Anjana Munshi* and Vandana Sharma
Institute Of Genetics and Hospital for Genetic Diseases,
Osmania University, Begumpet, Hyderabad,
India

1. Introduction

Alcoholism is a complex relapsing disorder of heterogeneous etiology, affecting people internationally. Alcohol dependence is a cumulative response of inability to stop drinking, craving and developing the symptoms of physical dependence and tolerance. In past two decades, mounting evidence has suggested that alcoholism or alcohol addiction is a host of major psychological, social, financial and health problems (Poznyak et al., 2005). According to World Health Organization, alcoholism is responsible for 4% of global disease burden and is the third major preventable risk factor for premature death and disability in developed nations (World Health Organization, 2002). Although, the exclusive biological mechanisms underlying the development of alcoholism are still uncertain, the major risk factors contributing towards the development of alcoholism are age (adolescents are at higher risk of developing alcoholism), gender (men are more prone to develop alcoholism as compared to women due to depression), personality (experience seeking), and psychiatric or behavioral disorders. The prevalence, age of onset, clinical symptoms and outcome of alcoholism differs from individual to individual and varies according to ethnicity (Kenneth et al., 2011). In addition to this, lower social status and low education have also been found to be associated with alcoholism in cross sectional and longitudinal studies (Fukuda et al., 2005; Poznyak et al., 2005; Subramanian et al., 2005; Wray et al., 2005).

According to World Health Organization report on global alcohol status, it has been found that approximately 2 billion people consume alcoholic beverages and there are about 76.3 million people with diagnosable alcohol disorder (World Health Organization, 2004). In India the prevalence of alcoholism has been found to be 21.4% as recoded by epidemiological surveys (Benegal, 2005).The deleterious effects of alcohol on central nervous system can be observed in the form of changes in mood and personality, anxiety and depression. Although, it affects all the organs in the body, brain neurotransmitters are the main target sites of alcohol (Wertheimer et al., 2003). The specific physiological effects of alcohol depend on dose, concentration in blood, absorption, distribution, metabolism, excretory conditions, prior drinking experience, concurrent use of other drugs, and

---

* Corresponding Author

comorbid conditions. The body adapts metabolically and neurally to repeated exposure of alcohol so as to develop tolerance (Zaleski et al., 2004).

Recent advances in the field of neurobiology have improved our understanding about associated risk factors and neurochemical mechanisms responsible for the development of alcoholism. Evidences suggest that there is large inter-individual variation in terms of development of alcohol dependence and treatment of alcoholism. People consume alcohol and respond to its effects in a number of ways e.g. some develop no side effects even in moderate to higher levels and some may develop problems even when consumed in smaller doses. This variation is the result of individual's genetic makeup directly influencing the metabolism of alcohol (Strat et al., 2008).

Genetic factors have been found to play a critical role in the etiology of alcoholism (Heath et al., 2001; Sloan et al., 2008; Kenneth et al., 2011). Researchers have suggested that 50-60% of alcohol dependence is determined by genetics (Goldman and Bergen 1998; McGue et al., 1999). Based on results of adoption, twin, and family studies it is now clear that the vulnerability to alcoholism is determined by genetic factors as well as by environmental factors (Moussas et al., 2009). However, it is difficult to determine the individual determinant of alcoholism (Flensborg-Madsen et al., 2007). The candidate gene approach has revealed a number of biomarkers, which are responsible for alcoholism. Certain variants of alcohol dehydrogenase and aldehyde dehydrogenase genes (genes encoding for alcohol metabolizing enzymes) have been found to alter the metabolism of alcohol in a dramatic way (Nurnberger et al., 2004). In addition to this, polymorphisms in neurotransmitter genes (target receptor genes) such as gamma amino butyric acid and opioid receptor genes have also been reported to be associated with marked risk of alcohol dependence (Strat et al., 2008). Current treatment approaches to alcoholism are moderately effective with perhaps as many as half of the patients receiving treatment due to abstinent or significantly reducing episodes of binge drinking (Group, 1997). Pharmacotherapy and behavioral therapy including psychosocial support are two main types of treatment in alcoholism. The pharmacological agents approved by FDA prescribed in the treatment of alcoholism are disulfiran (antabuse), naltrexone (revia), acamprosate (campral) and Vivitrol (Krishnan-Sarin & O'Malley et al., 2008).

The major drawback of ineffectiveness of pharmacotherapy of alcoholism is inter-individual variation in response to medication (Radel and Goldman, 2001). There are individuals, showing lesser/no therapeutic efficacy of a drug prescribed, known as non-responders. Another group of individuals showing high therapeutic efficacy towards the same drug are known as responders (McLeod et al., 2000).

Recent advances in the area of molecular biology have increased our knowledge of understanding the influence of genetic variants on pharmacokinetic and pharmacodynamic profile of alcohol and neurobiology of alcoholism (Ray et al., 2010a). The unavoidable alcohol withdrawl symptoms, depression, unpredicted death, medical complications, socioeconomic repercussions of alcoholism suggest that the treatment strategies should be improved with new and targeted approach of pharmacogenetics.

Pharmacogenetics is a measure of predicting individual's genetic profile responsible for variable drug responses. The genetic analysis along with consideration of other factors of alcoholic patients can lead to the identification of clinical subtypes of patients with specific treatments. This will improve the treatment of alcoholism. Alcohol pharmacogenetics has great potential in improving treatment strategies for alcoholism (Radel and Goldman, 2001; Quickfall and el-Guebaly, 2006). The treatment strategy of combining clinician's views based on genotypic information would individualize and optimize the treatment for alcoholism with best possible outcome of individual's good health free of alcohol dependence. Pharmacogenetics is expected to add new dimensions and would tailor the therapeutic treatment of alcoholism.

The chapter provides an overview of the molecular, pharmacological and neurological aspects of alcoholism with main emphasis on pharmacogenetics of alcoholism treatment.

2. Metabolism of alcohol

Alcohol is generally taken orally, absorbed unchanged through the whole length of digestive tract. Almost 20% absorption takes place rapidly through stomach and 80% through small gut (Caballeria, 2003). The rate of absorption depends on volume, concentration, nature of alcoholic drink, presence and absence of food in stomach, permeability of gastric and intestinal tissues and genetic variation. After absorption into the blood-stream, alcohol is distributed quickly throughout the total body fluid (Pawan, 1972). The distribution of alcohol is accelerated by vascularization and blood flow e.g. organs rich in blood supply such as brain and lungs achieve the higher initial concentrations of alcohol.

Liver is the main site of alcohol metabolism. In hepatocytes three systems are involved in alcohol metabolism located in three different cellular compartments. These are alcohol dehydrogenase (ADH) located in cytosol, microsomal ethanol oxidizing system (MEOS) situated in endoplasmic reticulum and catalase in peroxisomes (Caballeria, 2003). These are involved in conversion of alcohol to acetaldehyde (Figure 1).

The metabolic pathway involves conversion of alcohol (ethanol) to acetaldehyde via oxidation catalyzed by ADH in cytoplasm of hepatocytes, a rate limiting step. The second reaction is catalyzed by aldehyde dehydrogenases (ALDH), acetaldehyde is converted to acetic acid and finally to carbon dioxide and water through citric acid cycle into circulation. Acetaldehyde plays central role in the toxicity produced by alcohol consumption as in liver it reaches to saturation point and escapes into blood circulation. Further it impairs mitochondrial functions and reactions leading to damage of hepatocytes. The rate of metabolism of alcohol differs from person to person because it is influenced by genetic variants of metabolizing enzymes mentioned above (Quertemont, 2004).

2.1 Alcohol dehydrogenase system

Alcohol dehydrogenase (ADH) occurs in multiple forms and is encoded by 7 different genes. These are ADH1A, ADH1B, ADH1C, ADH4, ADH5, ADH6 and ADH7. These genes are aligned along a small region of chromosome 4. ADH enzymes encoded by ADH gene function as dimers i.e. the active forms are composed of two subunits. On the basis of their similar amino acid sequences and kinetic properties, these seven ADH types have been divided into five classes. The class I genes ADH1A, ADH1B and ADH1C are closely related. These encode for α, β and γ subunits respectively, which form homodimers or heterodimers and account for most of the alcohol oxidizing capacity in liver (Hurley et al., 2002; Lee et al.,

2006). Further, ADH1A, ADH1B and ADH1C are mainly present in liver and linings of stomach. ADH4 encodes π-ADH which has been reported to contribute significantly to ethanol oxidation at higher concentration. The ADH5 gene encodes for χ-ADH, a ubiquitously expressed formaldehyde dehydrogenase, which has low affinity for ethanol. ADH6 mRNA is found in fetal and adult liver. Since the enzyme has not been isolated from tissues so far, therefore little is known about it. ADH7 encodes for σ-ADH, which oxidizes both ethanol and retinol (Edenberg, 2007).

2.2 Aldehyde dehydrogenase

These enzymes rapidly convert acetaldehyde to acetate using cofactor NAD^+ via oxidation. ALDH is divided into nine major categories. Some of these are significantly involved in acetaldehyde metabolism, and others metabolize a variety of substrates. Two main ALDH enzymes reported to be involved in metabolization of acetaldehyde during the oxidation of ethanol are ALDH1 and ALDH2. ALDH1 encoded by ALDH1A1 gene is found in fluid filling cells (the cytosol) while ALDH2 is found in mitochondria and is encoded by the ALDH2 gene. The two genes are 52 kb and 43 kb in length and are present on chromosome 9 and chromosome 12 respectively. Both genes have a similar structure with 13 exons and the protein encoded by both the genes is 70% similar in sequence and structure (Hurley et al., 2002). ALDH1A1, ALDH1B1 and ALDH2 are mainly involved in acetaldehyde oxidation.

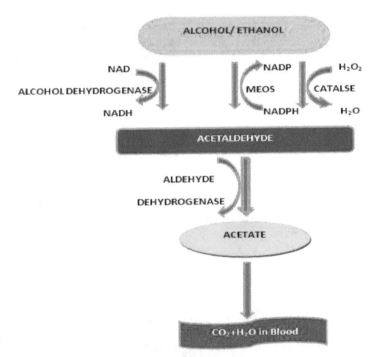

Fig. 1. Metabolism of alcohol in liver hepatocytes using 3 systems, (i) Alcohol dehydrogenase, (ii) Microsomal ethanol oxidizing enzyme (iii) Catalase and finally Aldehyde dehydrogenase converts acetaldehyde into acetate

2.3 Microsomal ethanol oxidizing enzymes

Apart from ADH which accounts for greater part of ethanol oxidation, a quantitatively small portion of alcohol is catalyzed by microsomal ethanol oxidizing system involving CYP2E1 (Edenberg, 2007). Studies have shown that CYP2E1 is induced by high ethanol concentration and by chronic intake of alcohol or ethanol (up to 10 fold) (Quertemont, 2004). It has been found that after chronic ethanol consumption CYP2E1 increases the rate of ethanol clearance and this may result in development of ethanol tolerance (Lieber et al., 1968; 1988; Takahashi et al., 1993; Tsutsumi et al., 1989). CYP2E1 induction may further lead to higher concentrations of acetaldehyde leading to injuries in hepatocytes.

2.4 Catalase

Catalase oxidizes alcohol to acetaldehyde within the peroxisomes (Oshino et al., 1973). This reaction is hydrogen peroxide (H_2O_2) dependent. Under normal conditions catalase plays a minor role in ethanol oxidation. However, the functional activity of catalase is accelerated in the presence of reactive oxygen species and H_2O_2 (Quertemont, 2004). Zimatkin et al. (1997) have suggested that catalase may be one of alternative metabolic pathways for ethanol oxidation in brain where CYP2E1 and ADH appear to be of minor importance. However, the precise role of catalase in brain ethanol oxidation is still not clear.

2.5 Nonoxidative ethanol metabolism

Apart from oxidative metabolism of alcohol, nonoxidative metabolism also takes place in organs lacking oxidative metabolism such as heart (Beckemeier et al., 1998). A minor extent of alcohol is metabolized by nonoxidative pathway using enzyme fatty acid ethyl synthases resulting in the formation of fatty acid ethyl esters (Caballeria 2003). Further, these esters have been found to be involved in alcohol-induced organ injuries (Beckemeier et al., 1998).

3. Genetic variants affecting alcohol metabolism

Genes encoding for alcohol metabolizing enzymes are supposed to have major influence on development of alcoholism. There are multiple ADH and ALDH enzymes encoded by different genes. Some of these genes have been reported to occur in several variants or alleles. The enzymes encoded by different alleles can differ in the rate at which they metabolize ethanol (Edenburg, 2007).

3.1 Genetic variants of alcohol dehydrogenase

Researchers have studied the genetic variants of ADH1B and ADH1C genes that result in the production of enzymes with different kinetic properties and have been implicated in the susceptibility to develop alcoholism. These genetic variants or SNPs and their effects have been widely studied in different populations and three different alleles have been reported which alter the amino acid sequence of the encoded beta subunit. ADH1B*1 allele, (reference allele) encodes for β1 subunit that has arginine at positions 48 and 370. ADH1B*1 is the predominant allele in most populations. ADH1B*2 encodes for β2 subunit with histidine at position 48 and is commonly found in Asians. ADH1B*3 encodes for β3 subunit that has cysteine at position 370 and is prevalent in people of African descent. In β2 and β3 subunits, amino acid substitutions occur at an amino acid which contacts with coenzyme nicotineamide dinucleotide (required for ethanol oxidation) (Hurley et al., 2002). The substitution results in enzymes, which have 70- to 80- fold higher turnover rate than the β1 subunit. This is because the coenzyme is released more rapidly at the end of reaction.

For ADH1C gene, there are 3 alleles ADH1C*1 encoding γ1 subunit with arginine at position 272 and isoleucine at position at position 350. ADH1C*2 encodes the γ2 subunit which has glutamine (Gln) at position 272 and a valine (Val) at position 350. These two SNPs occur together (i.e., are in very high linkage disequilibrium). It has been found that the ADH with two γ1 subunits (i.e., the γ1γ1 homodimeric enzyme) has a turnover rate that is about 70 percent higher than that of the γ2γ2 enzyme (Edenberg, 2007). ADH1C*Thr352 encodes for a subunit with threonine at position 352 and has been found in Native Americans (Osier et al., 2002). However, the studies on this protein are still lacking. Researchers have identified the differences in the rate of metabolism of ethanol in liver on the basis of difference in amino acid sequence resulting in difference in kinetic properties of encoded enzyme. If a person carries two copies of reference allele i.e. ADH1B*1 and ADH1C*1 alleles (homozygous for ADH1B*1and ADH1C*1) the enzyme (together α, β, γ subunits) together accounts for liver's 70% ethanol oxidizing capacity, additionally π ADH accounts for 30% (Hurley et al., 2002). ADH1B*1 allele has been reported to reduce the occurrence of alcohol abuse and alcoholism in Asians, in Whites and in Jewish populations where this allele has a relatively high prevalence (Carr et al., 2002; Neumark et al., 1998). ADH1B*2 has been found to occur in a higher frequency in nonalcoholics and in moderate drinkers relative to heavy drinkers. As far as ADH1B*2 is concerned, this allele has been found to be associated with lower rates of heavy drinking and alcohol dependence in Native Americans (Quertemont, 2007).

A meta-analysis conducted by Whitfield has concluded that ADH1B*1 allele is associated with a threefold increase in risk of alcoholism in comparison with ADH1B*2 allele.ADH1B*2 allele encodes for an enzyme with a faster ethanol oxidation rate (Whitfield, 1997). It has been assumed that this allele protects against alcoholism and alcohol abuse because of the unpleasant effects associated with acetaldehyde accumulation (Yin, 1994). The frequency of ADH1C*1 allele has been reported to about 50% in European population and up to 90% in some Asian and African populations (Goedde et al., 1992; Osier et al., 2002). This allele has also been shown to provide a protection against alcohol abuse and alcoholism since a higher frequency of this allele has been found in nonalcoholics especially from Asian population.

Gene-gene interactions have also been found to play an intricate role in development of alcoholism. Oseir et al. (2004) found that there is potential epistatic interaction between ADH1B and ADH7 which leads to protective effect against alcoholism among Han Chinese population (Oseir et al., 2004).

3.2 Genetic variants of aldehyde dehydrogenase (ALDH)

The best known variation of alcohol metabolizing enzymes has been associated with ALDH2 gene. A variant of this gene known as ALDH2*2 allele leads to the substitution of lysine to glutamine at 504 position (Chou et al., 1999). This substitution results in the production of a nearly inactive ALDH2 enzyme which no longer oxidizes acetaldehyde to acetate. Studies have demonstrated that this variant is dominant because people who are heterozygous (ALDH2*1 and ALDH2*2) have almost no detectable activity of ALDH2 enzyme in the liver. People with an ALDH2*2 allele show an alcohol flush reaction even when they consume alcohol in relatively small amounts (Harada et al., 1981). The presence of even a single ALDH2*2 allele has been shown to be strongly protective against alcohol dependence. The protective effect of ALDH2*2 is the most widely reproduced association of a specific gene with alcoholism (Chen et al., 1999; Hurley et al., 2002; Luczak et al., 2006; Thomasson et al., 1991).

3.3 Genetic variants of microsomal ethanol oxidizing system

Another enzyme, microsomal ethanol oxidizing enzyme involved in alcohol metabolism is encoded by CYP2E1 gene. CYP2E1 is induced (increase in activity up to 10 fold) by chronic alcohol drinking and may contribute to development of metabolic tolerance in alcoholics. Studies have revealed that polymorphism in CYP2E1 (CYP2E1*1D) has been found to be significantly associated with alcohol dependence in Canadian native Indians (Howard et al., 2003; Itoga et al., 1999). Another rare mutant named as c2 allele (CYP2E1*5B) in CYP2E1 gene has been found to be associated with higher transcriptional activity leading to elevated level of the enzyme as compared to wild type c1 allele i.e. CYP2E1*5A (Hayashi et al., 1991).

3.4 Genetic variants of catalase

Studies have revealed that subjects with positive family history of alcoholism have a higher mean activity of catalase as compared to control subjects (Koechling and Amit et al., 1992). A significant positive correlation was observed in brain and blood catalase activity in rats (Amit and Aragon., 1988). Koechling and Amit (1992) have reported a significant coorelation between blood catalase activity with alcohol consumption. However, there are no studies on the association of genetic polymorphism of catalase with alcoholism.

4. Neuropharmacological aspects of chronic alcoholism

The neuropharmacological actions of alcohol such as cognitive impairment and other behavioral changes are mediated via their interaction with brain neurotransmitters. Neurotransmitters are the chemicals involved in communication of neurons in brain and may be inhibitory or excitatory depending upon their mechanism of action. Although alcohol does not have any specific target neurotransmitter, it acts on multiple neurotransmitter systems (Deitrich and Erwin, 1996; Tabakoff and Hoffman, 1992).

Chronic alcohol consumption may cause cognitive impairment, tolerance and physical dependence due to changes in neurotransmitter system in brain. The neuropharmacological changes caused by chronic alcoholism involve monoamine oxidase, neurotransmitter amino acids and calcium ion channels and some other pathways leading to neuroadaptations and development of tolerance (Zaleski et al., 2004). The complex mechanism of action involving neurochemical changes explains why even moderate doses of alcohol may lead the subject to develop psychiatric complications and alcohol dependence. The addictive and alcohol seeking behavior can be explained by understanding the neurotransmitter involved in the processes (Vengeliene et al., 2006).

Few of the neurotransmitters involved in alcohol dependence are as follows:

4.1 Alcohol and monoamines

Ethanol affects the release of the main neurotransmitters present in central nervous system, such as dopamine, gamma amino butyric acid (GABA), serotonin, noradrenaline and opioid peptides (Kianmaa &Tabakoff, 1983; Tabakoff, 1977, 1983). Alcohol activates the firing of dopaminergic neurons in the ventral tegmental area and nucleus accumbens structures which together are a part of mesolimbic pathway and play an important role for the rewarding effect of ethanol (Diana et al., 1992). Studies have demonstrated that the stimulation of dopaminergic neurons may indirectly activate serotonergic pathways. The low levels of serotonin have been reported to be a risk factor for development of alcoholism (Lovinger, 1991).

4.2 Alcohol and neurotransmitter amino acids

Several studies have demonstrated the actions of ethanol on neurotransmitter amino acids which consist of glutamate-main excitatory neurotransmitter in the central nervous system. It has N-methyl-D-aspartate (NMDA) and amino-3-hydroxy-5-methyl-4-isoxazoleproprionate (AMPA), and kainate receptors. The NMDA receptors are controlled by several regulatory sites. To open the channel of NMDA receptor, presence of glycine is required. Glycine is an amino acid which has its own site, acting as a coagonist. Alcohol has been reported to act on glycine binding site therefore, inhibiting the function of NMDA receptor (Woodword, 1994). The receptor has been found to play an important role in learning and memory and in development of alcohol tolerance (Longo et al., 2002). Glutamate, a neurotransmitter has been found to play a significant role in the pathogenesis of alcohol dependence by mediating excitatory pathways (Sander et al., 2000). Chronic alcohol use has been found to be associated with upregulation of NMDA receptors. Alcohol shows lower affinity for AMPA and kainate glutamate receptors (Ferreira & Morato, 1997). In case of acute ethanol withdrawal, NMDA receptor releases increased amount of glutamate which is associated with tremors, anxiety, ataxia, and convulsions.

Alcohol produces sedative-hypnotic effects mediated via GABA, an inhibitory neurotransmitter. There are three types of GABA receptors, GABA A, GABA B, and GABA C in brain. GABA A receptors are responsible for the intoxicating effects of alcohol such as motor incoordination, anxiolysis and sedation. The neurobehavioral effects of ethanol mediated via neurotransmitter GABA are directly dose-dependent. The effects of alcohol at GABA A receptors vary across brain regions. This might be due to the differential expression of GABA A receptor subunits (Loh et al., 1999).

Another neurotransmitter, Neuropeptide Y (NPY) is an amino acid peptide which has been associated with reward, appetite and anxiety. The association of NPY has also been reported with alcohol dependence in animal models. NPY-deficient mice have been reported to show higher alcohol consumption as compared with wild type mice (Thiele et al., 1998).

4.3 Alcohol and calcium ion channels

Voltage sensitive calcium channels (VSCCs) play a major role in gating synaptic calcium influx and thereby modulating a range of calcium dependent intracellular processes, membrane potential, and neurotransmitter release (Kennedy & Liu, 2003). The types of

VSCC are of L-type (dihydropyridine-sensitive), N-type (neuronal), P-type (Purkinje), R-type (Resistant), and T type (transient) channels. It has been found that alcohol (ethanol) blocks L-type channels. The L-type VSCC antagonists show some ethanol, like effects in rats. Evidence suggested that chronic administration of alcohol in mice up-regulates the number and function of N-type calcium channels. Ethanol actions at VSCCs may modulate its behavioral effects in humans (Zaleski et al., 2004). It has been reported that there is an increase in the inflow of Calcium ions through these channels, contributing to the development of withdrawal symptoms such as seizures and craving.

4.4 Alcohol and other mechanisms of actions

Studies assessing cognitive functions have associated the chronic ingestion of ethanol with the reduction in concentration of acetylcholine in humans as well as mice, caused by the degeneration of brain tissues which seems to be related to the development of tolerance of alcohol. Chronic consumption of alcohol may affect opioid receptor system thus exerting neurobehavioral effects such as reinforcement. The three major classes of opioid system are μ, δ and κ. Alcohol may stimulate the release of certain opioid peptides such as endorphins and enkephalins, which in turn, could interact with the centers (mesolimbic dopamine pathway) of the brain, associated with reward and positive reinforcement and may lead to further alcohol consumption (Vengeliene et al., 2008). Human and animal studies have suggested that μ opioid receptor is mainly involved in initial sensitivity and response to alcohol. The increased activity of brain opioid peptide systems, in response to ethanol exposure, may be important for initiating and maintaining high alcohol consumption and for mediating the positive reinforcing effects of alcohol (Gianoulakis et al., 1996).

5. Genetic variants of neurotransmitters

Alcohol exerts its effects such as reward and reinforcement by acting on a number of neurotransmitter in the brain. Studies have revealed that polymorphisms in genes encoding for neurotransmitter may increase the risk of developing alcoholism (Radel & Goldman, 2001; Foley et al., 2006). The knowledge of gene variants affecting neurotransmitters is very important as it serves the basis for developing novel and targeted therapeutic agents in treatment of alcoholism. A few of the genetic variants of neurotransmitters associated with alcohol dependence are as:

5.1 Glutamate

Candidate gene studies have shown that individuals bearing G603A polymorphism of glial glutamate transporter gene (EAAT2) are at increased risk of alcoholism (Sander et al., 2000). The individuals with genetic variants of NMDA (subunit NR2A) and glutamate receptor metabotropic gene (mGLUR5) have been studied in a hospital based study in Germany (Schumann et al., 2008). It was found that carriers of the NR2A risk genotypes for rs2072450 CC and rs9924016 Del/Del had higher risk of developing alcohol dependence as compared to the individuals with protective genotypes rs2072450 AC and rs9924016 Del/Ins (Schuman et al., 2008). In the case of mGLUR5 gene, individuals of the risk genotypes rs3824927 C/C and rs 3462 G/G have been found to be at higher risk of developing alcohol dependence when compared with individuals bearing the protective genotypes rs3824927 CA and rs3462 GA.

5.2 Gamma amino butyric acid

Association of genetic variants of GABARA1 and GABAR6 with alcoholism has been reported in Korean population (Park et al., 2006).The GG genotype of GABAA1 receptor has been found to be significantly associated with early onset and severity of alcoholism in Korean population (Park et al., 2006). It has been also been reported that Pro385Ser substitution in GABA A6 is associated with alcohol dependence and with antisocial alcoholism (Sander et al., 1999).

5.3 Norepinephrine

Studies have suggested that alcohol produces biphasic effects on norepinephrine turnover in the brain, with low doses increasing turnover and higher doses depressing turnover. The sensitivity of noradrenergic systems to ethanol effects varies among brain regions. A few studies have been attempted to see the effect of genetic variants of norepinephrine on alcoholism. Huang et al. (2008) reported that norepinephrine transporter polymorphisms T-182C and G1287A are not associated with alcohol dependence and its clinical subgroups in Han Chinese population.

5.4 Dopamine

Research studies have revealed that there is a positive association between polymorphism in Dopamine receptor gene (DRD) with alcoholism. Ponce et al. (2008) reported that the two SNPs (-141C Ins/Del) and TaqI A, present on DRD2 gene locus were associated with alcoholism in North Indian population. Studies from South Indian population have reported no association between TaqI A polymorphism and alcoholism.

The -141 Ins/Del polymorphism in DRD2 gene has been found to be associated with alcoholism in several studies across different populations, but with inconsistent results. This promoter polymorphism plays a significant role in D2 receptor expression via altering the transcriptional activity. Johann et al. (2005) studied the association of -141I Del variant (-141C) SNP in German alcoholics. It was found that -141 Del C variant of DRD2 gene might be a protective factor against development of alcoholism. On the other hand the -141 Ins allele has been found to be a genetic risk factor for alcoholism in Mexican-Americans. This can be correlated with decreased DRD2 receptor density in alcoholic patients which in turn stimulates craving-reward pathway- thereby promoting alcoholism.

Another polymorphism in DRD2 gene Taq I A in Ankyrin repeat and Kinase Domain containing (ANKK1)(rs 1800497) is one of the most frequently studied mutations. The DRD2 gene is actually not located on DRD2 but rather within the protein coding region exon 8 of the adjacent ANKK1gene (Neville et al., 2004). TaqI A SNP causes an amino acid substitution within the 11th ankyrin repeat of the putative protein and has been found to affect the substrate binding specificity (Ponce et al., 2008). In a meta-analysis, the single nucleotide variant TaqIA (rs 1800497) of the DRD2 gene has been found as a vulnerability gene for alcoholism in more than 40 studies, but with conflicting results.

5.5 Serotonin

The genetic variants of serotonin receptor gene for example rs1042173   may influence alcohol dependence (Jhonsan et al., 2011). The presence of genetic variation may lead to manipulation of serotonergic transmission therefore affecting the rate of development of tolerance and alcohol dependence (Yoshimoto et al., 1996).

5.6 Cholinergic and nicotinic receptor gene

Evidence from genetic studies suggested that alcohol dependence as well as cigarette smoking in families share the genetic vulnerability. Research studies have identified a missense mutation (rs16969968) in exon 5 of the nicotinic receptor (CHRNA5) gene and a variant in the 3'-UTR of the CHRNA3 gene in association with alcoholism and nicotine dependence (Wang et al., 2009). Cholinergic muscarinic 2 receptor (CHRM2) SNP (rs1824024) has been significantly associated with the pathogenesis of depression and alcohol dependence disorders (Jung et al., 2011; Luo et al., 2005).

5.7 Opioids

Bart et al. (2005) have identified positive association between A118G polymorphism and increased risk of alcohol dependence in individuals from Sweden. The single nucleotide polymorphism A118G in exon 1 of opioid receptor gene (OPRM1) results in increase in 3 fold binding capacity of beta endorphin. However, the results of a number of research studies are contradictory. Few studies have failed to find the association between the A118 G allele and alcoholism (Bergen et al., 1997; Franke et al., 2001; Gelernter et al., 1999; Kim et al., 2004; Kranzler et al., 1998; Schinka et al., 2002), while few others have found positive association between the A118 allele and alcoholism (Town et al., 1999). The explanations for these conflicting reports may be small sample size of the populations under study and the ethnic variation.

5.8 Other neurotransmitters (Neuropeptide Y)

In Humans, Leu7Pro polymorphism in NPY gene has been established to affect the release of mature NPY. Individuals with Pro7/Leu7 allele have 42% higher plasma concentration of NPY as compared with Leu7/Leu7 variant. Kauhanen et al. (2000) reported that Pro7allele is associated with more (34% higher) alcohol consumption in a cohort of Finnish middle aged men. Lappalainnen and others have reported that NPYPro7 allele significantly contributes towards the heritability of alcohol dependence in European American population (Lappalainnen et al., 2002).

6. Pharmacotherapy of alcoholism

The first step in the treatment of alcoholism is detoxification assisted by medical treatment (Wertheimer and Chaney 2003). Detoxification is required to manage the clinical and psychological symptoms of alcoholism. After detoxification there is need for counseling or psychotherapy and rehabilitation (Williams, 2001). The pharmacological agents or medicines in use for alcoholism treatment act on specific neurotransmitter systems. The treatment is aimed at normalizing the alcohol specific neuroadaptations (Krishnan-Sarin et al., 2008). The selection criteria for treatment of alcoholism is based on the length of illness and additional amount of alcohol related problems (Wertheimer &Chaney, 2003).

6.1 FDA approved drugs for treatment of alcoholism

Some of the drugs approved by FDA for treatment of alcoholism are as follows (Krishnan-Sarin et al., 2008).

6.1.1 Disulfiram

Disulfiram has been in use to treat alcoholism since 1940. Disulfiram produces an aversive effect by disrupting alcohol metabolism. The proposed mechanism of action of disulfiram on alcohol use has been found to be primarily related to the inhibition of liver aldehyde dehydrogenase (metabolizing enzyme of alcohol) and secondarily related to central nervous system actions, via modulation of catecholamine neurotransmission. It blocks ALDH activity by forming intermolecular disulfide bridges resulting in acetaldehyde accumulation. Excessive buildup of acetaldehyde results in many unpleasant effects including lowered blood pressure, palpitation, nausea, vomiting, headache and difficulty in breathing.

In clinical doses, disulfiram inhibits the enzyme dopamine–β–hydroxylase, which converts dopamine to norepinephrine, leading to increase in dopamine levels in brain (Goldstein & Nakajima, 1967; Goldstein et al., 1964). It has been found in clinical trials of disulfiram that there are lower rates of relapse to drinking in those who are compliant with the medication (Fuller et al., 1986). However, due to aversive nature of this drug, noncompliance is one of the biggest problems encountered with its use. The use of disulfiram is supervised in many clinical settings.

6.1.2 Naltrexone

Naltrexone is a drug used mainly for the treatment of alcohol dependence, and is available as oral medication and in injectable form. The drug is well tolerated with primary gastrointestinal side effects (O'Malley et al., 1992; Volpicelli et al., 1992). The efficacy of naltrexone in reducing alcohol drinking is mediated via interactions between the endogenous opioid system and dopamine systems, specifically through antagonism of the μ–opioid receptors. The studies on animal models suggested that alcohol increases release of β–endorphins in certain portions of the brain known to be involved in alcohol reward (Marinelli et al., 2003; Zalewska-Kaszubska et al., 2006). Nalotrexane blocks the release of these endorphins. Naltrexone has also been shown to reduce drinking in animal models (Froehlich et al. 2003; Swift, 2000).

A number of clinical trials indicate that alcoholics receiving naltrexone treatment in combination with behavioral intervention have lower levels of relapse and reduced levels of alcohol craving (O'Malley et al., 1992). Recent reports (Bouza et al., 2004; Srisurapanont & Jarusuraisin, 2002) suggest that naltrexone has modest efficacy in preventing relapse to drinking. Although, naltrexone is well tolerated, the potential risk of toxicity of liver at high doses is the major cause of concern in patients with liver disease.

6.1.3 Acamprosate

Acamprosate is available in an oral, delayed release formula, Camprel. The mechanism of action is through antagonizing of the N-methyl D-aspartate (NMDA) glutamate receptor site or via modulation of glutamate neurotransmission (DeWitte et al., 2005; Harris et al., 2002).

It has been found that acamprosate reduces neuronal hyperexcitability during alcohol withdrawal, due to reductions in glutamate levels, so as to normalize the balance between excitatory and inhibitory neurotransmitters produced in chronic alcohol consumption (Spanagel et al., 1996; Dahchour et al., 1998; Littleton & Zieglgansberger, 2003).

6.2 Other promising medicines

In addition to the drugs approved by FDA for treating alcoholism there are other medications which are in use because of some clinical evidence of efficacy.

6.2.1 Ondansetron

Ondansetron is a 5HT3 receptor antagonist used mainly as antinausea medicine after postoperative nausea and as anticraving medicine in alcoholism. Human laboratory studies have demonstrated that ondansetron decreases alcohol preference and desire to drink (Johnson et al., 1993). The efficacy of ondansetron in reducing drinking behavior has also been reported in Clinical trials, especially in drinkers with early onset alcoholism (Kranzler et al., 2003).

6.2.2 Baclofen

Baclofen, a GABA B receptor antagonist is used clinically for the treatment of muscle spasticity. The preclinical trials have shown the effectiveness of baclofen in reducing chronic alcoholism (Colombo et al., 2004). In a recent clinical trial, it was found that the drug is well tolerated in alcohol dependent patients with liver cirrhosis and has some efficacy in improving abstinence rates. However, more clinical research is needed to establish its efficacy and tolerability in alcoholic patients.

6.2.3 Topiramate

Topiramate is an antiseizure medication which has been shown to be effective in reducing alcohol use in recent clinical trials. Its action is mediated via antagonizing α amino-3-hydroxy 5-methylisoxazole 4-propionic acid (AMPA) and kainate glutamate receptors as well as inhibition of GABA A receptors, L type calcium channels, and voltage dependent sodium channels (SCN). Topiramate has been shown to reduce alcohol use in animal models (Farook et al., 2007). It also helps in reducing alcohol withdrawl induced convulsions. It has some side effects such as numbness, anorexia, cognitive difficulty, and taste distortion, as well as some rare incidents of visual side effects including myopia, glaucoma, and increased intraocular pressure. The clinical trials used a slow titration over several weeks to the desired dose to reduce the incidence of side effects.

6.2.4 Selective serotonin reuptake inhibitors (SSRI)

Selective serotonin reuptake inhibitors such as fluoxetine, citalopram, and sertraline are used in the treatment of alcoholism because existing evidence has shown that lowering brain serotonin levels decrease preference for alcohol and SSRI. SSRI's are basically used in the treatment of depression, therefore the effectiveness has been found in depressed alcoholics in some clinical trials.

7. Pharmacogenetics of alcoholism

The sequencing of the human genome has become the foundation for one of the most significant scientific contribution, the idea that although all human individuals are genetically similar, each retains a unique genetic identity. The publication of the human blueprint has triggered an explosion in pharmaceutical research to utilize this knowledge in the prescription of drugs for various ailments including alcoholism to be tailored according to the genetic makeup of susceptible individuals or in other words personalized medicine.

Just before half a century ago the Human Genome Project, scientists had realized that inheritance was an important factor which accounts for individual variation in drug response (Kalow, 1962; Venter et al., 2001). This led to the birth of the term Pharmacogenetics. Pharmacogenetics is the study of the role of inter-individual genetic variation in drug response. Although human beings are 99.9% similar in their genetic makeup, 0.1% variability in terms of single-nucleotide polymorphisms is significantly accountable for an individual's susceptibility to diseases and inter- and intra-individual variation of drug response (Brooks, 1999).

On the basis of our current understanding of neurobiology numerous candidate genes have been implicated in the etiology and response to treatments for different addictions including alcoholism. The focus is on functional genetic variants of proteins involved in the neural response to alcohol including alcohol sensitivity, reward and tolerance and variants of the enzyme involved in metabolism of alcohol.

8. Genetic predictors of medication response

The inter-individual variation in drug response results in categorization of alcoholic patients into responders and nonresponders. The responders experience therapeutic efficacy with a particular drug given in therapeutic range without any toxicity or adverse effects. The nonresponders do not show any therapeutic effect, even when the administered drug reaches to peak level in blood, leading to ineffective treatment, known as poor as poor metabolizers. Therefore the traditional approach of one dose fits for all is no longer helpful in predicting the therapeutic efficacy of a drug. The pharmacogenetics focuses on identifying genetic factors that is with are responsible responsible for variability in pharmacotherapeutic effect both in terms of pharmacodynamics and efficacy (Evans &Johnson, 2001). The field has greatly benefitted from advances in molecular genetic tools, developments in bioinformatics and functional genomics for identifying genetic variants.

Genetic factors can account for interindividual differences in drug toxicity and efficacy in many ways e.g. the variability in genes may lead to differences in drug metabolism and disposition through functional differences in activity of enzymes or drug transporters (Ray et al., 2010a). Alternatively genetic variation may impact a drug's target such as particular receptor. Genetic variants that may modulate the effects of naltrexane have been identified in the gene coding for μ OPRM1, which is the primary target of naltrexaone (Oslin et al., 2003). One of the most widely studied SNPs in OPRM1 is +118A/G (rs 1799971) located in the +118 position of exon1 one which encodes for Asn40Asp substitution (Bond et al., 1998). This A/G substitution has been reported to affect the receptor affinity for endogenous ligands, β-endorphin leading to gain in function such that the G variant was thought to bind β-endorphin with greater affinity than A allele. However, some recent studies have shown that G allele has a loss of function rather than a gain. Further, the results of the study testing the relationship between this SNP of the OPRM1 gene and alcoholism have shown inconsistent results, some support the association of this SNP and alcohol dependence while others have failed to replicate this association (Schinka et al., 2002; Kranzler et al., 1998; Town et al., 1999). Further, this SNP of OPRM1 gene has also been associated with a differential response in clinical trials of naltrexone. Oslin et al. (2003) has reported that this SNP is associated with clinical response to naltrexaone among alcohol dependent patients such that individuals with at least one copy of the G allele, coding for more potent OPRM1 receptor reported lower relapse rates and longer time to return to heavy drinking after treatment with naltrexone, in comparison with individuals who were homozygous for the A allele.

It has been reported that persons of Asian descent possess an ALDH2*2 genetic variant (Quertemont et al., 2004). ALDH2*2 genetic variant of the ALDH enzyme metabolizes slowly and leads to accumulation of acetaldehyde (Edenberg, 2007). When the individuals bearing this variant drink alcohol they develop high acetaldehyde blood concentration and experience of flushing reaction similar to that seen in combination of ethanol and disulfiram. ALDH2*2 variation is the best characterized genetic factor protecting against the development of alcohol dependence. Pharmacogenomic studies suggest that it is highly unlikely that disulfiram will be helpful in treating the patients who have genetically compromised ALDH.

In addition disulfiram chelates copper and thus inhibits copper containing enzyme dopamine beta hydroxylase which further inhibits norepinephrine and dopamine in brain (Haile et al., 2009). The individuals harboring TT allele of dopamine beta hydroxylase (DβH) gene with C1021T polymorphism respond better to disulfiram treatment and need less dose whereas carriers (CT) would need intermediate dose and those with CC allele need maximum concentration to reach the efficacy level.

Acamprosate, is a drug used for abstinence and maintenance as it reduces craving in alcoholic patients who have undergone detoxification (De Witte et al., 2005). The effective acamprosate response in alcohol dependent subjects may be influenced by genetically controlled variation of NMDA receptor and the type of glutaminergic mGLU5 receptor. Confirmation of this hypothesis could lead to development of effective individualized treatment and recommendation for alcohol dependent patients based on pharmacogenetically relevant genetic variant.

Ondansetron, an antagonist of serotonin is important in the treatment of alcoholism. Serotonin transporter gene is an important regulator of neuronal 5-HT's function. The genetic difference in this gene may modulate the severity of alcohol consumption and predict the therapeutic response to 5-HT3 receptor antagonist ondansetron. A variable tandem repeat polymorphism (5-HTT LPR) is common in the promoter region of 5-HTT gene which alters the transcriptional activity. Two important variants are long (insertion LL) and short (SS) version. It has been reported in a randomized clinical trial that individuals with LL genotype (Homozygous for the long version) of 5-HTT gene showed significant results in improvements of alcoholism with treatment of ondansetron as compared to LS and SS genotype (Johnson et al., 2011).

Another functional T/G polymorphism (rs1042173) as in the 3/ untranslated region of the 5-HTT gene may alter the therapeutic response in alcoholism treatment with ondansetron in alcohol addiction treatment (Jhonsan et al., 2011). The effect of ondensateron will be higher in individuals possessing the combination of LL genotype and TT genotype of 5-HTT gene.

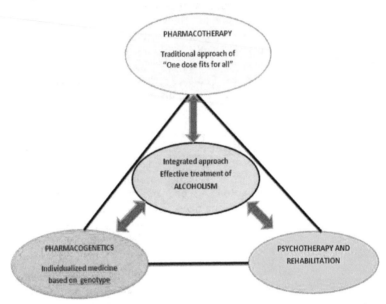

Fig. 2. Alcoholism Treatment: A Treatment approach to use a trio of Pharmacotherapy using pharmacological agents, where a traditional approach of "One dose for all" is used and Psychotherapy – an important part of treatment in alcoholism and Pharmacogenetics based on Genetic makeup of the Individual for better and effective treatment in alcoholism

9. Conclusion

Lot of work still needs work still needs to be done in order to improve our understanding of the genetic and environmental factors underlying alcohol dependence and also utilizing the genetic information in prescribing the drugs as per the genetic architecture of the individuals. The integrated approach of incorporating a trio of pharmacogenetic, pharmacotherapy and psychotherapy would be more promising in treatment of alcoholism (Fig 2). As the genetic testing becomes more common in the practice of medicine variety of ethical and practical challenges unique to alcohol addiction, will also need to be addressed.

10. References

Amit, Z. Aragon, C.M. (1988). Catalase activity measured in rats naive to ethanol correlates with later voluntary ethanol consumption: possible evidence for a biological marker system of ethanol intake. *Psychopharmacology*, Vol. 95. pp. 512–515

Bart, G. Kreek, M.J. Ott, J. LaForge, K.S. Proudnikov, D. Pollak, L. Heilig, M. (2005). Increased attributable risk related to a functional mu-opioid receptor gene polymorphism in association with alcohol dependence in central Sweden. *Neuropsychopharmacology*, Vol. 30, No. 2, pp. 417-422

Beckemeier, M.E. Bora, P.S. (1998). Fatty acid ethyl esters: potentially toxic products of myocardial ethanol metabolism. *J Mol Cell Cardiol,* Vol. 30, pp. 2487-2494

Benegal, V. (2005). India alcohol and public health.*Addiction* August vol.100 No. 8, pp. 1051-1056

Bergen, A.W. Kokoszka, J. Peterson, R. Long, J.C. Virkkunen, M. Linnoila, M. Goldman, D. (1997). Mu-opioid receptor gene variants: lack of association with alcohol dependence. *Mol Psychiatry,* Vol. 2, pp. 490–494

Bond, C. LaForge, K.S. Tian, M. Melia, D. Zhang, S. Borg, L. Gong, J. Schluger, J. Strong, J.A. Leal, S.M. Tischfield, J.A. Kreek, M.J. Yu, L. (1998). Single-nucleotide polymorphism in the human mu opioid receptor gene alters beta-endorphin binding and activity: possible implications for opiate addiction. *ProcNatlAcadSci,* Vol. 95, pp. 9608-9613

Bouza, C. Angeles, M. Muñoz, A. Amate, J.M. (2004). Efficacy and safety of naltrexone and acamprosate in the treatment of alcohol dependence: A systematic review. *Addiction,* Vol. 99, No.7, pp. 811– 828

Brooks, A.J. (1999). The essence of SNPs. *Gene,* Vol. 234, pp. 177–186

Caballeria, J. (2003). Current concepts in Alcoholmetabolism.*Annals of Hepatology,* Vol. 2, No. 2, pp. 60-68

Carr, L.G. Foroud, T. Stewart, T. Castellucio, P. Edenberg, H.J. Li, T. (2002). Influence of ADH1B polymorphism on alcohol use and its subjective effects in a Jewish population.*Am J Med Genet,* Vol. 112, pp. 138-143

Chen, C.C. Lu, R.B. Chen, Y.C. Wang, M.F. Chang, Y.C. Li, T.K. Yin, S.J. (1999). Interaction between the functional polymorphisms of the alcohol-metabolism genes in protection against alcoholism.*American Journal of Human Genetics,* Vol. 65, No. 3, pp. 795–807

Chou, W.Y. Stewart, M.J. Carr, L.G. Zheng, D. Stewart, T.R. Williams, A. Pinaire, J. Crabb, D.W. (1999). AnA/G polymorphism in the promoter of mitochondrial aldehyde dehydrogenase (ALDH2): Effects of the sequence variant on transcription factor binding and promoter strength. *Alcohol Clin and Experimental Res,* Vol. 23, No. 6, pp. 963–968

Colombo G, Addolorato G, Agabio R, Carai MA, Pibiri F, Serra S, Vacca G, Gessa GL. (2004). Role of GABA(B) receptor in alcohol dependence: Reducing effect of baclofen on alcohol intake and alcohol motivational properties in rats and amelioration of alcohol withdrawal syndrome and alcohol craving in human alcoholics. *Neurotoxicity Research,* Vol. 6, No. 5, pp. 403–414

Dahchour, A. De Witte, P. Bolo, N. Nedelec, J.F. Muzet, M. Durbin, P. Macher, J.P. (1998). Central effects of acamprosate: Part 1. Acamprosate blocks the glutamate increase in the nucleus accumbens microdialysate in ethanol withdrawn rats. *Psychiatry Research,* Vol. 82, No. 2, pp. 107–114

De Witte, P. Littleton, J. Parot, P. Koob, G. (2005). Neuroprotective and abstinence-promoting effects of acamprosate: elucidating the mechanism of action. *CNS drugs,* Vol. 19, No. 6, pp. 517–537

Deitrich, R.A.&Erwin, V.G. E. (1996).Pharmacological Effects of Ethanol on the Nervous System.*Hand book of Pharmacology and toxicology,* CRC Press, ISBN: 9780849383892

Diana, M. Gessa, G.L. Rossetti, Z.L. (1992). Lack of tolerance to ethanol-induced stimulation of dopamine mesolimbic system. *Alcohol,* Vol. 2, No. 4, pp. 329-333

Edenberg, H.J. (2007). The Genetics of Alcohol Metabolism.Role of Alcohol Dehydrogenase and Aldehyde dehydrogenase variants.*Alcohol Research and Health*, Vol. 30, No.1, pp. 5-13

Evans, W.E. Johnson, J.A. (2001). Pharmacogenomics the inherited basis for inter-individual differences in drug response. *Annu Rev Genomics Hum Genet.* Vol. 2, pp. 9-39

Farook, J.M. Morrell, D.J. Lewis, B. Littleton, J.M. Barron, S. (2007). Topiramate (Topamax) reduces conditioned abstinence behaviors and handling-induced convulsions (HIC) after chronic administration of alcohol in Swiss-Webster mice. *Alcohol and Alcoholism*, Vol. 42, No. 4, pp. 296–300

Ferreira, V.M.M. Morato, G.S. (1997). D-Cycloserine blocks the effects of ethanol and HA-906 in rats tested in the elevated plus-maze. *Alcohol Clin Exp Res*, Vol. 21, No. 9, pp. 1638-1642

Flensborg-Madsen, T. Knop, J. Mortensen, E. L. Becker, U.&Gronbek, M. (2007). Amount of Alcohol consumption and risk of developing alcoholism in men and women. *Alcohol and Alcoholism*, Vol. 42, No.5 pp. 442-447

Foley, P.F.Loh, E.W. Innes, D.J. Williams, S.M. Tannenberg, A.E. Harper, C.G. Dodd, P.R. (2004).Association studies of neurotransmitter gene polymorphisms in alcoholic Caucasians.*Ann N Y AcadSci*, Vol 1025pp39-46.

Franke, P. Wang, T. Nothen, M.M. Knapp, M. Neidt, H. Albrecht, S. Jahnes, E. Propping, P. Maier, W. (2001). Nonreplication of association between μ-opioid-receptor gene (OPRM1) A118G polymorphism and substance dependence.*Am J Med Genet*, Vol. 105, pp. 114 –119

Froehlich J, O'Malley S, Hyytia P, Davidson D, Farren C. (2003). Preclinical and clinical studies on naltrexone: What have they taught each other? Alcoholism: *Clinical and Experimental Research*, Vol. 27, No. 3, pp. 533–539

Fukuda, Y. Nakamura, K. Takano, T. (2005). Accumulation of health risk behaviours is associated with lower socioeconomic status and women's urban residence: a multilevel analysis inJapan. *BMC Public Health*, Vol.5, No. 53.doi:10.1186/1471-2458-5-53,ISSN 1755-7682

Fuller, R.K. Branchey, L. Brightwell, D.R. (1986). Disulfiram treatment of alcoholism: A Veterans Administration cooperative study. *Journal of the American Medical Association*, Vol. 256, No. 11,pp. 1449–1455

Gelernter, J. Kranzler, H. Cubells, J. (1999). Genetics of two μ-opioid receptor gene (OPRM1) exon I polymorphisms: population studies, and allele frequencies in alcohol- and drug-dependent subjects. *Mol Psychiatry*, Vol. 4, pp. 476–483

Gianoulakis,C. (1996). Implications of endogenous opioids and dopaminein alcoholism: human and basic science studies. *Alcohol AlcoholSuppl*, Vol. 1, pp. 33–42

Goedde, H.W. Agarwal, D.P. Fritze, G. Meier-Tackmann, D. Singh, S. Beckmann, G. Bhatia, K, Chen, L.Z. Fang, B. Lisker, R. (1992). Distribution of Adh2 and Aldh2 Genotypes in Different Populations.*Hum Genet*, Vol. 88, pp. 344–346

Goldman, D. & Bergen, A. (1998).General and specific inheritance of substance abuse and alcoholism.*Archives of General Psychiatry*, Vol.55, pp. 964–965

Goldstein, M. &Nakajima, K. (1967). The effect of disulfiram on catecholamine levels in the brain. *Journal of Pharmacol and Exp Therap*, Vol. 157, No. 1, pp. 96–102

Goldstein, M. Anagnoste, B. Lauber, E. &Mckeregham, M.R. (1964).Inhibition of dopamine-beta-hydroxylase by disulfiram.*Life Sciences*, Vol. 3, pp. 763–767

Group, P.M.R. (1997).Matching Alcoholism Treatments to Client heterogeity: Project MATCH posttreatment drinking outcomes.*J Stud Alcohol,* Vol.58, No.1, pp. 7-29

Haile, C.N. Kosten, T.R. Kosten, T.A. (2009). Pharmacogenetic treatments for drug addiction: cocaine, amphetamine and methamphetamine. *Am J Drug Alcohol Abuse,* Vol. 35, No. 3, pp.161-77

Harris, B.R. Prendergast, M.A. Gibson, D.A. Rogers, D.T. Blanchard, J.A. Holley, R.C. Fu, M.C. Hart, S.R. Pedigo, N.W. Littleton, J.M. (2002). Acamprosate inhibits the binding and neurotoxic effects of trans-ACPD, suggesting a novel site of action at metabotropic glutamate receptors. *Alcohol Clin Exp Res,* Vol. 26, No.12, pp. 1779–1793

Hayashi, S. Watanabe, J. Kawajiri, K. (1991). Genetic polymorphisms in the 5'-flanking region change transcriptional regulation of the human cytochrome P450IIE1 gene. *J Biochem,* Vol. 110, pp. 559–565

Heath, A.C. Madden, P.A.F. Bucholz, K.K. Bierut, L.J. Whitefild, J.B. Dinwiddie, W.S. Slutske, D.B. Statham, D.B.&Martin, N.G. (2001). Towards a molecular epidemiology of alcohol dependence: analyzing the interplay of genetic and environmental risk factors. *British Journal of Psychiatry,* Vol. 178, No.40, pp. s33-s40

Hoerner, M. Behrens, U. Worner, T. Lieber, C.S. (1986). Humoralimmuneresponses to acetaldehyde adducts in alcoholic patients. *Res CommunChemPathol Pharmacol,* Vol. 54, pp. 3-12

Howard, L.A. Ahluwalia, J.S. Lin, S.K. Sellers, E.M. Tyndale, R.F. (2003). CYP2E1*1D regulatory polymorphism: association with alcohol and nicotine dependence. *Pharmacogenetics,* Vol. 13, No. 7, pp. 441-442

Huang, S.Y. Lu, R.B. Ma, K.H. Shy, M.J. Lin, W.W. (2008). Norepinephrine transporter polymorphisms T-182C and G1287A are not associated with alcohol dependence and its clinical subgroups. *Drug Alcohol Depend,* Vol. 92, No. 1-3, pp. 20-26

Hurley, T.D. Edenberg, H.J. Li, T.K. (2002). The pharmacogenomics of alcoholism. In: *Pharmacogenomics: The Search for Individualized Therapies.*Weinheim, Germany: Wiley-VCH, pp. 417–441

Itoga, S. Nomura, F. Harada, S. Tsutsumi, M. Takase, S. Nakai, T. (1999).Mutations in the exons and exon–intron junction regions of human cytochrome P-4502E1 gene and alcoholism.*Alcohol Clin Exp Res,* Vol. 23, pp. 13s–16s

Jessica, E. Sturgess, J.E. George, T.P. Kennedy J.L. Heinz, A.& Müller, D.J.(2011). Pharmacogenetics of alcohol, nicotine and drug addiction treatments.*Addiction Biology,* Vol. 16, No.3, pp. 357-376

Johann, M. Putzhammer, A. Eichhammer, P. Wodarz, N. (2005). Association of the -141C Del variant of the dopamine D2 receptor (DRD2) with positive family history and suicidality in German alcoholics.*Am J Med Genet B Neuropsychiatr Genet,* Vol. 132, No.1, pp. 46-49

Johnson, B.A. Ait-Daoud, N. Seneviratne, C. Roache, J.D. Javors, M.A. Wang, X.Q. Liu, L. Penberthy, J.K. DiClemente, C.C. Li, M.D. (2011). Pharmacogenetic approach at the serotonin transporter gene as a method of reducing the severity of alcohol drinking.*Am J Psychiatry,* Vol. 168, No. 3, pp. 265-275

Johnson, B.A. Campling, G.M. Griffiths, P. Cowen, P.J. (1993). Attenuation of some alcohol-induced mood changes and the desire to drink by 5-HT3 receptor blockade: A preliminary study in healthy male volunteers. *Psychopharmacology*, Vol. 112, No.1, pp.142–144

Jung, M.H. Park, B.L. Lee, B.C. Ro, Y. Park, R. Shin, H.D. Bae, J.S. Kang, T.C. Choi, I.G. (2011).Association of CHRM2 polymorphisms with severity of alcohol dependence.*Genes Brain Behavior,* Vol. 10, No. 2, pp. 253-256

Kalow, W. (1962). Pharmacogenetics: Heredity and the response to drugs. Philadelphia, W.B. Saunders.

Kauhanen, J. Karvonen, M.K. Pesonen, U. Koulu, M. Tuomainen, T.P. Uusitupa, M.I.J. Salonen, J.T. (2000). Neuropeptide Y polymorphism and alcohol consumption in middle-aged men.*Am J Med Genet,* Vol. 93, pp. 117-121

Kennedy, R.H.& Liu, S.J. (2003). Sex differences in L-type calcium current after chronic ethanol consumption in rats.*ToxicolApplParmacol,* Vol. 15, No. 3, pp. 196-203

Kenneth, S. Kendler, M.D. Andrew, C. Heath, D. Michael, C. Neale. Kessler R.D.& Eaves L.J. (2011). A population - based Twin study of Alcoholism in Women. *JAMA,* Vol. 268, No.14, pp. 1877-1882

Kianmaa, K. Tabakoff, B. (1983).   Neurochemical correlates of tolerance and strain differences in the neurochemical effects of ethanol. *Pharmacol BiochemBehav,* Vol. 8, pp. 383-388

Kim, S.G. Kim, C.M. Kang, D.H. Kim, Y.J. Byun, W.T. Kim, S.Y. Park, J.M. Kim M.J. Oslin, D.W. (2004). Association of functional opioid receptor genotypes with alcohol dependence in Koreans.*Alcohol Clin Exp Res,* Vol. 28, pp. 986–990

Koechling, U.M. Amit, Z. (1992). Relationship between blood catalase activity and drinking history in a human population, a possible biological marker of the affinity to consume alcohol.*Alcohol,* Vol. 27, pp. 181–188

Kranzler, H.R. Gelernter, J. O'Malley, S. Hernandez-Avila, C.A. Kaufman, D. (1998). Association of alcohol or other drug dependence with allelesofthe μ-opioid receptor gene (OPRM1). *Alcohol Clin Exp Res,* Vol. 22, pp. 1359–1362

Kranzler, H.R. Pierucci-Lagha, A. Feinn, R. Hernandez-Avila, C. (2003). Effects of ondansetron in early- versus late-onset alcoholics: A prospective, open-label study. *Alcoholism: Clinical and Experimental Research*, Vol. 27, No. 7, pp. 1150–1155

Krishnan-Sarin, S. O'Malley, S. &Krystal, J.H. (2008). Treatment Implications: Using Neuroscience to Guide the development of new Pharmacotherapies for Alcoholism. *Alcohol, Res &Health,*pp. 400-407

Lappalainen, J. Kranzler, H.R. Malison, R. Price, L.H. Van Dyck, C. Rosenheck, R.A. Cramer, J. Southwick, S. Charney, D. Krystal, J. Gelernter, J. (2002). A functional neuropeptide Y Leu7Pro polymorphism associated with alcohol dependence in a large population sample from the United States.*Arch Gen Psychiatry,* Vol. 59, No. 9, pp. 825-831

Lee, S.L.Chau, G.Y. Yao, C.T. Wu, C.W. Yin, S.J. (2006). Functional assessment of human alcohol dehydrogenase family in ethanol metabolism: Significance of first-pass metabolism. *Alcoholism: Clinical and Experimental Research,* Vol. 30, No.7 pp.1132–1142

Lieber, C.S. DeCarli, L.M. (1968). Ethanol oxidation by hepatic microsomes: adaptive increase after ethanol feeding. *Science,* Vol.162, pp. 917–918

Lieber, C.S. Lasker, J.M. DeCarli, L.M. Saeli, J. Wojtowicz, T. (1988).Role of acetone, dietary fat, and total energy intake in the induction of the hepatic microsomal ethanol oxidizing system.*J Pharmacol Exp Ther,* Vol. 247, pp. 791–795

Lieber, C.S. (1999). Microsomal ethanol-oxidizing system: the first 30 years (1968–1998) a review. *Alcohol Clin Exp Res,* Vol. 23, pp. 991–1007

Littleton, J. &Zieglgänsberger, W. (2003).Pharmacological mechanisms of naltrexone and acamprosate in the prevention of relapse in alcohol dependence.*American Journal on Addictions,* Vol. 12, No. 1, pp. S3–S11

Loh, E.W. Smith, I. I. Murray, R. McLaughlin, M. McNulty, S. Ball, D. (1999). Association between variants at the GABAAbeta2, GABAAalpha6 and GABAAgamma2 gene cluster and alcohol dependence in a Scottish population.*Mol Psychiatry,* Vol. 4, No.6, pp. 539–544

Longo, L.P. Campbell, T. Hubatch, S. (2002). Divalproex sodium (Depakote) for alcohol withdrawal and relapse prevention.*J Addict Dis,* Vol. 21, No. 2, pp. 55-64

Lovinger, D.M. (1991).Ethanol potentiation of 5HT3 receptor-mediated ion current in NCB-20 neuroblastoma cells.*Neurosci Lett,* Vol. 122, pp. 57-60

Luczak, S.E. Glatt, S.J. & Wall, T.J. (2006).Meta-analyses of ALDH2 and ADH1B with alcohol dependence in Asians. *Psychological Bulletin,* Vol. 132, No. 4, pp. 607–621

Luo, X. Kranzler, H.R. Zuo, L. Wang, S. Blumberg, H.P. Gelernter, J. (2005). CHRM2 gene predisposes to alcohol dependence, drug dependence and affective disorders: results from an extended case-control structured association study. *Human Molecular Genetics,* Vol. 14, No.16, pp. 2421-2434

Marinelli, P.W. Quirion, R. Gianoulakis, C. (2003). A microdialysis profile of beta-endorphin and catecholamines in the rat nucleus accumbens following alcohol administration.*Psychopharmacology,* Vol. 169, No.1, pp. 60–67

McGue, M. (1999).The behavioral genetics of alcoholism.*Current Directions in Psychological Science,* Vol. 8, pp. 109–115

McLeod, H.L.Krynetski, E.Y.Relling, M.V. Evans, W.E. (2000). Genetic polymorphisms of thiopurinemethyltransferase and its clinical relevance for childhood lymphoblastic leukemia.*Leukemia,* Vol. 14, pp. 567–572

Moussas, G. Christodoulou, C.Douzenis, A. (2009). A Short review on the etiology of alcoholism. *Annals of General Psychiatry,* Vol. 8, No.10, doi:10.1186/1744-859X-8-10

Neumark, Y.D. Friedlander, Y. Thomasson, H.R. Li, T.K. (1998). Association of the ADH2*2 allele with reduced ethanol consumption in Jewish men in Israel: a pilot study. *J Stud Alcohol,* Vol. 59, pp. 133–139

Neville, M.J. Johnstone, E.C. Walton, R.T. (2004). Identification and characterization of ANKK1: a novel kinase gene closely linked to DRD2 on chromosome band 11q23.1.*Human Mutation,* Vol. 23, pp. 540-545

Nurnberger, J.I. Wiegand, R. Bucholz, K. O'Connor, S. Meyer, E.T. Reich, T. Rice, J. Schuckit, M. King, L. Petti, T. Bierut, L. Hinrichs, A.L. Kuperman, S. Hesselbrock, V.&Porjesz, B. (2004). A Family Study of Alcohol Dependence - Coaggregation of Multiple Disorders in Relatives of Alcohol- Dependent Probands.*Arch Gen Psychiatry,* Vol. 61, pp. 1246-1256

O'Malley, S.S.Jaffe, A.J. Chang, G. Rode, S.Schottenfeld, R. Meyer, R.E.Rounsaville, B. (1992). Naltrexone and coping skills therapy for alcohol dependence: A controlled study. *Archives of General Psychiatry,* Vol. 49, No.11, pp. 881–887

Oshino, N. Oshino, R. Chance, B. (1973). The characteristics of the peroxidatic reaction in ethanol oxidation.*Biochem J*, Vol. 131, pp. 555-567

Osier, M.V. Pakstis, A.J.Soodyall, H. Comas, D. Goldman, D. Odunsi, A.Okonofua, F.Parnas, J. Schulz, L.O.Bertranpetit, J. Bonne-Tamir, B. Lu, R.B. Kidd, J.R. Kidd, K.K. (2002). Aglobal perspective on genetic variation at the ADH genes reveals unusual patterns of linkage disequilibrium and diversity. *Am J Genet*, Vol. 71, pp. 84-99

Osier, M.V. Lu, R.B. Pakstis, A.J. Kidd, J.R. Huang, S.Y. Kidd, K.K. (2004). Possible epistatic role of ADH7 in the protection against alcoholism.*American Journal of Medical Genetics*. Part B *Neuropsychiatric Genetics*, Vol. 126, pp.19-22

Oslin, D.W. Berrettini, W. Kranzler, H.R. Pettinati, H. Gelernter, J Volpicelli, J.R. O'Brien, C.P. (2003). A functionalpolymorphism of the mu-opioid receptor gene is associated withnaltrexone response in alcohol-dependent patients. *Neuropsychopharmacology*, No. 28, pp.1546-1552

Park, C.S. Park, S.Y. Lee, C.S. Sohn, J.W. Hahn, G.H. Kim, B.J. (2006). Association between Alcoholism and the Genetic polymorphism of the GABA A receptor genes on chromosome 5q33-34 in Korean population.*J Korean Med Sci*, Vol. 21, No. 3, pp. 533-538

Pawan, G.L.S. (1972). Meatbolism of Alcohol (ethanol) in Man. *ProcNutrSoc*, Vol. 3I, pp. 83-89

Ponce, G. Hoenicka, J. Jiménez-Arriero, M.A. Rodríguez-Jiménez, R. Aragüés, M. Martín-Suñé, N. Huertas, E. Palomo, T. (2008). DRD2 andANKK1 genotype in alcohol-dependent patients with psychopathic traits: association and interaction study.*Br J Psychiatry*, Vol. No. 2, pp. 121-125

Poznyak, V. Saraceno, B. Obot, I.S. (2005). Breaking the vicious circle of determinants and consequences of harmful alcohol use.*Bulletin of the World Health Organization*.Vol.83, pp 803

Quertemont, E. (2004). Genetic polymorphism in ethanol metabolism: acetaldehyde contribution to alcohol abuse and alcoholism.*MoleculPsychiat*, Vol. 9, pp. 570-581

Quickfall, J.& el-Guebaly, N. (2006). Genetics and Alcoholism: How close are we to potential clinical applications? *Can Journal of Psychiatry*, Vol. 51, No.7, pp. 461-467

Radel, M. Goldman, D. (2001). Pharmacogenetics of alcohol response and alcoholism: the interplay of genes and environmental factors in thresholds for alcoholism.*DrugMetabDispos*, Vol. 29, No. 4, pp. 489-494

Ray, L.A. Mackillop, J.&Monti, P.M. (2010a). Subjective responses to alcohol consumption as endophenotypes: Advancing behavioral Genetics in etiological and treatment models of Alcoholism. *Substance Use and Misuse*, Vol. 45, pp. 1742-1765

Ray, L.R. Chin, P.F. Miotto, K. (2010b). Naltrexone for the treatment of Action and Pharmacogenetics.*CNS & Neurological Disorders Drug Targets*. Vol. 9, pp. 13-22

Sander, T. Ball, D. Murray, R. Patel, J. Samochowiec, J. Winterer, G.Rommelspacher, H. Schmidt, L.G. Loh, E.W.(1999). Association analysis of sequence variants of GABA(A) alpha 6, beta 2, and gamma 2 gene cluster and alcohol dependence. *Alcohol Clin Exp Res*, Vol.23, No. 3, pp. 427-431

Sander, T. Ostapowicz, A. Samochowiec, J. Smolka, M. Winterer, G. Schmidt, L.G. (2000).Genetic variation of the glutamate transporter EAAT2 gene and vulnerability to alcohol dependence.*Psychiatry Genet*, Vol. 10, No. 3, pp. 103-107

Schinka, J.A. Town, T. Abdullah, L. Crawford, F.C. Ordorica, P.I. Francis, E. (2002).A functional polymorphism within the μ-opioid receptor gene and risk for abuse of alcohol and other substances.*Mol Psychiatry*, Vol. 7, pp. 224 –228

Schumann, G. Johann, M. Frank, J. Preuss, U. Dahmen, N. Laucht, M. Rietschel, M. Rujescu, D. Lourdusamy, A. Toni-Kim, C. Krause, K. Dyer, A. Depner, M. Wellek, S. Treutlein, J. Szegedi, A. Giegling, I. Cichon, S. Blomeyer, D. Heinz, A. Heath, S. Lathrop, M. Wodarz, N. Soyka, M. Spanagel, R. Mann, K. (2008). Systematic analysis of glutaminergic neurotransmission genes in alcohol dependence and adolescent risky drinking behavior.*Arch Gen Psychiatry*, Vol. 65, No.7, pp. 826-838

Sloan, C.D. Sayarath, V.&Moore, J.H. (2008). Systems Genetics of Alcoholism.*Alcohol Research and Health,*Vol. 31,No.1, pp. 14-25

Spanagel, R. Putzke, J. Stefferl, A. Schöbitz, B. Zieglgänsberger, W. (1996). Acamprosate and alcohol: II. Effects on alcohol withdrawal in the rat.*Europ Journal of Pharmacol*, Vol. 305, No. 1–3, pp. 45–50

Srisurapanont, M. &Jarusuraisin, N. (2002).Opioid antagonists for alcohol dependence. *Cochrane Database Syst Rev*. No. 1, CD001867

Strat, Y.L. Ramoz, N. Schumann, G.&Gorwood, P.(2008).Molecular Genetics of Alcohol Dependence and Related endophenotypes. *Current Genomics*, Vol. 9, pp. 444-451.

Subramanian, S.V.Nandy, S. Irving, M. Gordon, D. Davey, Smith, G. (2005) Role of socioeconomic markers and state prohibition policy inpredicting alcohol consumption among men and women in India:a multilevel statistical analysis. *Bulletin of the World Health Organization*, Vol. 83, pp. 829–836

Swift, R.M. (2000). Opioid antagonists and alcoholism treatment.*CNS Spectrums,*Vol. 5, No. 2, pp. 49–57

Tabakoff, B. Hoffman, P.L. Moses, F.(1977). Neurochemical correlates of ethanol withdrawal: alterations in serotonergic function. *J Pharm Pharmacol*, Vol. 29, pp. 471-476

Tabakoff, B. (1983). Current trends in biologic research on alcoholism.*Drug Alcohol Depend*, Vol. 11, No. 1, pp. 33-37

Tabakoff, B.&Hoffman, P.L. (1992). Alcohol: Neurobiology. *Substance Abuse*, 2nd edition, pp. 152–185

Takahashi, T. Lasker, J.M. Rosman, A.S. Lieber, C.S. (1993). Induction of cytochrome P-4502E1 in the human liver by ethanol is caused by a corresponding increase in encoding messenger RNA. *Hepatology*, Vol. 17, pp. 236–245

Thiele, T.E. Marsh, D.J. Ste Marie, L. Bernstein, I.L. Palmiter, R.D. (1998). Ethanol consumption and resistance are inversely related to neuropeptide Y levels. *Nature*, Vol. 396, pp. 366–369

Thomasson, H.R. Edenberg, H.J. Crabb, D.W. Mai, X.L. Jerome, R.E. Li, T. K. Wang, S.P. Lin, Y.T. Lu, R.B. Yin, S.J. (1991).Alcohol and aldehyde dehydrogenase genotypes and alcoholism in Chinese men. *American Journal of Human Genetics*, Vol. 48, No. 4, pp. 677–681

Town, T. Abdullah, L. Crawford, F. Schinka, J. Ordorica, P.I. Francis, E. Hughes, P. Duara, R. Mullan, M. (1999). Association of a functionalμ-opioid receptor allele (+118A) with alcohol dependency.*Am J Med Genet*, Vol. 88, pp. 458–461

Tsutsumi, M. Lasker, J.M. Shimizu, M. Rosman, A.S. Lieber, C.S. (1989). Theintralobular distribution of ethanol-inducible P-450IIE1 in rat and human liver.*Hepatology*, Vol. 10, pp. 437–446

Vengeliene, V. Bilbao, A. Molander, A.&Spanagel, R. (2006). Neuropharmacology of Alcohol addiction.*British Journal of Pharmacology*, Vol. 154, pp. 299-315

Vengeliene, V. Bilbao, A. Molander, A. Spanagel, R. (2008).Neuropharmacology of alcohol addiction. *Br J Pharmacol*, Vol. 154, No. 2, pp. 299-315

Venter, J.C. Adams, M.D. Myers, E.W.Li, P.W. Mural, R.J. Sutton, G.G (2001). The sequence of the human genome.*Science*, Vol. 291, pp. 1304-1351

Volpicelli, J.R. Alterman, A.I. Hayashida, M. O'Brien, C.P. (1992). Naltrexone in the treatment of alcohol dependence. *Archives of General Psychiatry*, Vol. 49, No.11, pp. 876-880

Wang, J.C. Grucza, R. Cruchaga, C. Hinrichs, A.L. Bertelsen, S. Budde, J. P. Fox, L. Goldstein, E. Reyes, O. Saccone, N. Saccone, S. Xuei, X. Bucholz, K. Kuperman, S. Nurnberger, J. Rice, J.P. Schuckit, M.J. Tischfield, J. Hesselbrock, V. Porjesz, B. Edenberg, H.J. Bierut, L.J. Goate, A.M. (2009). Genetic variation in the CHRNA5 gene affects mRNA levels and is associated with risk for alcohol dependence Association of CHRNA5 with alcohol dependence. *Molecul Psychiatry*, Vol.14, pp. 501-510

Wertheimer, A.I.& Chaney, N.M. (2003). The full extent of Alcoholism: A WorldwideEconomic and Social Tragedy. *Malaysian Journal of Pharmacy*, Vol.1, No.3, pp. 54-58

Whitfield, J.B. (1997). Meta-analysis of the effects of alcohol dehydrogenase genotype on alcohol dependence and alcoholic liver disease.*Alcohol*, Vol. 32, pp. 613-619

Williams, S. (2001). Introducing an in-patient treatment for alcohol detoxification into community settings. *J Clin Nursing*, Vol. 10, pp. 635-642

Woodward, J.J. (1994). A comparison of the effects of ethanol and the competitiveglycine agonist 7-chlorokynurenic acid on N-methyl-D-aspartate acid-inducedneurotransmitter release from rat hippocampal slices. *J Neurochem*, Vol. 62, No. 98, pp. 7-91

World Health Organization.(2002). The World Health Report 2002- Reducing risks, Promoting Healthy Life.*World Health Organization, Geneva*, pp. 65-67.

World Health Organization.(2004). *WHO Global Status Report on Alcohol.* pp. 1-68

Yin, S.J. (1994). Alcohol dehydrogenase: enzymology and metabolism. *Alcohol AlcoholSuppl*, Vol. 29, No. 2, pp. 113-119

Wray, L.A. Alwin, D.F. &McCammon, R.J. (2005). Social statusand risky health behaviors: results from the health and retirement study. *Journals of Gerontology Series B-Psychological Sciences and Social Sciences*, Vol.60, No 2, pp. 85-92.

Yoshimoto, K. Yayama, K. Sorimachi, Y. Tani, J. Ogata, M. Nishimura, A. Yoshida, T. Ueda, S. Komura, S. (1996). Possibility of 5-HT3 receptor involvement in alcohol dependence: a microdialysisstudy of nucleus accumbens dopamine and serotonin releasein rats with chronic alcohol consumption. *Alcohol Clin Exp Res*, Vol. 20, No. 9, pp. 311A-319A

Zaleski, M. Morato, G.S. da Silva V.A. Lemos, T. (2004). Neuropharmacological aspects of chronic alcohol use and withdrawl symptoms. *Rev Brain Psiquiater*, Vol. 26, pp. 40-42

Zalewska-Kaszubska, J. Gorska, D. Dyr, W. Czarnecka, E. (2006). Effect of acute administration of ethanol on beta-endorphin plasma level in ethanol preferring and non-preferring rats chronically treated with naltrexone. *Pharmacol, Biochemistry, and Behavior*, Vol. 85, No.1, pp. 155-159

Zimatkin, S.M. Deitrich, R.A. (1997). Ethanol metabolism in the brain.*Addict Biol*, Vol. 2, pp. 387-399

11

Future of Pharmacogenetics in Cardiovascular Diseases

Rianne M.F. Van Schie#, Talitha I. Verhoef#
and Anke-Hilse Maitland-Van Der Zee et al.*
Utrecht University
The Netherlands

1. Introduction

Pharmacogenetics is the study of variations in DNA sequence as related to drug response (European Medicines Agency [EMA], 2007). Several gene-drug interactions have been discovered in the field of cardiovascular diseases (CVDs). These gene-drug interactions can help to identify nonresponse to drugs, estimate dose requirements or identify an increased risk of developing adverse drug reactions. An individualized approach based on pharmacogenetic testing will provide physicians and pharmacists with tools for decision making about pharmacotherapy. While pharmacogenetic testing is already part of everyday practice in oncology, it is not widely implemented in the field of CVDs. However, in the near future, pharmacogenetics will probably also play a valuable role in this field as well.

1.1 Complexity of pharmacogenetics of CVDs

Prophylaxis and treatment of CVD is complex. Patients often have more than one cardiovascular risk factor (e.g. hypertension and hypercholesterolemia) and/or CVD, or other comorbidities such as diabetes mellitus. Frequently, more than one drug is used by the patient and this may potentially lead to serious drug interactions with adverse health outcomes. Therefore, not only the comorbidities but also the interaction between co-medications should be taken into account if a pharmacogenetics based dosing strategy is developed.

1.2 The aim of this book chapter

The aim of this book chapter is to describe and explore several examples of gene-drug interactions in CVD, the factors that affect the implementation in clinical practice, the cost-effectiveness analysis of pharmacogenetic testing, and the development of new technologies that could improve research of pharmacogenetic interactions in CVD.

---

* Anthonius de Boer[1], Tom Schalekamp[1], Felix J.M. Van Der Meer[2],
William K. Redekop[3] and Rahber Thariani[4]
# These authors contributed equally
[1]*Utrecht University, The Netherlands*
[2]*Leiden University Medical Center, The Netherlands*
[3]*Erasmus University Rotterdam, The Netherlands*
[4]*University of Washington, USA*

2. Examples of pharmacogenetics for cardiovascular diseases

Cardiovascular drugs are widely used for prevention or treatment of CVD. Gene-drug interactions were demonstrated in the treatment with platelet inhibitors, anticoagulants, antihypertensive drugs and statins. The findings of the many studies that have been conducted on pharmacogenetics of antihypertensive drugs, are not suitable for clinical implementation, often because the results could not be replicated or the clinical relevance was low (Arnett & Claas, 2009). The most commonly prescribed drugs in the management of CVD with important gene-drug interactions are statins, clopidogrel and coumarin derivatives. These three drugs are candidates for pharmacogenetic testing in everyday practice and will be discussed in more detail below.

2.1 Statins

Patients with hypercholesterolemia have an increased risk of CVD. Statins are widely used to treat hypercholesterolemia and prevent CVD. This treatment, often accompanied by lifestyle changes, has been proven to be effective and safe, but the efficacy varies among patients (Pearson et al., 2000). The effect of statins depends on the statin concentration at the site of action, the liver. This concentration can be altered by several factors, like diet and concomitant medication (Romaine et al., 2010). Muscle symptoms are a common problem during statin use ranging from mild myalgia to severe rhabdomyolysis (Law & Rudnicka, 2006). Although muscle symptoms are generally not life-threatening, they can negatively affect the patient's quality of life and also his or her adherence to statin therapy (Peters et al., 2009).

Several transporters play a role in the access of statins in the liver. Multiple studies have demonstrated a role for statin transportation by the organic anion transporter polypeptide 1B1 (OATP1B1) (Niemi, 2007; Pasanen et al., 2006), which is encoded by the *SLCO1B1* gene. An impaired hepatic uptake of several statins has been shown for patients with a specific single nucleotide polymorphism (SNP) in this gene, namely the *SLCO1B1* c.521T>C SNP. A decreased effect of statins is therefore seen in patients with this variant allele. This effect was shown in users of atorvastatin, pitavastatin, pravastatin and rosuvastatin in some studies, while others could not find a significant or clinically relevant effect (SEARCH Collaborative Group, 2008; Voora et al., 2009).

The impaired hepatic uptake causes an increased plasma concentration of statins, which probably causes a higher rate of adverse events. Carriers of a c.521C allele show an increased risk of developing myopathy after simvastatin use. Because this SNP does not seem to influence plasma concentration of fluvastatin, this could be an alternative for patients at risk of simvastatin induced muscle symptoms (Niemi et al., 2006). Genotyping before starting statin therapy might help to choose the right statin. Carriers of a variant allele could then be identified and treated with a *SLCO1B1* genotype independent statin, for example fluvastatin. In this way, genotyping for this *SLCO1B1* SNP may increase the safety of statin therapy. This approach of determining the most optimal therapy has not yet been investigated in a clinical trial.

2.2 Clopidogrel

Clopidogrel is a platelet inhibitor (PI), used together with aspirin to treat patients after percutaneous coronary interventions. This dual antiplatelet therapy reduces the risk of stent thrombosis, myocardial infarction, stroke and cardiovascular death. Clopidogrel monotherapy may be used for secondary prevention of atherosclerotic complications, in case aspirin can not be used, for example due to allergy (Anderson et al., 2010).

Clopidogrel is administered to patients as a prodrug. It needs to be metabolized by several hepatic cytochrome P450 (CYP) enzymes in order to form the active platelet aggregation inhibiting metabolite. This is done in two steps. During the first step, the intermediate 2-oxo-clopidogrel metabolite is formed. In this step three isoenzymes (CYP1A2, CYP2B6 and CYP2C19) are involved. During the second step this metabolite is hydrolyzed into the active thiol derivative R-130964, which blocks the ADP P2Y12 receptors on the platelet surface, causing inhibition of platelet aggregation. This step is catalyzed by four isoenzymes (CYP2B6, CYP2C9, CYP2C19 and CYP3A4) (Yukhanyan et al., 2011).

Although the effectiveness of clopidogrel has been demonstrated in many trials, variation in response is still an issue. Some patients experience cardiovascular events despite dual antiplatelet therapy (Yukhanyan et al., 2011). This difference in risk of cardiovascular events is genetically determined. In addition, response-variability is also caused by a genetically determined difference in platelet aggregation (Harmsze et al., 2010a). The interindividual variability in response to clopidogrel can be explained by multiple genetic and environmental factors. Variation in response to clopidogrel related to genetic variability in the *CYP2C19* gene has been investigated thoroughly, as the CYP2C19 enzyme plays an important role in both metabolizing steps (Anderson et al., 2010). In several studies a relationship between carriage of a loss-of-function allele in the *CYP2C19* gene and the occurrence of adverse cardiovascular events has been demonstrated. Up to now, more than 33 alleles of the *CYP2C19* gene have been identified. Most of these are rare in the general population. The most common allele in the European population is *CYP2C19*1*. The enzyme encoded by this allele enables extensive metabolizing of clopidogrel into the active metabolite. A common variant allele is the *2 allele. Patients carrying at least one of this variant allele have a decreased activity of the CYP2C19 enzyme. This leads to a reduced plasma concentration of the active metabolite and possibly to an increased risk of recurrent cardiovascular events. Knowledge of the *CYP2C19*2* genotype can explain approximately 12% of the variation in response to clopidogrel. An increased risk of stent thrombosis has been demonstrated in carriers of a *CYP2C19*3* allele. Both carriers of a *2 of a *3 allele have a decreased enzyme activity, resulting in a lower amount of active metabolite (Harmsze et al., 2010b). The *CYP2C19*17* allele however, encodes for a more active enzyme. Carriers of this allele therefore have an increased antiplatelet response to clopidogrel. This might be associated with an increased risk of bleeding (Yukhanyan et al., 2011; Zabalza et al., 2011).

Pharmacogenetic testing for the *2 or *3 variant alleles could identify patients that are less likely to respond to clopidogrel and who might benefit more from treatment with an alternative, more expensive PI such as prasugrel or ticagrelor. Prasugrel and ticagrelor have less variability in response than clopidogrel, mainly due to a smaller influence of genetic variations. However, patients using prasugrel or ticagrelor have an increased risk of bleeding compared to patients using clopidogrel (Jakubowski et al., 2011; Collet & O'Connor, 2011). At the moment, randomized controlled trials (RCTs) are ongoing to evaluate the (cost) effectiveness of pre-treatment genotyping (Crespin et al., 2011). Based on the results of these trials, physicians can decide whether or not to prescribe clopidogrel or another PI on the patient's genotype.

2.3 Coumarin derivatives

Oral anticoagulants of the coumarin type are used to treat and prevent thromboembolic events in patients with different conditions, including venous thromboembolism and atrial fibrillation (Ansell et al., 2008). The effect is monitored by the International Normalized Ratio (INR), which should be kept within a certain range (for example, the range for atrial fibrillation is between 2.0 and 3.0). Wide interpatient variability in dose requirement means that the dosage is difficult to predict and frequent monitoring of the INR is necessary. INR values below the therapeutic range increase the risk of thromboembolic events while a supratherapeutic INR leads to an increased risk of bleeding events. These bleeding events can range from minor bleedings to major, life-threatening bleedings such as intracranial hemorrhage (James et al., 1992).

The wide variability in dose requirement is caused by several factors. Dietary intake of Vitamin K, comorbidities (e.g. altered thyroid function), concomitant medication, sex, age, height and weight all influence the required coumarin dose. Also genetic factors are shown to have an important role (Custodio das Dores et al., 2007; Penning-van Beest et al., 2001; Torn et al., 2005). First the influence of the CYP2C9 gene, encoding the main metabolizing enzyme, cytochrome P450 2C9 (CYP2C9) was discovered. Carriers of a *2 or *3 allele require a lower dose and have an increased risk of overanticoagulation, which is associated with an increased risk of bleedings (Schalekamp, 2004). A few years later was discovered that with the VKORC1 gene, encoding the target enzyme vitamin K epoxide reductase multiprotein complex 1, even a larger part of dose requirement variability could be explained. CYP2C9 and VKORC1 together explain approximately half of the variation in coumarin dose requirement (Schalekamp & de Boer, 2010; van Schie et al., 2011).

Currently, most patients receive an identical initial coumarin dosage. After a few days, the response is evaluated by INR measurement. The dose can then be adapted to the patient's needs. If patients are genotyped before starting coumarin therapy, they can receive a genotype-guided dose from day 1 on. This is suggested to prevent overanticoagulation in carriers of a variant allele and to reach a stable dose earlier. RCTs are currently ongoing to provide evidence for the (cost) effectiveness of pre-treatment genotyping for coumarin derivatives (van Schie et al., 2009; French et al., 2010).

In addition to the three mentioned examples, we expect more pharmacogenetic interactions will be found to be clinically relevant in CVD therapy.

3. Pharmacogenetic testing

Pharmacogenetic testing is thought to increase the efficacy and safety of drugs. However, for CVD, pharmacogenetic testing is not yet established in daily practice. Currently ongoing RCTs will hopefully provide evidence to implement pharmacogenetic testing in daily practice. However, implementation of a pharmacogenetic approach of a treatment depends on many different factors that extend beyond the outcomes of RCTs. These factors will be discussed in this paragraph.

3.1 Clinical trials to provide evidence

At this moment, a pharmacogenetic approach to determine the appropriate therapy for an individual patient is not yet widely used. There are currently only a few therapies where genotyping is used to establish the right dose or make a decision about which drug to use. Pharmacogenetic testing has not yet been used extensively since physicians are still hesitant about genotyping. Although physicians are willing to customize the therapy for an individual patient based on the patient's genetic profile, their capacity to do so is limited by their time and complexity of the procedure (Levy & Young, 2008). However, genotyping may provide physicians with tools for optimizing drug treatment for the individual patient. In other words, it could provide the physician with information on the individual reaction of the patient to the medication or the dose, comparable to what liver- and kidney function tests provide them with. These function tests were implemented in clinical practice without evidence for their added value from clinical trials. However, it is unlikely that pharmacogenetic tests would be implemented without RCTs, because of considerable uncertainty surrounding their efficacy and overall health outcome impact. These RCTs are therefore needed to convince physicians of the added value of genotyping the patient.

Currently, a number of RCTs are underway to hopefully provide evidence of improved efficacy and safety by genotyping the patient and using this information to individualize the treatment. Use of the search term "pharmacogenetics" on clinicaltrials.gov, a website where clinical trials are registered, produced a list of 361 studies (performed on 15 August 2011). Of these studies, 117 studies were interventional studies seeking new volunteers. In contrast, use of the term "cardiovascular" produced a list of 20,123 studies. However, only 61 studies were found after combining the search term "pharmacogenetics" with "cardiovascular". Of those 61 studies, 4 were being performed for statins, 4 for clopidogrel and 18 for the coumarin derivatives. This suggests that pharmacogenetics is currently only a minor research field in clinical trials and that most of the activity in that field is on coumarin derivatives.

Although thorough research is currently being performed to investigate the added value of genotyping on the efficacy and safety of drugs, it is not feasible to conduct a clinical trial for each newly found gene-drug interaction. There are several reasons for this. The first reason is that it is not always ethical to perform a clinical trial, for example in a situation in which observational studies have already shown that patients will be at a risk for an adverse event if they have a certain genotype (Peters, 2010). Secondly, costs and resource use would be prohibitive (e.g. study personnel, insurance). Thirdly, clinical trials are time-consuming. The length of the actual follow-up period is only one factor here; clinical trials take substantial time to initiate (e.g. writing the protocol, instructing study personnel), perform and analyse. For obvious gene-drug interactions, it is not ethical to waste money and time for performing clinical trials instead of implementing them directly. This would mean that we expect, in the future, that some observational studies should provide sufficient evidence to implement the findings in clinical practice. However, replication of the results in observational pharmacogenetic studies is often not obtained. Therefore, strict guidelines should be developed to define which evidence is necessary to implement the investigated pharmacogenetic interaction into clinical practice. Factors to consider are:

- Have the results been replicated in different studies with independent researchers?
- Are the results valid for various countries and ethnicities?
- Is the estimated improvement large enough?
- Is the estimated improvement cost-effective (see also paragraph 4)?
- Is it feasible to implement it in clinical practice? For example:
  - Are the genotyping results available in time?

- Are all facilities available?
- Are the parties involved trained to perform the implementation?

3.2 Parties involved in implementation

Once studies have shown that a pharmacogenetic approach of determining the optimal treatment for a patient is superior to the conventional therapy, it can be implemented in clinical practice. There are multiple parties involved in the implementation of pharmacogenetic based therapies in everyday clinical situations. In this paragraph, we will discuss all different parties involved and their rationales.

3.2.1 Patients

Successful implementation of pharmacogenetic testing in everyday practice heavily depends on patient attitudes. Without the cooperation of patients, development of new pharmacogenetic strategies or guidelines is futile. Fortunately, research has shown that this group is willing to provide a sample for genotyping. Van Wieren-De Wijer et al. examined the reasons for non-response in a pharmacogenetic case-control study. They approached 1871 myocardial infarction cases and 14,102 controls of which 794 and 4997 responded, respectively. Only 1.1% of the non-responding participants were unwilling to provide a DNA sample (van Wieren et al., 2009). Moreover, since this study used a case-control design where all cardiovascular events had occurred before testing, the participants could not benefit from the test outcome. In case their drug treatment would be personalized by their genetic profile, this percentage is expected to decrease.

3.2.2 Health care professionals

The attitude of health care providers towards pharmacogenetic guided therapies is important in making their decision about the treatment the patient will receive. Although the FDA updated the warfarin label already in 2008 (Teichert et al., 2009a; Food and Drug Administration [FDA], 2007), genotyping preceding the anticoagulation therapy with coumarin derivatives is not commonly performed. Currently, health care professionals' attitudes are reserved towards pharmacogenetic dosing. Not many therapies need pharmacogenetic testing at the moment, so health care professionals need to get familiarized with the idea of genetic testing, like they are familiarized with performing liver and kidney function tests. Different approaches are thought to help with familiarizing health care professionals with pharmacogenetic testing:

- Clinical trials are needed to convince the health care professional and make genetic testing as normal as liver and kidney function tests.
- Recommendations in guidelines and drug labels of pharmacogenetic testing to improve treatment quality are required, such as the FDA did for warfarin.
- Education of the health care profession on how to perform and use the pharmacogenetic tests is desired.
- Favourable experiences will stimulate the health care professional to use pharmacogenetic testing in everyday clinical practice.
- Facilities for genotyping need to be available at the right place and time.
- Consistency and standards for pharmacogenetic testing are needed.

The focus of the process should not only be on the physician but also pharmacists should be involved. To enhance the implementation of pharmacogenetic testing, the Royal Dutch Association for the Advancement of Pharmacy developed pharmacogenetic-based therapeutic (dose) recommendations (Swen et al., 2011; Wilffert et al., 2010). In addition, the pharmacist could be involved in genotyping the patient with easy to use point-of-care tests that will be available soon. The results of, for example, CYP-enzymes, could be used for decision making in multiple therapies. The pharmacist is not the only candidate to genotype the patient; others such the GP or a nurse in the hospital could also genotype the patient. Therefore, dissemination of the genotyping results (e.g., by means of electronic dossiers) is important.

3.2.3 Regulatory authorities

Regulatory authorities will also play an important role in the implementation of pharmacogenetic guided therapies in daily practice. They have the power to develop guidelines which health care professionals are obligated to follow. They can also adjust the label information of the medication.

In order to harmonize approaches to drug regulation, a guideline was developed to ensure that consistent definitions of terminology are applied across all constituents of the International Conference on Harmonisation (ICH) (EMA, 2007; FDA, 2008). This guideline contains nonbinding recommendations. The Committee for Human Medicinal Products (CHMP) facilitated an informal process of sharing scientific and technical information between applicants and regulators by releasing a concept paper on "Briefing Meetings on Pharmacogenetics". The Pharmacogenetics Working Party was set up to support discussions regarding the implementation of pharmacogenetic testing. In April 2006, a guideline on Pharmacogenetics Briefing Meetings was adopted by the CHMP. This guideline provides guidance for starting the discussion with the Pharmacogenetics Working Party and provides considerations on the submission of pharmacogenetic data in informal regulatory submissions. Briefing meetings take place when new pharmacogenetic information becomes available during the development of a new medicinal product or when a new indication is explored based on recent developments in pharmacogenetics (EMA, 2006). The Food and Drug Administration (FDA) developed a guideline called "Guidance for Industry, Pharmacogenomic Data Submissions". This guideline facilitates the scientific pharmacogenomics process and the use of pharmacogenomic data in drug development (U.S. Department of Health and Human Services et al., 2005). The FDA and European Medicinal Agency (EMA) have joint Voluntary Genomic Data Submissions (VGDSs). This is not part of the regulatory decision-making process, but gains an understanding of genomic data and provides options for sponsors to have joint FDA-EMA briefing meetings (Goodsaid, 2006). A consistent regulatory environment is also helpful in encouraging industry to develop pharmacogenetic products, and for consumers (including patients and physicians) to use the product.

3.2.4 Health insurance companies

Implementation of pharmacogenetic guided approaches to plan therapy will depend on whether it is reimbursed by health insurance companies. If the patient needs to pay for the genotyping kit, it is less likely that pharmacogenetic testing will be implemented in clinical practice than when health insurance companies will pay for it. However, these companies will likely only pay for genetic tests if their use leads to more cost-effective care. Health insurers would be very interested in genotyping if it improved treatment effectiveness but also reduced total health care costs (including the cost of genotyping). There are different ways in which genotyping results could lead to lower health care costs, for example:

- Fewer visits to the GP or hospital for therapy adjustments, i.e. improved patient response or efficacy
- Better prophylaxis resulting in lower costs
- Fewer side effects, especially serious side effects resulting in expensive hospital admissions.

In some cases, health insurers may reimburse genotyping even if it is believed to increase overall costs. For example, if the genotyping approach is more costly and more effective compared to the non-genotyping approach, the health insurer could consider the greater effectiveness worth the extra cost. All in all, this means that pharmaco-economic evaluations are of importance in pharmacogenetic studies. See also paragraph 4 on cost-effectiveness analysis.

3.2.5 Researchers (public and private industry)

Sound scientific research is needed to develop new strategies of pharmacogenetic guided therapies. Without research, new ideas of pharmacogenetic guided therapies will not arise. Both the public as well as the private industry could perform this research. There are different focus points that researchers could have. First, they could investigate new pharmacogenetic interactions. Interactions could be of different value. They could look for common SNPs that have a small effect, but since the SNPs are common, many patients might benefit. On the other hand, they could investigate rare SNPs that might cause major effects, in which case there could be a huge benefit for relatively few patients. However, this last area of research would require big sample sizes to have enough power to investigate the effect of a rare SNP. Second, studies to develop better and faster genotyping methods will be required if pharmacogenomic testing is to be used just as extensive as liver and kidney function tests. An example of a user-friendly and quick genotyping system is Optisense's Genie 1 with HyBeacon® assays (Howard et al., 2011). See also paragraph 5. Third, the industry could develop new drug therapies for a subpopulation. For example, a new drug that does not have the desired effect in the whole population might benefit patients with a certain genotype. Although only for this subpopulation, this new medication could then still enter the market. Forth, scientists should aim to develop genotype guided therapies that do not require large and time-consuming clinical trials. Currently, clinical trials are needed to convince health care professionals, but in the future, cohort studies could be used for the implementation of pharmacogenetic testing. It is important that the results are replicated in various external datasets before being implemented in clinical practice. After implementation, it remains important to validate the process and, if necessary, adjust the pharmacogenetic based guidelines if it does not seem to be working satisfactorily.

3.3 Facilities

Several facilities should be in place before pharmacogenetic testing can be implemented in clinical practice.

3.3.1 Availability of genotyping results

Genotyping results should be available quickly. If results are available before the therapy starts, they are of greater value than when they become available after treatment start. However, in the current clinical situation, health care professionals need to collect blood samples from a number of patients to be able to genotype a batch of samples. Therefore, it can sometimes take a few weeks before the genotype is known. Currently, new techniques are being developed, and will continue to be developed in the coming years, to make genotyping results more rapidly available (Howard et al., 2011). The need to collect samples from many patients will diminish, since one assay can be run using a Point-Of-Care Test (POCT) for a single patient. By increasing the number of tests needed, the availability of POCTs will increase (Huang, 2008) and the price per POCT assay will probably decrease (see also paragraph 5).

3.3.2 Authority guidelines

The authorities can assist in implementing pharmacogenetic testing in clinical practice by developing guidelines and ensuring that health care professionals follow them. In 2008, the FDA updated the warfarin label (Teichert et al., 2009a; Food and Drug Administration [FDA], 2007) and advised pharmacogenetic testing before the coumarin therapy starts. However, at that time no guidelines were provided as to how the dosages should be changed based on the genetic profile of the patient. This illustrates that guidelines should contain information on how to adjust drug therapy based on genotype. It also underlines the importance that different parties work closely together.

4. Cost-effectiveness analysis of pharmacogenetic testing

Many would argue that clinical practice guidelines should just focus on whether pharmacogenetic testing improves effectiveness and ignore cost considerations. However, decision making about the widespread use of genotyping also depends on its cost-effectiveness. This means that even if authorities were to recommend genotyping patients prior to cardiovascular therapy based on proof of effectiveness, the recommendation might not easily be implemented without the support of other stakeholders. One important stakeholder is the payer, such as a health insurance company and its attitude can be an instrumental factor in the successful implementation of pharmacogenetic testing. Health insurance companies may require proof of cost-effectiveness - and some estimates of budget impact - before considering reimbursement.

A cost-effectiveness analysis (CEA) compares the total costs and effectiveness of two or more different treatment strategies. All sorts of costs must be considered here, including not just the cost of genotyping, but also the cost of monitoring and the cost of cardiovascular events that occur later in time. While costs are all expressed in the same way (money!), effectiveness can be defined in different ways. The definition of effectiveness determines how cost-effectiveness is expressed. For example, effectiveness can focus on the risk of an adverse event and the difference in effectiveness between two treatments can be expressed as the absolute reduction in risk of an event. The cost-effectiveness of one treatment versus another will then be expressed as the extra cost to avoid one adverse event (calculated by dividing the difference in costs by the reduction in risk). However, since this expression of cost-effectiveness is very disease-specific, it is difficult, if not impossible, to compare the cost-effectiveness of different treatments for different diseases with each other and this comparability is valuable when making budget allocation decisions. For this reason, some authorities or health insurance companies require a cost-utility analysis. In a cost-utility analysis (CUA), the health gains acquired by a new treatment are expressed in Quality Adjusted Life Years (QALYs), which can be compared more easily with other treatments, also in other diseases, than the cost per adverse event avoided.

Several economic evaluations (such as CEAs and CUAs) have been performed for coumarin derivatives. The problem with these analyses is that no robust data on the effectiveness of genotyping are available yet; the large RCTs that can provide this data are still ongoing (van Schie et al., 2009; French et al., 2010). This current lack of evidence results in a wide variability in cost-effectiveness ratios among the studies that have been done, ranging from dominance (where use of genotyping reduces costs and increases health) to a very high incremental cost of $347,000 per QALY gained (Verhoef et al., 2010). The costs of genotyping are also not clear yet. In literature, the estimated cost of genotyping for *CYP2C9* ranges from $67 to $350 and the estimated cost of genotyping both *CYP2C9* and *VKORC1* ranges from $175 to $575. Recently, a Point-Of-Care Test (POCT) for genotyping *CYP2C9* and *VKORC1* has been developed. With this test, the patient's genotype can be determined in the physician's office within 2 hours and this is estimated to cost less than $50 per patient for both *CYP2C9* and *VKORC1* (Howard et al., 2011). The costs of genotyping are expected to decrease even further, with increased usage. This will also influence the chance that pharmacogenetic testing is cost-effective.

Decisions about whether or not to implement pharmacogenetic testing in clinical practice will differ among different countries. This difference can be caused by several factors. Firstly, the amount of money society is willing to pay varies among different countries. For example, this 'willingness to pay' is approximately $50,000 per QALY gained in the US or £20,000–30,000 (approximately $33,000-50,000) per QALY gained in the UK (National Institute for Health and Clinical Excellence [NICE], 2008). Secondly, the costs, not only of genotyping but also of the consequences like bleeding events, are not identical in all countries. Next to this, the effectiveness of genotyping can also be higher in one country than in another. This is for example possibly the case with coumarin derivatives. In some countries the standard care is already of very high quality, with specialized anticoagulation clinics to monitor the effect of the drug, while in other countries this is not the case and there is still room for further improvement.

As mentioned before, the use of pharmacogenetics in treatment with a certain drug can only be recommended if information on effectiveness and costs of genotyping is available, although it is not clear what level of evidence is needed for a valid decision. Obviously, it is impossible to obtain perfect evidence. Therefore, value of information (VOI) analyses could be performed to establish the cost–effectiveness of further research on the efficiency of the strategy. If the costs of performing this research are greater than the benefits of the additional information, then it would not be worthwhile to conduct this research (Sculpher & Claxton, 2005). The parameters that have the greatest influence on the uncertainty regarding the cost–effectiveness of genotyping should be the main focus of future studies in this area. The costs of conducting these studies should also be considered. However, this will also depend upon the regulatory environment, and VOI forms only a part of the picture.

5. Pharmacogenetic developments

Until now, only the most obvious gene-drug interactions have been detected since these are least complicated to detect when researchers are looking for causal SNPs. However, rare SNPs with large effects might as well be of importance, but it is a challenge to find large numbers of cases that are required to obtain enough power in pharmacogenetic studies when looking at smaller effects or lower allele frequencies (Daly, 2010). A trend is observed that larger studies are being performed and meta-analyses are carried out to investigate these less frequent genetic profiles. Several techniques are further developed and might lead to new insights in the pharmacogenetic research field. We will discuss them in this paragraph.

5.1 Candidate-gene studies

This type of study investigates the association between drug response and previously identified candidate genes. These candidate genes might play a relevant role in the pharmacokinetics or pharmacodynamics of the drug and might therefore be, for example, the metabolizing enzyme or the target protein. An example is the use of candidate gene approaches for the understanding of the overall drug response to coumarins. (Daly, 2010). In 1992, Rettie *et al.* indicated *CYP2C9* as main metabolizing enzyme of warfarin (Rettie et al., 1992). A few years later, Furuya *et al.* first reported that SNPs in this gene affect the stable coumarin maintenance dose (Furuya et al., 1995). A decade later, VKORC1 was identified as the target enzyme of the coumarins (Rost et al., 2004; Li et al., 2004) and studies confirming the association between *VKORC1* genotypes and stable coumarin maintenance dose followed. Another example is the role of the *CYP2C19* genotype on the clopidogrel (Hulot, 2006) therapy response and how the treatment with tamoxifen is influenced by the *CYP2D6* genotype (Hoskins, 2009).

5.2 Genome-wide association studies

Since 2007, genonome wide association (GWA) studies have become more frequently applied in the pharmacogenetics field. This resulted in novel identified associations between drug response and variations in DNA (Daly, 2010). In CVD, GWA studies resulted in confirmation of the already available knowledge, rather than in newly identified interactions. For clopidogrel, the influence of *CYP2C19* was confirmed (Schuldiner et al., 2009) and for statin induced muscle symptoms an association with *SLCO1B1* was found (SEARCH Collaborative Group, 2008) in a GWA study. In a GWA study on acenocoumarol maintenance dose, an additional effect was found for polymorphisms in *CYP4F2* and *CYP2C18* (Teichert et al., 2009b). These GWA studies led to more knowledge about several drug-gene interactions, but the causality of the relationship is not always clear in these studies. Another difficulty with this type of analyses is the need of large patient numbers because of the correction for multiple testing.

5.3 Sequencing

DNA sequencing is the determination of the nucleotide bases in DNA. In contrast to GWA studies, where tag SNPs are used to cover as much of the variation within the gene as possible, this technique will determine the exact order of nucleotides in DNA. Instead of tag SNPs that are usually markers for the causal SNP - and thereby introduce noise because they are not always in complete linkage disequilibrium - the causal SNPs can be identified. Therefore, this technique might provide new insights in associations between drug response and pharmacogenetic parameters that are not observed when performing a candidate-gene study or a GWA study. It is possible to sequence a whole genome or whole exome. In addition, there is an option 'targeted sequencing' which means that a candidate gene is sequenced. This technique is relatively new and gaining interest in the last few years, but the same issues (i.e. causality of the relationship is not always clear and large patient numbers are needed) as with the GWA studies occur with sequencing. This warrants that the functionality of the SNP should be studied (Sadee, 2011).

5.4 Point-of-care testing

As discussed earlier, point-of-care tests can be used as mobile genotyping instruments in different settings, including the pharmacy, anticoagulation clinic and physician's office. It avoids the need to collect multiple samples and the genotyping results are available within 2 hours. This technique might be used to genotype the patient before the start of the therapy. However, the applicability of a point-of-care test may be different from centralized laboratory testing because of different sensitivity and specificity parameters. Also, it is not attractive to use such a test in research where large patient groups are needed to find a pharmacogenetic interaction, since that would be very labor intensive.

6. Conclusion

There is considerable potential for pharmacogenetic based drug dosing in CVD, but at the moment, these are not widely implemented in clinical practice. Convincing evidence was found for several CVD drugs. Carriers of a variant allele of the *SLCO1B1* gene could be treated with a *SLCO1B1* independent statin to increase the safety of the treatment. Clopidogrel is less metabolized into its active form by patients carrying a variant allele of *CYP2C19*, resulting in a less effective therapy. Information about the patient's *VKORC1* and *CYP2C9* genotype could be used when defining the appropriate dose during the anticoagulation therapy with coumarins to enhance the efficacy and increase the safety of the treatment. However, implementation of this knowledge is challenging and depends on multiple factors. First, clinical trials are needed to provide evidence for and enhance the implementation of pharmacogenetic testing. However, it is not feasible to perform a clinical trial for every newly found gene-drug interaction. Therefore it is desirable to develop guidelines to which observational studies should apply before implementing the gene-drug interaction in clinical practice. Secondly, multiple parties are involved, such as patients, health care professionals, regulatory authorities, health insurance companies and researchers. We discussed the different parties involved and their rationales. Thirdly, several facilities should be in place before pharmacogenetic testing can be implemented in clinical practice, such as availability of genotyping results and authority guidelines. Lastly, before it comes to implementation, the cost-effectiveness of the pharmacogenetic approach should be investigated. Health insurance companies may require proof of cost-effectiveness before considering reimbursement and therefore implementation of pharmacogenetic testing.

For the coming years, researchers will continue to develop the different genotyping methods. Larger studies will be performed and meta-analyses will be carried out to investigate less frequent genetic profiles. Analysis of GWA studies and sequencing is challenging due to the enormous amount of data obtained by this technique.

In the field of oncology, pharmacogenetic testing already is part of daily practice. We expect that pharmacogenetic testing will also be implemented in CVD in the near future.

7. References

Anderson, C., Biffi, A., Greenberg, S. & Rosand, J. (2010). Personalized approaches to clopidogrel therapy: are we there yet? *Stroke* 41, 12, (Dec 2010), 2997-3002.

Ansell, J., Hirsh, J., Hylek, E., Jacobson, A., Crowther, M. & Palareti, G. (2008). Pharmacology and management of the vitamin K antagonists: American College of Chest Physicians Evidence-Based Clinical Practice Guidelines (8th Edition). *Chest* 133, 6 suppl, (Jun 2008), 160S-198S.

Arnett, D. & Claas, S. (2009). Pharmacogenetics of antihypertensive treatment: detailing disciplinary dissonance. *Pharmacogenomics* 10, 8, (Aug 2009), 1295-1307.

Collet, J. & O'Connor, S. (2011). Clinical effects and outcomes with new P2Y12 inhibitors in ACS. *Fundam. Clin. Pharmacol.* (Sep 2011).

Crespin, D., Federspiel, J., Biddle, A., Jonas, D. & Rossi, J. (2011). Ticagrelor versus genotype-driven antiplatelet therapy for secondary prevention after acute coronary syndrome: a cost-effectiveness analysis. *Value Health.* 14, 4, (Jun 2011), 483-491 (2011).

Custodio das Dores, S., Booth, S., Martini, L., de Carvalho Gouvea, V., Padovani, C., de Abreu Maffei, F., Campana, A. & Rupp de Paiva, S. (2007). Relationship between diet and anticoagulant response to warfarin: a factor analysis. *Eur J Nutr* 46, 3, (Apr 2007), 147-154.

Daly, A. (2010). Genome-wide association studies in pharmacogenomics. *Nat. Rev. Genet.* 11, 4, (Apr 2010), 241-246.

European Medicines Agency [EMA]. (2006). Guideline on pharmacogenetics briefing meetings.

European Medicines Agency [EMA]. (2007). ICH Topic E15 Definitions for genomic biomarkers, pharmacogenomics, pharmacogenetics, genomic data and sample coding categories.

Food and Drug Administration [FDA]. (2007). Transcript of the FDA press conference on Warfarin held on 16 August.

Food and Drug Administration [FDA]. (2008). Guidance for Industry E15 Definitions for Genomic Biomarkers, Pharmacogenomics, Pharmacogenetics, Genomic Data and Sample Coding Categories

French, B., Joo, J., Geller, N., Kimmel, S., Rosenberg, Y., Anderson, J., Gage, B., Johnson, J., Ellenberg, J. & COAG investigators. (2010). Statistical design of personalized medicine interventions: the Clarification of Optimal Anticoagulation through Genetics (COAG) trial. *Trials* 11, (Nov 2010), 108.

Furuya, H., Fernandez-Salguero, P., Gregory, W., Taber, H., Steward, A,, Gonzalez, F. & Idle, J. (1995) Genetic polymorphism of CYP2C9 and its effect on warfarin maintenance dose requirement in patients undergoing anticoagulation therapy. *Pharmacogenetics.* 5(6), (dec 1995), 389-392.

Goodsaid, F. (2006). 42nd annual meeting; Joint USFDA-EU Pharmacogenomic Initiatives.

Harmsze, A., van Werkum, J., Ten Berg, J., Zwart, B., Bouman, H., Breet, N., van 't Hof, A., Ruven, H., Hackeng, C., Klungel, O., de Boer, A. & Deneer, V. (2010a). CYP2C19*2 and CYP2C9*3 alleles are associated with stent thrombosis: a case-control study. *Eur. Heart J.* 31, 24, (Dec 2010) 3046-3053.

Harmsze, A., van Werkum, J., Bouman, H., Ruven,H., Breet, N., Ten Berg, J., Hackeng, C., Tjoeng, M., Klungel, O., de Boer, A. & Deneer, V. (2010b). Besides CYP2C19*2, the variant allele CYP2C9*3 is associated with higher on-clopidogrel platelet reactivity in patients on dual antiplatelet therapy undergoing elective coronary stent implantation. *Pharmacogenet Genomics* 20, 1, (Jan 2010), 18-25.

Howard, R., Leathart, J., French, D., Krishan, E., Kohnke. H., Wadelius, M., van Schie, R., Verhoef, T., Maitland-van der Zee, A., Daly, A. & Barallon, R. (2011). Genotyping for CYP2C9 and VKORC1 alleles by a novel point of care assay with HyBeacon(R) probes. *Clin. Chim. Acta*, (Jul 2011).

Hoskins, J., Carey, L. & McLeod, H. (2009). CYP2D6 and tamoxifen: DNA matters in breast cancer. *Nature Rev. Cancer*, 9, 576-586.

Huang, S. (2008). Warfarin Pharmacogenetic Testing is Now Ready for Prime Time, AACC Annual Meeting, Washington DC, July 28, 2008.

Hulot, J., Bura, A., Villard, E., Azizi, M., Remones, V., Goyenvalle, C., Aiach, M., Lechat, P. & Gaussem, P. (2006) Cytochrome P450 2C19 loss-of-function polymorphism is a major determinant of clopidogrel responsiveness in healthy subjects. *Blood* 108, 2244-2247

Jakubowski, J., Riesmeyer, J., Close, S., Leishman, A. & Erlinge, D. (2011). TRITON and Beyond: New Insights into the Profile of Prasugrel. *Cardiovasc. Ther.* (Feb 2011).

James, A., Britt, R., Raskino, C. & Thompson, S. (1992). Factors affecting the maintenance dose of warfarin. *J Clin Pathol* 45, 8, (Aug 1992), 704-6.

Law, M. & Rudnicka, A. (2006). Statin safety: a systematic review. *Am. J. Cardiol.* 97, 8A, (Apr 2006), 52C-60C.

Levy, H. & Young, J. (2008). Perspectives from the clinic: will the average physician embrace personalized medicine? *Clin. Pharmacol. Ther.* 83, 3, (Mar 2008), 492-493.

Li, T., Chang, C., Jin, D., Lin, P., Khvorova, A., & Stafford, D. (2004). Identification of the gene for vitamin K epoxide reductase. *Nature*, 427, 541-544.

Nice. (2008). Guide to the methods of technology appraisal.

Niemi, M., Pasanen, M. & Neuvonen, P. (2006). SLCO1B1 polymorphism and sex affect the pharmacokinetics of pravastatin but not fluvastatin. *Clin. Pharmacol. Ther.* 80, 4, (Oct 2006), 356-366.

Niemi, M. (2007). Role of OATP transporters in the disposition of drugs. *Pharmacogenomics* 8, 7, (Jul 2007), 787-802.

Pasanen, M., Neuvonen, M., Neuvonen, P. & Niemi, M. (2006). SLCO1B1 polymorphism markedly affects the pharmacokinetics of simvastatin acid. *Pharmacogenet Genomics* 16, 12 (Dec 2006), 873-879.

Pearson, T., Laurora, I., Chu, H. & Kafonek, S. (2000). The lipid treatment assessment project (L-TAP): a multicenter survey to evaluate the percentages of dyslipidemic patients receiving lipid-lowering therapy and achieving low-density lipoprotein cholesterol goals. *Arch. Intern. Med.* 160, 4, (Feb 2000), 459-467.

Penning-van Beest, F., van Meegen, E., Rosendaal, F. & Stricker, B. (2001). Drug interactions as a cause of overanticoagulation on phenprocoumon or acenocoumarol predominantly concern antibacterial drugs. *Clin Pharmacol Ther* 69, 6, (Jun 2001), 451-457.

Peters, B., Klungel, O., Visseren, F., de Boer, A. & Maitland-van der Zee, A. (2009). Pharmacogenomic insights into treatment and management of statin-induced myopathy. *Genome Med.* 1, 1, (Dec 2009), 120.

Peters, B. (2010). Thesis: "Methodological approaches to the pharmacogenomics of statins"

Rettie A., Korzekwa, K., Kunze, K. , Lawrence, R. Eddy, A., Aoyama, T., Gelboin, J., Gonzalez, F. & Trager, W. (1992) Hydroxylation of warfarin by human cDNA-expressed cytochrome P-450: A role for P-4502C9 in the etiology of (S)-warfarin-drug interactions. *Chem. Res. Toxicol.* 5, 54-59.

Romaine, S., Bailey, K., Hall, A. & Balmforth, A. (2010). The influence of SLCO1B1 (OATP1B1) gene polymorphisms on response to statin therapy. *Pharmacogenomics J.* 10, 1, (Feb 2010), 1-11.

Rost, S., Fregin, A., Ivaskevicius, V., Conzelmann, E., Hörtnagel, K., Pelz, H., Lappegard, K., Seifried, E., Scharrer, E., Tuddenham, E., Müller, C., Strom, T. & Oldenburg, J. (2004). Mutations in VKORC1 cause warfarin resistance and multiple coagulation factor deficiency type 2. *Nature*, 427, 537-541.

Sadee, W., (2011). Pharmacogenomic biomarkers: validation needed for both the molecular genetic mechanism and clinical effect. *Pharmacogenomics*, 12, 5, (May 2011), 675-80.

Schalekamp, T., Oosterhof, M., van Meegen, E., van Der Meer, F., Conemans, J., Hermans, M., Meijerman, I. & de Boer, A. (2004). Effects of cytochrome P450 2C9 polymorphisms on phenprocoumon anticoagulation status. *Clin. Pharmacol. Ther.* 76, 5, (Nov 2004), 409-417.

Schalekamp, T. & de Boer, A. (2010). Pharmacogenetics of oral anticoagulant therapy. *Curr Pharm Des* 16, 2, (2010) 187-203.

van Schie, R., Wadelius, M., Kamali, F., Daly, A., Manolopoulos, V., de Boer, A., Barallon, R., Verhoef, T., Kirchheiner, J., Haschke-Becher, E., Briz, M., Rosendaal, F., Redekop, W., Pirmohamed, M. & van der Zee, A. (2009) Genotype-guided dosing of coumarin derivatives: the European pharmacogenetics of anticoagulant therapy (EU-PACT) trial design. *Pharmacogenomics* 10, 10, (Oct 2009), 1687-1695.

van Schie, R., Wessels, J., le Cessie, S., de Boer, A., Schalekamp, T., van der Meer, F., Verhoef, T., van Meegen, E., Rosendaal, F. & Maitland-van der Zee, A., for the EU-PACT Study Group (2011) Loading and maintenance dose algorithms for phenprocoumon and acenocoumarol using patient characteristics and pharmacogenetic data. *Eur Heart J.* 32,15, (Aug 2011), 1909-1917.

Sculpher, M. & Claxton, K. (2005). Establishing the cost-effectiveness of new pharmaceuticals under conditions of uncertainty--when is there sufficient evidence? *Value Health*, 8, 4, (Jul 2005), 433-446.

SEARCH Collaborative Group. (2008). SLCO1B1 variants and statin-induced myopathy--a genomewide study. *N. Engl. J. Med.* 359, 8, (Aug 2008), 789-799.

Shuldiner, A., O'Connell, J., Bliden, K., Gandhi, A., Ryan, K., Horenstein, R., Damcott, C., Pakyz, R., Tantry, U., Gibson, Q., Pollin, T., Post, W., Parsa, A., Mitchel, B., Faraday, N., Herzog, W. & Gurbel, P. (2009). Association of cytochrome P450 2C19 genotype with the antiplatelet effect and clinical efficacy of clopidogrel therapy. *JAMA*, 302, 8, (Aug 2009), 849-857.

Swen, J., Nijenhuis, M., de Boer, A., Grandia, L., Maitland-van der Zee, A., Mulder, H., Rongen, G., van Schaik, R., Schalekamp, T., Touw, D., van der Weide, J., Wilffert, B., Deneer, V. & Guchelaar, H. (2011). Pharmacogenetics: from bench to byte- an update of guidelines. *Clin. Pharmacol. Ther.* 89, 5, (May 2011), 662-673.

Teichert, M., van Schaik, R., Hofman, A., Uitterlinden, A., de Smet, P., Stricker, B. & Visser, L. (2009a). Genotypes associated with reduced activity of VKORC1 and CYP2C9 and their modification of acenocoumarol anticoagulation during the initial treatment period. *Clin. Pharmacol. Ther.* 85, 4, (Apr 2009), 379-386.

Teichert, M., Eijgelsheim, M., Rivadeneira, F., Uitterlinden, A., van Schaik, R., Hofman, A., De Smet, P., van Gelder, T., Visser, L. & Stricker, B. (2009b). A genome-wide association study of acenocoumarol maintenance dosage. *Hum. Mol. Genet.* 18, 19, (Oct 2009), 3758-86.

Torn, M., Bollen, W., van der Meer, F., van der Wall, E. & Rosendaal, F. (2005). Risks of oral anticoagulant therapy with increasing age. *Arch Intern Med* 165, 13, (Jul 2011) 1527-1532.

U.S. Department of Health and Human Services, Food and Drug Administration, Center for Drug Evaluation and Research (CDER), Center for Biologics Evaluation and Research (CBER) & Center for Devices and Radiological Health (CDRH). (2005). Guidance for Industry, Pharmacogenomic Data Submissions.

Verhoef, T., Redekop, W., Darba, J., Geitona, M., Hughes, D., Siebert, U., de Boer, A., Maitland-van der Zee, A. & EU-PACT group. (2010). A systematic review of cost-effectiveness analyses of pharmacogenetic-guided dosing in treatment with coumarin derivatives. *Pharmacogenomics* 11, 7, (Jul 2010), 989-1002.

Voora, D., Shah, S., Spasojevic, I., Ali, S., Reed, C., Salisbury, B. & Ginsburg, G. (2009). The SLCO1B1*5 genetic variant is associated with statin-induced side effects. *J. Am. Coll. Cardiol.* 54, 17, (Oct 2009), 1609-1616.

van Wieren-de Wijer, D., Maitland-van der Zee, A., de Boer, A., Kroon, A., de Leeuw, P., Schiffers, P., Janssen, R., Psaty, B., van Duijn, C., Stricker, B. & Klungel, O. (2009). Reasons for non-response in observational pharmacogenetic research. *Pharmacoepidemiol. Drug Saf.* 18, 8, (Aug 2009), 665-671.

Wilffert, B., Swen, J., Mulder, H., Touw, D., Maitland-van der Zee, A., Deneer, V. & KNMP working Group Pharmacogenetics (2010). From evidence based medicine to mechanism based medicine. Reviewing the role of pharmacogenetics. *Pharm. World Sci.* (Nov 2010).

Yukhanyan, L., Freynhofer, M., Siller-Matula, J., Schror, K. & Huber, K. (2011). Genetic variability in response to clopidogrel therapy and its clinical implications. *Thromb. Haemost.* 105 Suppl 1, (May 2011), S55-9.

Zabalza, M., Subirana, I., Sala, J., Lluis-Ganella, C., Lucas, G., Tomas, M., Masia, R., Marrugat, J., Brugada, R. & Elosua, R. (2011). Meta-analyses of the association between cytochrome CYP2C19 loss- and gain-of-function polymorphisms and cardiovascular outcomes in patients with coronary artery disease treated with clopidogrel. *Heart*, (Jun 2011).

12

Warfarin Enantiomers Pharmacokinetics by CYP2C19

Yumiko Akamine and Tsukasa Uno
Department of Hospital Pharmacy, Faculty of Medicine,
University of the Ryukyus, Okinawa,
Japan

1. Introduction

Warfarin, a coumarin vitamin K antagonist, is the most widely prescribed anticoagulant agent for the control and prevention of atrial fibrillation-related thrombus formation, stroke, and arterial and venous thrombembolism (Hirsh J et al., 1998). The recommend warfarin therapy consists of the lowest dose required to maintain the target international normalized ratio (INR) because of the drug's narrow therapeutic window. However, there can be a 20-fold difference in the dose required by patients to achieve this target INR. It is well known that cytochrome P450 (CYP), predominantly CYP2C9, activity is an important source of variability (Kaminsky LS and Zhang ZY, 1997) . Additionally, Rieder et al. (2005) have reported that an effect of the vitamin K epooxide reductase complex subunit 1 gene (VKORC1) has an important role on dose requirement. However, Takahashi et al. (2006) shows that Caucasians and African-Americans have high frequencies of VKORC1 and CYP2C9 genotypes, which lead to either reduced metabolic activity or attenuated sensitivity to warfarin, whereas only about 20% of the Japanese population possesses these genotypes. Therefore, further study of sources of variability in warfarin dose requirements among Japanese patients is warranted.

Warfarin is administered clinically as a racemic mixture of the *S*- and *R*-enantiomer (Fig. 1), however *S*-warfarin is 3–5 times more potent than *R*-enantiomer. Both enantiomers are extensively metabolized in the liver (Chan E et al., 1994; Takahashi H and Echizen H, 2001). The more potent *S*-enantiomer is metabolized mainly to *S*-7-hydroxywarfarin by CYP2C9, whereas *R*-enantiomer is metabolized to *R*-6, *R*-7, *R*-8 and *R*-10-hydroxywarfarin by several CYPs involving CYP1A2, CYP3A4 and CYP2C19 (Kaminsky LS and Zhang ZY, 1997). Among these CYPs, it has been shown that both CYP2C9 and CYP2C19 are subject to single nucleotide polymorphisms (SNPs). In Japanese, because the heterozygous frequency of the CYP2C9 Leu359 allele is 3.5% (Takahashi H et al., 1998) and the frequency of the defective CYP2C19 alleles is 18.8% (Kubota T et al., 1996), the latter may be more closely associated with the clinical effect of warfarin. In this chapter, we therefore focus on the effect of CYP2C19 genotypes on the pharmacokinetics and pharmacodynamics of warfarin enantiomers. In addition, we characterize the impact of omeprazole, a CYP2C19 inhibitor, on the stereoselective pharmacokinetics and pharmacodynamics of warfarin between CYP2C19 genotypes.

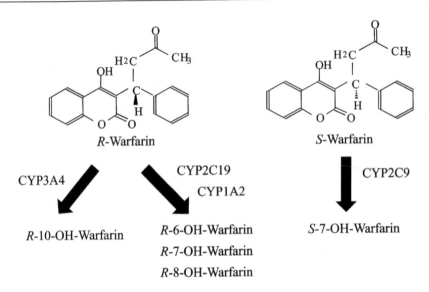

Fig. 1. Metabolic pathways of *R*-warfarin and *S*-warfarin.

2. Analytical methods

2.1 Genotypic identification

17 healthy Japanese volunteers (12 males and 5 females) were enrolled in this study after giving written informed consent. All subjects were enrolled in this study after giving written informed consent. Each Subject underwent a CYP2C19 genotyping test by use of a polymerase chain reaction-restriction fragment length polymorphism (PCR-RFLP) method with allele–specific primer for identifying the *CYP2C19* wild-type (*1) gene and the 2 mutated alleles, *CYP2C19*2 (*2) in exon 5 and *CYP2C19*3 (*3) in exon 4 (De Morais SM et al., 1994), and they were classified into 2 genotype groups as follows: homozygous extensive metabolizers (hmEMs, *1/*1, 10 subjects), poor metabolizers (PMs, *2/*2 or *2/*3, 7 subjects). Similarly, CYP2C9 genotyping test by use of a PCR-RFLP method with allele–specific primer was performed for identifying the *CYP2C9* wild-type (*1) gene and the 2 mutated alleles, *CYP2C9*2 (Arg144Cys) and *CYP2C9*3 (Ile359Leu) (Yasar U et al., 1999). Alleles in which neither *CYP2C9*2 nor *CYP2C9*3 variants were identified were regarded as wild type in all subjects.

2.2 Assay

Plasma concentrations of warfarin enantiomers and S-7-hydroxywarfarin were determined using high performance liquid chromatography (HPLC) method developed in our laboratory (Uno T et al., 2007). In brief, warfarin enantiomers, S-7-hydroxywarfarin and an internal standard, diclofenac sodium, were extracted from 1 ml of plasma sample using diethyl ether-chloroform (80:20, v/v). The extract was injected onto column I (TSK precolumn BSA-C8, 5 μm, 10 mm x 4.6 mm i.d.) for clean-up and column II (Chiralcel OD-RH analytical column, 150 mm x 4.6 mm i.d.) coupled with a guard column (Chiralcel OD-

RH guard column, 10 mm x 4.6 mm i.d.) for separation. The mobile phase consisted of phosphate buffer-acetonitrile (84:16 v/v, pH 2.0) for clean-up and phosphate buffer-acetonitrile (45:55 v/v, pH 2.0) for separation. The peaks were monitored with an ultraviolet detector set at a wavelength of 312 nm, and total time for chromatographic separation was about 25 minutes. The retention times of S-7-hydoxywarfarin, R-warfarin, I.S. and S-warfarin were 17.6 min, 19.1 min, 20.0 min and 21.2 min, respectively. The validated concentration ranges of this method were 3-1000 ng/ml for R- and S-warfarin, and 3-200 ng/ml for R- and S-7-hydroxywarfarin, respectively. Intra- and inter-day coefficients of variation were less than 4.4 and 4.9% for R-warfarin and 4.8 and 4.0% for S-warfarin, and 5.1 and 4.2% for R-7-hydroxywarfarin and 5.8 and 5.0% for S-7-hydroxywarfarin at the different concentrations. The limit of quantification was 3 ng/ml for both warfarin and 7-hydroxywarfarin enantiomers. Plasma samples for the pharmacokinetic study were stored at -20 ˚C and analyzed within 3 months after sampling, and then were stable at -70 ˚C for 12 months.

Plasma concentrations of omeprazole and 5-hydroxyomeprazole were quantitated using HPLC method developed in our laboratory (Shimizu M et al., 2006). In brief, after alkalization with 0.1 mL of 0.5 M disodium hydrogen phosphate, 1 mL plasma was extracted with 4 mL of diethyl ether-dichloromethane (55:45, v/v). The organic phase was evaporated at 60 ˚C to dryness. The residue was dissolved with 30 μL of methanol and 100 μL of 50 mM disodium hydrogen phosphate buffer (pH 9.3), and then a 30-μL aliquot was injected to an HPLC system (SHIMADZU CLASS-VP, SHIMADZU Corporation, Kyoto, Japan), with a Inertsil ODS-80A column as an analytical column (particle size 5 μm; GL Science Inc, Tokyo, Japan). The mobile phase consisted of phosphate buffer-acetonitrile-methanol (65:30:5 v/v/v, pH6.5). Flow rate was 0.8 mL/min and wavelength was set at 302 nm. Limit of quantification was 3 ng/mL for omeprazole and 5-hydroxyomeprazole. Intra- and inter-day coefficient variations were less than 5.1 and 6.6% for omeprazole concentrations ranging from 4 to 1600 ng/mL and 4.6 and 5.0% for 5-hydroxyomeprazole concentration ranging from 4 to 400 ng/mL, respectively.

3. Pharmacokinetics of warfarin enantiomers

We examined the pharmacokinetics of warfarin enantiomers by administering 10 mg of racemic warfarin to 17 healthy volunteers (Uno T et al., 2008). Blood samples were obtained before and over the course of 120 hours after dosing for the determination plasma warfarin enantiomer concentrations and prothrombin time-INR (PT-INR). Fig. 2 shows the mean plasma concentration-time curves for R- and S-warfarin between the CYP2C19 genotypes. The mean pharmacokinetic parameters of these compounds are summarized in Table 1.

In this study, the area under the plasma concentration-time curve (AUC$_{0-\infty}$) and the elimination half-life (t$_{1/2}$) of R-warfarin were about 2-fold greater than those of S-warfarin in 17 subjects (Table 1). These values of R- and S-warfarin were in line with a previous report in which the same dose of racemic warfarin was administered (Lilja JJ et al., 1984). Additionally, AUC$_{0-\infty}$ and t$_{1/2}$ of R-warfarin in PMs were significantly greater than those in hmEMs ($P < 0.001$ and $P = 0.010$, respectively). Similarly, there is a significant difference ($P = 0.007$) in the apparent oral clearance (CL) in hmEMs compared with that in PMs. The S/R ratios of AUC$_{0-\infty}$ of warfarin enantiomers were 0.51 in hmEMs and 0.37 in PMs ($P = 0.005$). Whereas, no difference was found in all pharmacokinetic parameters of S-warfarin and S-7-hydroxywarfarin in hmEMs compared with PMs of CYP2C19.

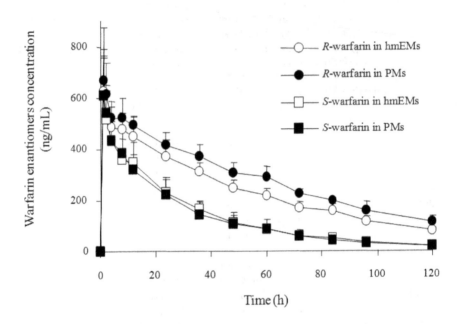

Fig. 2. Plasma concentrations-time curves (mean + S.D.) of *R*-warfarin or *S*-warfarin in hmEMs (*R*-; open circles, *S*-; open square) and PMs (*R*-; closed circles, *S*-; closed square) after a single dose of 10 mg warfarin.

4. Drug interaction between omeprazole and warfarin enantiomers

Omeprazole 20 mg/daily was given orally to 17 healthy volunteers for 11 days, and on day 7, a single dose of racemic warfarin 10 mg was added (Uno T et al., 2008).

The pharmacokinetic parameters are summarized in Table 1. In hmEMs, the omeprazole treatment significantly increased *R*-warfarin $AUC_{0-\infty}$ ($P = 0.004$), and prolonged its $t_{1/2}$ ($P = 0.017$) without any effect on *R*-warfarin C_{max} or t_{max}. However, the omeprazole treatment did not alter any pharmacokinetic parameters of *S*-warfarin in both hmEMs and PMs as well as those of *R*-warfarin in hmEMs. Consequently, the omeprazole treatment decreased the *S/R* enantiomer ratio of warfarin $AUC_{0-\infty}$ from 0.51 to 0.43 in hmEMs ($P = 0.010$), but not in PMs.

In addition, significant differences were found in mean C_{max} ($P < 0.001$), $t_{1/2}$ ($P = 0.005$), and AUC_{0-24} ($P < 0.001$) of omeprazole between different CYP2C19 genotypes, though there was no difference in mean C_{max} or AUC_{0-24} of 5-hydroxyomeprazole between hmEMs and PMs.

Variable	hmEMs			PMs		
	Control	Omeprazole	Fold change	Control	Omeprazole	Fold change
R-warfarin						
C_{max} (ng/mL)	692 (616, 768)	629 (556, 702)	0.92 (0.70-1.18)	706 (599, 813)	589 (474, 703)	0.84 (0.55-1.08)
t_{max} (h)	1.4 (0.8, 2.0)	3.3 (1.3, 5.3)	3.02 (0.25-12)	2.6 (0.6, 4.5)	3.6 (0.6, 6.5)	2.79 (0.5-12)
$t_{1/2}$ (h)	40.8 (36.1, 45.6)	46.4 (44.2, 48.7)†	1.12 (0.96-1.27)	49.6 (46.9, 52.3)*	48.8 (42.5, 55.0)	0.97 (0.63-1.18)
$AUC_{0-\infty}$ (ng*h/mL)	34613 (32702, 36524)	41387 (37221, 45552)††	1.19 (1.02-1.39)	42938 (39342, 46533)**	39100 (34802, 43399)	0.92 (0.74-1.08)
CL (mL*kg/h)	2.4 (2.1, 2.5)	2.1 (1.8, 2.2)††	0.87 (0.72-1.09)	1.9 (1.6, 2.3)**	2.1 (1.6, 2.6)	1.12 (0.93-1.36)
S-warfarin						
C_{max} (ng/mL)	659 (570, 748)	600 (528, 673)	0.93 (0.62-1.36)	630 (520, 739)	554 (469, 638)	0.90 (0.69-1.12)
t_{max} (h)	1.3 (0.7, 1.9)	1.7 (1.1, 2.3)	1.63 (0.25-2)	1.1 (0.9, 1.4)	1.1 (0.9, 1.4)	1.07 (0.5-2)
$t_{1/2}$ (h)	25.4 (22.0, 28.9)	27.0 (21.3, 32.8)	1.13 (0.50-1.80)	22.7 (19.7, 25.8)	25.4 (21.7, 29.0)	1.13 (0.82-1.37)
$AUC_{0-\infty}$ (ng*h/mL)	16968 (15233, 18701)	18166 (15705, 20628)	1.07 (0.87-1.54)	15851 (12686, 19016)	14756 (11768, 17745)	0.93 (0.78-1.03)
CL (mL*kg/h)	5.0 (4.6, 5.4)	4.7 (4.1, 5.3)	0.95 (0.65-1.13)	5.6 (4.7, 6.4)	6.0 (4.9, 7.1)	1.08 (0.97-1.28)
The S/R ratios of $AUC_{0-\infty}$	0.51 (0.47, 0.54)	0.43 (0.40, 0.46)††	0.82 (0.76-0.88)	0.37 (0.31, 0.43)***	0.38 (0.31, 0.44)	1.05 (0.98-1.12)
S-7-hydroxywarfarin						
C_{max} (ng/mL)	69.8 (61.7, 77.8)	72.0 (62.8, 81.2)	1.03 (0.91-1.18)	68.1 (63.1, 73.1)	67.6 (63.0, 72.2)	1.00 (0.83-1.08)
t_{max} (h)	18.0 (13.0, 23.0)	26.0 (19.7, 32.3)	2.35 (1.0-12.0)	24.0 (16.7, 27.5)	18.9 (9.1, 28.6)	0.74 (0.3-1.5)
$t_{1/2}$ (h)	28.8 (19.3, 38.2)	25.2 (20.5, 30.0)	1.07 (0.33-2.14)	22.1 (16.7, 27.4)	24.6 (16.3, 33.0)	1.24 (0.39-2.41)
$AUC_{0-\infty}$ (ng*h/mL)	2584 (1997, 3171)	2695 (2101, 3289)	1.06 (0.87-1.21)	2471 (1982, 2959)	2429 (2065, 2792)	1.00 (0.85-1.13)
The metabolic ratio	0.15 (0.12, 0.19)	0.16 (0.12, 0.19)	1.04 (0.89-1.11)	0.17 (0.11, 0.24)	0.18 (0.12, 0.24)	1.03 (0.97-1.22)

AUC, area under plasma concentration-time curve; C_{max}, peak concentration; t_{max}, time to C_{max}; $t_{1/2}$, elimination half-life; CL, apparent oral clearance. The S/R ratios of AUC; $AUC_{0-\infty}$ S-warfarin / $AUC_{0-\infty}$ R-warfarin. The metabolic ratio; $AUC_{0-\infty}$ of S-7-hydroxywarfarin / $AUC_{0-\infty}$ of S-warfarin. *P <0.05,**P <0.01, ***P <0.001, between hmEMs and PMs., †P <0.05,††P <0.01, between control and omeprazole phase. Data are shown as mean and 95% confidence interval ; t_{max} and fold change data are shown as a median wich a range.

Table 1. The summary of pharmacokinetics of warfarin enantiomers

5. Pharmacodynamics of warfarin

No significant difference was found between hmEMs and PMs in either the PT-INR AUC_{0-120} or the PT-INR max during the placebo phase, and the omeprazole treatment did not affect these parameters in both hmEMs and PMs (Uno T et al., 2008).

6. The effect of CYP2C19 genotypes on the pharmacokinetics

Previous studies in patients with different CYP2C19 genotypes reported not to affect plasma R-warfarin concentrations at the steady state in clinical studies, in which the concentrations were evaluated at a one sampling point (Obayashi K et al., 2006; Scordo MG et al., 2002; Takahashi et al., 1998). However, two of the reports (Obayashi K et al., 2006; Scordo MG et al., 2002) observed that the S/R ratio based on steady-state concentrations in PMs was smaller than that in hmEMs. The third study (Takahashi et al., 1998) compared PMs with EMs which included both hmEMs and heterozygous EMs with one mutated CYP2C19 allele. Therefore, the present study was designed to evaluate the elimination phase of warfarin and examine the effect of the CYP2C19 genotype on the pharmacokinetics of warfarin enantiomers. Although the pharmacokinetics was measured after a single administration in this study, our results indicated that the plasma concentrations and $t_{1/2}$ of R-warfarin in PMs were markedly higher compared with those of the corresponding R-enantiomer in hmEMs. In addition, the $AUC_{0-\infty}$ S/R ratio in PMs decreased significantly more than that in hmEMs, thereby showing that the pharmacokinetics of R-warfarin may be significantly affected by CYP2C19 polymorphism. In contrast, no difference was found in any pharmacokinetic parameters of S-warfarin between the hmEMs and the PMs. Consequently, these findings suggest that CYP2C19 activity is an important determinant of R-warfarin pharmacokinetics.

We also demonstrated that the reported interaction of R-warfarin with omeprazole was found only in the hmEMs of CYP2C19. In previous pharmacokinetic studies (Sutfin T et al., 1989; Unge P et al., 1992), omeprazole has been reported to cause a minor but significant increase in R-warfarin plasma concentrations [9.5% (Unge P et al., 1992) and 12% (Sutfin T et al., 1989)]. In our present study, although the pharmacokinetics of warfarin enantiomers of the PMs were not affected by the omeprazole treatment, mean R-warfarin $AUC_{0-\infty}$ and $t_{1/2}$ of the hmEMs increased after the omeprazole treatment to the levels comparable to those of the PMs. Mean R-warfarin $AUC_{0-\infty}$ of our hmEMs showed an 18 % increase, and the increase was greater than that of the previous studies (Sutfin T et al., 1989; Unge P et al., 1992), probably due to recruiting the same genotype in the present study. Omeprazole is known to be an inhibitor of some CYP enzymes including CYP2C9 and 2C19 (Ko JW et al., 1997; Li XQ et al., 2004). CYP2C9 is known to be responsible for the biotransformation from S-warfarin to S-7-hydroxywarfarin (Kaminsky LS and Zhang ZY, 1997), and the ratio of S-7-hydroxywarfarin AUC to S-warfarin AUC would reflect the *in vivo* activity of CYP2C9. Previous report suggested that the clearance of omeprazole is markedly reduced and plasma concentrations of omeprazole in CYP2C19 PMs are much more elevated than those in CYP2C19 EMs (Sohn DR et al., 1992). Increased plasma concentrations of omeprazole in CYP2C19 PMs might affect the pharmacokinetics of warfarin S-enantiomer, a substrate of CYP2C9 (Kaminsky LS and Zhang ZY, 1997), as well as its R-enantiomer, compared to those in CYP2C19 EMs. In this study, the inhibitory effect of omeprazole was noted only in the hmEMs of CYP2C19 despite higher omeprazole concentrations in the PMs, and the $AUC_{0-\infty}$ ratio of S-7-hydroxywarfarin to S-warfarin was relatively constant between the placebo and the omeprazole phases, suggesting that the 7-day administration of omeprazole 20 mg once daily would affect the CYP2C19 activity solely.

7. The effect of CYP2C19 genotypes on the pharmacodynamics

Interestingly, no significant difference was found in PT-INR between the hmEMs and PMs in both the control and the omeprazole phases even though the CYP2C19 genotypes affected the R-warfarin pharmacokinetic parameters. However, these findings are not surprising because the anticoagulant effect of S-enantiomer is 3-5 times more potent than that of R-enantiomer (Takahashi H and Echizen H, 2001), and a concentration rises of R-enantiomer was seemed to have little influence on the anticoagulant effect of warfarin. These results therefore suggest that altered pharmacokinetics of R-warfarin may play a minor role in determining the average clinical doses of warfarin. Moreover, these results also imply that inhibition of the *in vivo* CYP2C19 activity by the co-administration of a CYP2C19 inhibitor, such as omeprazole, lansoprazole or fluvoxamine (Hemeryck A and Belpaire FM, 2002; Ko JW et al., 1997; Li XQ et al., 2004), may scarcely modify the anticoagulant effects of warfarin. Recently, Rieder et al. (2005) have shown that there is an effect of the VKORC1 on dose requirement. Furthermore, Obayashi et al. (2006) reported that the genotyping of the vitamin K epooxide reductase complex subunit 1 gene (VKORC1) may be more predictive of the anticoagulant effect than genotyping of CYPs, which reflects the warfarin plasma concentrations. Therefore, these studies suggest that VKORC1 activity may be an important determinant of the pharmacodynamics of warfarin in Japanese patients.

8. Conclusion

These results indicate that CYP2C19 activity is important in the pharmacokinetics of R-warfarin because the pharmacokinetics of warfarin enantiomers were different between the CYP2C19 genotypes and the omeprazole affected the R-warfarin pharmacokinetics of CYP2C19 in only hmEMs. However, these affects are not translated into any significant effect in the pharmacodynamics of warfarin.

9. References

Chan E, McLachlan AJ, Pegg M, MacKay AD, Cole RB, Rowland M. (1994). Disposition of warfarin enantiomers and metabolites in patients during multiple dosing with rac-warfarin. *Br J Clin Pharmacol*, Vol. 37, pp. 563-569.

De Morais SM, Wilkinson GR, Blaisdell J, Meyer UA, Nakamura K, Goldstein JA. (1994). Identification of a new genetic defect responsible for the polymorphism of (S)-mephenytoin metabolism in Japanese. *Mol Pharmacol*, Vol. 46, pp. 594-598.

Hemeryck A, Belpaire FM. (2002). Selective serotonin reuptake inhibitors and cytochrome P-450 mediated drug-drug interactions: an update. *Curr Drug Metab*, Vol.3, pp. 13-37.

Hirsh J, Dalen JE, Anderson DR, Poller L, Bussey H, Ansell J, Deykin D, Brandt JT. (1998). Oral anticoagulants: mechanism of action, clinical effectiveness, and optimal therapeutic range. *Chest*, Vol. 114, pp. 445S-469S.

Kaminsky LS, Zhang ZY. (1997). Human P450 metabolism of warfarin. *Pharmacol Ther*, Vol. 73, pp. 67-74.

Ko JW, Sukhova N, Thacker D, Chen P, Flockhart DA. (1997). Evaluation of omeprazole and lansoprazole as inhibitors of cytochrome P450 isoforms. *Drug Metab Dispos*, Vol. 25, pp. 853-62.

Kubota T, Chiba K, Ishizaki T. (1996). Genotyping of S-mephenytoin 4'-hydroxylation in an extended Japanese population. *Clin Pharmacol Ther*, Vol. 60, pp. 661-666.

Lilja JJ, Backman JT, Neuvonen PJ. (2005). Effect of gemfibrozil on the pharmacokinetics and pharmacodynamics of racemic warfarin in healthy subjects. *Br J Clin Pharmacol*, Vol. 59, pp. 433-439.

Li XQ, Andersson TB, Ahlström M, Weidolf L. (2004). Comparison of inhibitory effects of the proton pump-inhibiting drugs omeprazole, esomeprazole, lansoprazole, pantoprazole, and rabeprazole on human cytochrome P450 activities. *Drug Metab Dispos*, Vol. 32, pp. 821-7.

Obayashi K, Nakamura K, Kawana J, Ogata H, Hanada K, Kurabayashi M. (2006). VKORC1 gene variations are the major contributors of variation in warfarin dose in Japanese patients. *Clin Pharmacol Ther*, Vol. 80, pp. 169-178.

Rieder MJ, Reiner AP, Gage BF, Nickerson DA, Eby CS, McLeod HL, Blough DK, Thummel KE, Veenstra DL, Rettie AE. (2005). Effect of VKORC1 haplotypes on transcriptional regulation and warfarin dose. *New England Journal of Med*, Vol. 352, pp. 2285-2293.

Scordo MG, Pengo V, Spina E, Dahl ML, Gusella M, Padrini R. (2002). Influence of CYP2C9 and CYP2C19 genetic polymorphisms on warfarin maintenance dose and metabolic clearance. *Clin Pharmacol Ther*, Vol. 72, pp. 702-710.

Shimizu M, Uno T, Niioka T, Yaui-Furukori N, Takahata T, Sugawara K, Tateishi T. (2006). Sensitive determination of omeprazole and its two main metabolites in human plasma by column-switching high-performance liquid chromatography: application to pharmacokinetic study in relation to CYP2C19 genotypes. *J Chromatogr B*, Vol. 832, pp. 241-248.

Sohn DR, Kobayashi K, Chiba K, Lee KH, Shin SG, Ishizaki T. (1992). Disposition kinetics and metabolism of omeprazole in extensive and poor metabolizers of S-mephenytoin 4'-hydroxylation recruited from an Oriental population. *J Pharmacol Exp Ther*, Vol. 262, pp. 1195-1202.

Sutfin T, Balmer K, Bostrom H, Eriksson S, Hoglund P, Paulsen O. (1989). Stereoselective interaction of omeprazole with warfarin in healthy men. *Ther Drug Monit*, Vol. 11, pp. 176-184.

Takahashi H, Wilkinson GR, Nutescu EA, Morita T, Ritchie MD, Scordo MG, Pengo V, Barban M, Padrini R, Ieiri I, Otsubo K, Kashima T, Kimura S, Kijima S, Echizen H. (2006). Different contributions of polymorphisms in VKORC1 and CYP2C9 to intra- and inter-population differences in maintenance dose of warfarin in Japanese, Caucasians and African-Americans. *Pharmacogenetics and Genomics*, Vol. 16, pp. 101-110.

Takahashi H, Echizen H. Pharmacogenetics of warfarin elimination and its clinical implications. (2001). *Clin Pharmacokinet*, Vol. 40, pp. 587-603.

Takahashi H, Kashima T, Nomizo Y, Muramoto N, Shimizu T, Nasu K, Kubota T, Kimura S, Echizen H. (1998). Metabolism of warfarin enantiomers in Japanese patients with heart disease having different CYP2C9 and CYP2C19 genotypes. *Clin Pharmacol Ther*, Vol. 63, pp. 519-528.

Unge P, Svedberg LE, Nordgren A, Blom H, Andersson T, Lagerstrom PO, Idstrom JP. (1992). A study of the interaction of omeprazole and warfarin in anticoagulated patients. *Br J Clin Pharmacol*, Vol.34, pp. 509-512.

Uno T, Sugimoto K, Sugawara K, Tateishi T. (2008). The role of cytochrome P2C19 in R-warfarin pharmacokinetics and its interaction with omeprazole.*Ther Drug Monit*, Vol. 30, pp.276-281.

Uno T, Niioka T, Hayakari M, Sugawara K, Tateishi T. (2007). Simultaneous determination of warfarin enantiomers and its metabolite in human plasma by column-switching high-performance liquid chromatography with chiral separation. *Ther Drug Monit*, Vol. 29, pp. 333-339.

Yasar U, Eliasson E, Dahl ML, Johansson I, Ingelman-Sundberg M, Sjoqvist F. (1999). Validation of methods for CYP2C9 genotyping: frequencies of mutant alleles in a Swedish population. *Biochem Biophys Res Commun*, Vol. 254, pp. 628-631.

Permissions

The contributors of this book come from diverse backgrounds, making this book a truly international effort. This book will bring forth new frontiers with its revolutionizing research information and detailed analysis of the nascent developments around the world.

We would like to thank Luca Gallelli, for lending his expertise to make the book truly unique. He has played a crucial role in the development of this book. Without his invaluable contribution this book wouldn't have been possible. He has made vital efforts to compile up to date information on the varied aspects of this subject to make this book a valuable addition to the collection of many professionals and students.

This book was conceptualized with the vision of imparting up-to-date information and advanced data in this field. To ensure the same, a matchless editorial board was set up. Every individual on the board went through rigorous rounds of assessment to prove their worth. After which they invested a large part of their time researching and compiling the most relevant data for our readers. Conferences and sessions were held from time to time between the editorial board and the contributing authors to present the data in the most comprehensible form. The editorial team has worked tirelessly to provide valuable and valid information to help people across the globe.

Every chapter published in this book has been scrutinized by our experts. Their significance has been extensively debated. The topics covered herein carry significant findings which will fuel the growth of the discipline. They may even be implemented as practical applications or may be referred to as a beginning point for another development. Chapters in this book were first published by InTech; hereby published with permission under the Creative Commons Attribution License or equivalent.

The editorial board has been involved in producing this book since its inception. They have spent rigorous hours researching and exploring the diverse topics which have resulted in the successful publishing of this book. They have passed on their knowledge of decades through this book. To expedite this challenging task, the publisher supported the team at every step. A small team of assistant editors was also appointed to further simplify the editing procedure and attain best results for the readers.

Our editorial team has been hand-picked from every corner of the world. Their multi-ethnicity adds dynamic inputs to the discussions which result in innovative outcomes. These outcomes are then further discussed with the researchers and contributors who give their valuable feedback and opinion regarding the same. The feedback is then collaborated with the researches and they are edited in a comprehensive manner to aid the understanding of the subject.

Apart from the editorial board, the designing team has also invested a significant amount of their time in understanding the subject and creating the most relevant covers. They scrutinized every image to scout for the most suitable representation of the subject and create an appropriate cover for the book.

The publishing team has been involved in this book since its early stages. They were actively engaged in every process, be it collecting the data, connecting with the contributors or procuring relevant information. The team has been an ardent support to the editorial, designing and production team. Their endless efforts to recruit the best for this project, has resulted in the accomplishment of this book. They are a veteran in the field of academics and their pool of knowledge is as vast as their experience in printing. Their expertise and guidance has proved useful at every step. Their uncompromising quality standards have made this book an exceptional effort. Their encouragement from time to time has been an inspiration for everyone.

The publisher and the editorial board hope that this book will prove to be a valuable piece of knowledge for researchers, students, practitioners and scholars across the globe.

List of Contributors

Gregory Stewart, Julie Kniazeff, Laurent Prézeau, Philippe Rondard, Jean-Philippe Pin and Cyril Goudet
Institut de Génomique Fonctionnelle, CNRS UMR5203 - INSERM U661 - Universités Montpellier 1&2, France

Hideaki Fujii, Shigeto Hirayama and Hiroshi Nagase
School of Pharmacy, Kitasato University, Japan

Alexandra Sideris
Department of Anesthesiology, New York University Langone Medical Center, New York, USA

Thomas Blanck
Department of Anesthesiology, Department of Physiology and Neuroscience, New York University Langone Medical Center, New York, USA

Esperanza Recio-Pinto
Department of Anesthesiology; Department of Pharmacology, New York University Langone Medical Center, New York, USA

Brian D. Herman and Nicolas Sluis-Cremer
University of Pittsburgh, Department of Medicine, Division of Infectious Diseases, Pittsburgh, USA

You-Hong Jin
Department of Anatomy the Affiliated Stomatological, Hospital of Nanchang University, Nanchang, Jiangxi Province, China

Motohide Takemura
Department of Oral Anatomy and Neurobiology, Osaka University Graduate School of Dentistry, Japan

Akira Furuyama
Departments of Oral Physiology, Japan

Norifumi Yonehara
Oral Medical Science (Division of Dental Pharmacology), Ohu University School of Dentistry, Koriyama, Fukushima, Japan

Jennifer Tremblay-Mercier
Université de Sherbrooke, Research Center on Aging, Canada

Heni Rachmawati
Pharmaceutics, Bandung Institute of Technology, Bandung, Indonesia

Heni Rachmawati, Adriana Mattos, Catharina Reker-Smit, Klaas Poelstra and Leonie Beljaars
University of Groningen, Dept. of Pharmacokinetics, Toxicology and Targeting, The Netherlands

Krzysztof Bryniarski
Jagiellonian University Medical College, Department of Immunology, Krakow, Poland

Bosun Banjoko
Obafemi Awolowo University, Ile-Ife, Nigeria

Anjana Munshi and Vandana Sharma
Institute Of Genetics and Hospital for Genetic Diseases, Osmania University, Begumpet, Hyderabad, India

Anthonius de Boer, Tom Schalekamp, Rianne M.F. Van Schie, Talitha I. Verhoef and Anke-Hilse Maitland-Van Der Zee
Utrecht University, The Netherlands

Felix J.M. Van Der Meer
Leiden University Medical Center, The Netherlands

William K. Redekop
Erasmus University Rotterdam, The Netherlands

Rahber Thariani
University of Washington, USA

Yumiko Akamine and Tsukasa Uno
Department of Hospital Pharmacy, Faculty of Medicine, University of the Ryukyus, Okinawa, Japan